BONNIE PRUDDEN'S AFTER FIFTY FITNESS GUIDE

BONNIE PRUDDEN's AFTER FIFTY FITNESS GUIDE

Bonnie Prudden

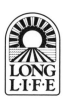

Photographs by Mort Engel
Foreword by Robert N. Butler, M.D., Series Editor

Published with the cooperation and consultation of the Gerald and
May Ellen Ritter Department of Geriatrics and Adult Development,
Mount Sinai School of Medicine, Mount Sinai Hospital.

BALLANTINE BOOKS • NEW YORK

To Dr. Desmond R. Tivy
a man for all seasons

Copyright © 1986 by Bonnie Prudden, Inc.
Photographs copyright © 1986 by Mort Engel
Illustrations copyright © 1986 Holly Johnson

Library of Congress Catalog Card Number: 86-92099

ISBN: 0-345-31807-2

This edition published by arrangement with Villard Books.

Design by Holly Johnson

Manufactured in the United States of America

First Ballantine Books Edition: October 1987

10 9 8 7 6 5 4 3 2 1

CONTENTS

ACKNOWLEDGMENTS

Without Dr. Butler, who has looked at "older Americans" through the eyes of eternal youth that see promise in every tomorrow, the future for that time of life would be bleak indeed.

He is affronted by those who would have us "fade away," "grow old gracefully," or live out our "*golden* years" in Sunny Wherever while turning our wonderfully experienced selves out to pasture.

He has demanded of himself extraordinary efforts in our behalf and therefore has the right to demand as much from us, the last fit Americans. To the degree we succeed in bringing comfort, excitement, and fulfillment to *all* of the After Fifty Crowd, we too will profit. For we will all grow old.

Without Enid "Beanie" Whittaker, my last two books, which were on controlling and erasing pain, would not have been written. Without those books, this one would have no meaning, since it is pain that ages, and painful aging is not meaningful living. "Beanie" did all the things that make a book possible and keep an author, drowning in information, sane. We all owe her a debt. Both you and I will be able to look forward to staying active, pain free, and productive because of "Beanie" . . . and when you find fun in these pages, it was she who triggered it.

Bonnie Prudden

FOREWORD

Some people are just "naturals": They seem to have a deep understanding of life processes and of people. Those who understand people have been called *Menschenkenners*. I don't know if there is a counterpart term for those who understand "things," beyond saying that they are mechanically gifted. Then, there are a few rare people who understand both; they understand people and they understand how the body works. Such a person is Bonnie Prudden.

The way our body works is a function of culture, personal history and behavior, and, of course, attitude. The history of "The After Fifty Crowd" has been more favorable than the history of those under fifty, as Bonnie Prudden shows. The after fifty crowd at least had a good beginning and they can maintain it or restore it to help achieve painless later years.

In this fine book, Bonnie Prudden gives us autobiography, fitness advice, and her experiences with Myotherapy. Myotherapy is a way to get rid of pain. It does not involve medications, it does involve an understanding of the body and the personality.

Bonnie Prudden is humble enough to acknowledge that she doesn't understand *how* myotherapy works, *only that it works*. One of the great destructive forces against a decent old age is muscle pain—in backs and shoulders, for example. Now that we have so dramatically extended life, we all recognize the desire to enhance its quality. Conventional medicine is contributing tremendously to that end and so too are those outside of the mainstream of medicine, such as Bonnie Prudden.

In recent times medicine has begun to recognize the contributions of people outside its formal structures. There are gifted people who have uncovered major insights and know how to apply them in direct and effective ways. I regard Bonnie Prudden as such a person.

This is a practical book with detailed recommendations about health, fitness, and pain-free living through myotherapy and exercise. There is one thing wrong with this book: It requires another one to be written for the crowd under fifty, for the kids that need to have fitness built into their lives. Perhaps we could persuade Bonnie Prudden to make this her next book.

Robert N. Butler, M.D.

INTRODUCTION

"It is pain that ages us—not years."

This is the first and only time in American history that five things will come together to turn out a remarkable group of people—*The Last Fit Americans*. This group is comprised of the last *naturally* fit generation of Americans, those whose childhood was spent at play out-of-doors. They are the last to walk to school no matter what the weather, the last to enjoy active, body-building play, and the last to use such play creatively.

Children who had finished elementary school by 1945—when riding a school bus replaced walking to and from school and running home and back at lunch time—are now fifty, pushing fifty, or past fifty. We fortunate people make up the after fifty crowd.

In addition to having energetic child-hoods (normal then, but lost for our grandchildren), we were the first generation to benefit from the explosions in the fields of biology and chemistry which delivered vaccines and antibiotics. *Natural* physical fitness, disease prevention, and infection control are responsible for the healthy maturing of our generation. Thirty years ago, penicillin was discovered, and that is why the eighty-five-and-up population of our group is increasing faster than teenagers. Today's Americans have been given the gift of time . . . time to grow into the Age of Reason and the Age of Leisure, neither of which is available long before the magic age of fifty.

The fourth factor contributing to the vigor of the after fifty crowd is the discovery *and acceptance* of the fact that exercise must be maintained as long as life is maintained.

The fifth—and quite as amazing and important as penicillin—is the development of Myotherapy.* Myotherapy can completely erase most pain and alleviate a great deal of the rest. Relief from pain opens up whole new vistas for the future. For the first time an after fifty crowd can look forward to a future free from the fear of pain that is said to be a possible concomitant of reaching fifty, a probable one by sixty, and frequently an incapacitating one by seventy.

For the after fifties who have already stepped over that invisible but very tangible border between pain and pain free, stiffness and flexibility, physical agility and physical limitation, Myotherapy can bring the added boon of "youth creep." This means "younging" instead of "ageing." It means all of the above positives and none of the negatives. It is a glass or two (and for some, a whole bottle) drawn from the long-sought Fountain of Youth. For it is pain that ages, not years.

Myotherapy can do something else: it can *prevent* pain. This aspect of pain relief will gain acceptance when athletes and dancers start using it to enhance performance; the rest of us will follow. People rarely attempt to prevent pain they do not already have, but that will come. It will come in the form of prevention magic for those who have erased pain and want to be sure it never troubles their bodies again.

Myotherapy will allow all of us to exercise, as we know we must, for one of its functions is to relieve muscles of

* Myotherapy[sm] is a service mark of Bonnie Prudden, Inc.

spasm and then to reeducate those muscles to serve us again as they did years ago, before stress and wear interfered with our freedom of movement.

Myotherapy, in combination with exercise, has a liberating effect on drug addiction and alcohol abuse. Drug addiction is the most destructive factor in modern-day life. Alcohol, tranquilizers, antidepressants, and psychogenic drugs cloud millions of minds. Steroids and NSAIDs (nonsteroid anti-inflammatory drugs) often destroy even as they relieve. There are more deaths from prescription drugs than from those bought from the pusher on the street. Twenty percent of our nation's wealth goes to buy over-the-counter drugs—painkillers, laxatives, cold medications, stomach palliatives, "arthritis" concoctions, sleeping pills, wake-up pills, and diet pills. And still the nation hurts, can't sleep, can't go to the bathroom, and is fatter than ever.

So give a cheer for the good fortune of the after fifty crowd. This most unusual generation will last well into the nineties, and many will celebrate their hundredth years. Over 300,000 are doing that now even without improved nutrition, improved lifestyle, and freedom from inactivity, pain, and drugs. This group will do it better, but the cutoff is right behind us.

The children who entered elementary school after buses had become a part of every school and the TV set a part of every home, have already lost out: they don't have *natural* physical fitness. The great development years are between birth and six; the honing years are between seven and eleven. Children today don't feel the way you did as a child. They lack the energy you had. The world is no longer so magical the way it was for you when the first robin appeared on your lawn in spring . . . and many of you had a lawn or a yard, or your grandparents did. Today's kids don't know the thrill of running in the wind and rolling down a hill of new-mown grass. Most of them have never felt *healthy*. Is it any wonder that they will try a little green, pink, brown, or white pill that will make them feel *different?*

For the after fifty crowd, this is about to be a golden time. I don't mean "The Golden Years," as in "Move over, Pop." It is going to be golden and magical because we really do come into wisdom with the years, and we really do store up experience. We begin to appreciate time and people and even our children, who, surprisingly, begin to appreciate us. Remember the old saying, "If youth but would and age but could . . ."? The implication is that youth is too callow, too inexperienced, too unaware for the

job, while age is too decrepit, too forgetful, too tired to accomplish it. Well it's time for a new saying. When you have read this book and learned that most of the demeaning myths about older people are *only* myths, you will feel differently about yourself and others. When you realize that you can feel at least twenty years younger, with all the strength and aggression that goes with being younger, you will look very differently at the future and your part in it. When you discover that the after fifty crowd is the cream of the crop and apt to maintain that place for some time, you may even look around and see what has been left undone. I can promise you that if you follow the directions on the package, you will be much younger, stronger, and more dangerous in a year.

It is important that we start to help each other, for our like will not be seen again.

PART ONE
WHO WE ARE

THE LAST FIT AMERICANS

As you know, we of the after fifty crowd are more fortunate than we have ever realized. The five developments that came together in our time will not only make us an interesting part of history, they will permit a goodly number of us to watch that history unfold. We are the last generation of Americans who are *naturally* fit.

Like most edifices, the human body needs to start with a strong base, and the human fetus begins to build that base at the moment of conception. We build steadily until around the age of six and we shape that edifice, our body, until around eleven. By then we have the almost-finished product. From that time on it can be painted, polished, and ornamented, but its base and frame, for good or not-so-good, is ours for the duration of our life.

It's no secret that shoddy workmanship yields an inferior product that stands up neither to time nor to wear. But *nature* is never shoddy, and we had nature as mother, teacher, friend, and playmate. If building strong, healthy bodies in our childhood had depended on parents as it does now, we would be as poorly put together as today's children. Had maintaining those bodies through adolescence depended as it does today on our schools, we would have fallen apart long ago. Had using those bodies well and wisely in our young and mid-adult years depended on intelligence and information alone, most of us would be like tomorrow's after fifty crowd—inadequate. But we didn't. We used our bodies hard for work and play, loving and laughing, because there was no other way to live.

Spectating was limited both by opportunity and distance. We experienced everything firsthand and a lot of it was out-of-doors in nature's lap. The rewards for doing what came naturally were ours for the claiming.

The easiest way to understand many things is to apply them to yourself. This book is all about you—a menu of choices and remembrances. One way to think about history is to tie yourself into the unrolling years. When I want to remember something I'm reading I write in the margins. I can bring recent history down to size by writing, for example, "I was three," or perhaps, "That was the year we were in Europe for the Olympics." If the event took place before my time, I use my father. "Dad ran away to war that year." History becomes my history and has personal meaning for me. It's like a memory budge. If you try it you will begin to notice how each bit of history changed things for you and your way of life. If you are to understand how exceptional you are and that your kind of future has never been provided for a whole generation before, you need to relate those important developments of your lifetime to yourself and your family.

HOW DID WE GET THIS WAY?

You still have the basics for an excellent body whether or not you know it, believe it, or understand what it could mean to you. Wherever you stand today, you have the potential to improve yourself far beyond anything most people would consider possible because of something over which you had no control: *you walked everywhere.* For most of us in the after fifty crowd if there was a family car in our childhood, it came out on Sundays—and father drove. Mother (in a hat) sat up front with him and the kids sat in back, hating every minute of confinement. What fun was looking at the passing scene compared to running and jumping in it!?

Our schools were in the neighborhood, and there was no need for a parking lot. Even teachers walked to school, which gave them a physical outlet for their tensions. That same guarantee applied to us, too. Our schoolyards were surfaced with packed dirt. You could get bumped, bruised, and skinned if you fell, but it wasn't like today's cement yards. Fractures, missing front teeth, and concussions were rare then. The only bad schoolyard accident I remember happened when I clobbered Martin O'Sullivan over the head with my sled. He had decided what was mine was his and I had decided differently. The principal in a rare dither shouted that I could have killed him. It didn't interest me much. I knew for certain that if he died he wouldn't be headed for heaven.

"Gym" may not have been everybody's favorite activity, but it was the rare child who didn't prefer marching-to-music, wand drills, and "setting-ups" to spelling, arithmetic, and finding the capital of Kansas on a map with no printing. To get excused from "gym" in those days you had to have something serious like tuberculosis, which my friend Gwen Fearing did have. She didn't have to go to school at all but was supposed to stay out-of-doors all day for three whole years. Not knowing that tuberculosis was responsible for 20 percent of the deaths in the western world, I thought it must be a wonderful disease to have. Gwen and I figured that if we spent enough time together maybe I'd catch it, like chicken pox, and then neither of us would have to go to school. With that in mind I spent a good portion of the fifth, sixth, and seventh grades outdoors with Gwen.

My family moved around a lot and no school was ever quite sure where I was at any given time. Besides, truant officers never looked in the woods which was where we spent our days. But I didn't get tuberculosis; instead, Gwen got better. Thus ended three wonderful, even educational years.

When we were in school we all raced home for a "hot lunch." Nutrition was beginning to have its followers, and the leaders in our parents' day were people like William Andrus Alcott and Sylvester Graham (he of the cracker which still has merit). The "hot lunch" was the positive essential for a healthy childhood, just as coffee ("It will stunt your growth") was the negative.

In spite of the fact that we had already expended considerable energy (occasionally and daringly called "animal spirits") running to school, home for lunch, and back again, once the doors banged open at 3:15 there was an explosive exodus of racing, skipping, hopping, laughing, screaming children. Most of us raced, skipped, hopped, laughed, and screamed all the way home, gathering playmates as we went.

For the sake of what you are going to do for yourself, try to remember the little boy or girl you were at that time. Get out the album and really *see* that strong little body. Then close your eyes and see it living still, but within you, right now.

"The childhood shows the man, as morning shows the day."
Milton, Paradise Regained

Children, in "The Olden Days," as my children call my childhood, had a lot more energy than kids today seem to have. Stop by any school at bus time or recess. They wander, meander, and cackle and have virtually nothing in common with the wild flocks that swooped and screeched when you were a kid. They suffer from the same problems that inflicted our generation: they have trouble at home; there is child abuse and alcoholism and sorrow; they too must sit for hours behind desks just as we did and they don't like it one bit better. But there is a staggering difference: they lack the physical outlets to balance those stresses. What is even worse, they lack the urge to release them physically. They don't even know how. This incredible lack is not merely the school's failure; the failure is total: family, nursery school, kindergarten, junior and senior high school, college, and government.

The American child's day is a perfect model for researchers who want to turn a colony of white mice into "sickies" for experimentation. They eat junk for breakfast, leave overheated houses in overheated buses and spend their days in overheated schools with sealed windows. They sit at breakfast, they sit in the bus, and they sit in classrooms until they transfer their overupholstered bottoms to the cafeteria where they sit some more. There they eat food that would have Graham twirling in his tomb. Recess (if there is a recess) is a perfect rendition of "Cows Returning at Eventide." They wander out the door and except for a few renegades (bless them!), lean against a wall until it's time to wander back in. If there has been a heavy dew they aren't even allowed out. At the end of a long sedentary day they ride back home in the same overheated buses to the same overheated houses where they will go straight to the refrigerators for the junk snacks that will keep their sugar levels up and cholesterol levels high.

The latest study released by the United States Department of Health and Human Services called "The Heckler Report" is discouraging enough if taken at face value, but it is far more encouraging than it has any right to be. It states that *The youth of today carry substantially more body fat than their counterparts in the 1960s did.*" The next statement could, with the assistance of a blind eye, be called merely erroneous, actually, it is an out-and-out falsification: "*About half don't receive appropriate physical activity to maintain effectively functioning cardiorespiratory systems.*" One has to wonder where they got their statistics on "physical activity" and what the word "about" really means. Truth would have been better served had they replaced "about half" with "over half." The facts come closer to 80 percent. At the very least that is the number denied real physical activity. They were not vague when it came to the medical aspects of the testing, however.

The report goes on to say that "*The minimum requirement of vigorous physical activity is generally accepted as 20 minutes at 60 percent of capacity three times a week.*" It may be "accepted" but who gets it? A few years ago an associate and I took the time to visit physical education classes in public schools in many states from El Paso, Texas, to Portland, Maine. As we observed the children we recorded their activity with hidden stopwatches. We gave our attention to every level from first grade through high school. We always used the same system: each of us would choose two children, one child eager and active, the second, lethargic and uninterested. We clocked our "samples" only when they were engaged in "productive movement" which meant running, jumping, climbing, dancing, tumbling, and anything else designed to improve muscle tone, strength, flexibility, coordination, and endurance. Our clocks were stopped when the children were sitting for attendance or explanations, waiting turns, or watching other children play. *The average time spent in "productive movement" in each 45-minute class was 3 minutes.* Most public schools provide two such classes a week. Some have well-equipped gyms, many do not, but the outcome from such a limited program is the same. In high school most physical education is optional after the first year and since the programs offered the nonvarsity student are utterly boring, most opt for something else—the band or study hall. Nothing we saw in our travels could have maintained a person even on the lowest rung of the fitness ladder. Three minutes of very mild activity twice a week adds up to six minutes a week. Sitting hours for each child—in school, in the bus, and in front of TV—add up to at *least* fifteen a day, or seventy-five sitting hours in a five-day week. What happens to American children over the weekend is another story.

The next statement hardly does credit to a government agency: "*Based on self reports of activity patterns and of exertion in exercise, approximately half* of today's youth do not meet these requirements year round." Now start with "self reports." From kids ten to sixteen? The questionnaires were probably preceded by a pep talk from a physical education teacher who knows all too well how to weight a speech and has many reasons for doing so. On top of that, the kids don't have any idea as to what the questions actually mean; they have never had any *real* physical education to use as a frame of reference. Few American kids (unless they are athletes, and their number is both miniscule and male) know what *normal capacity* is. They wouldn't know a good exercise from a disaster or a couple of hobbles around the track from a decent workout. Like many adults, they would hate to look like failures and dropouts when it came to things physical, so the answers to their questionnaires were undoubtedly creative ("creative" is a euphemism for "exaggerated").

What cannot be questioned, however, are the results of the medical tests to which the children under consideration were subjected. There was no self-evaluation there! The information showed that *The youngster's heart–lung fitness lags behind most middle-aged joggers. Forty-one percent of them have high levels of cholesterol in their blood."* That should come as no real surprise since as long ago as the Korean War, autopsies done on young men fallen in battle revealed similar statistics. We knew then that something should be done to protect our young men whose major peacetime danger lay in a heart attack. But we didn't follow through.

"Twenty-eight percent of them (the tested children) have higher than normal blood pressure and 98 percent present at least one major risk factor for developing heart disease." Mind you, these are kids between the ages of ten and sixteen.

Here is a statement you should consider when you realize that the average student gets six minutes a week of activity in school. *"The average youth gets more than 80 percent of his/her physical activities outside of the school physical education program. An average of 12 to 13 hours a week are spent in physical activity outside of class year round, compared to two to three hours in class."* Now *there* is creative reporting on the parts of both students and teachers. While the so-called fitness boom has hit college graduates and a fair number of young and middle-aged adults, it hasn't touched the teenagers or the pre-teens. If the reported two to three hours of class can be reduced to six minutes (when you deal with content rather than time elapsed), what will happen to those twelve to thirteen hours outside class? What is really happening? Remember—these children we are discussing are our own beloved grandchildren.

MY OWN STORY—SO FAR

The handwriting on the wall began to appear back in the forties and fifties when I had a school called The Bonnie Hirschland Conditioning Classes. In actuality these were exercise classes, but my very first day as a would-be exercise teacher taught me a lesson about the road America had taken since the twenties and thirties. My two little daughters were athletes long before they ever went to school. They swam before they walked, rode horses, climbed mountains, skied, and went to dancing school. When the first one went to school I began to notice a change—she put on weight, both fore and aft. I, the kid who loved "gym" with a passion, went to the school to see what they were doing since my child wasn't sure what it was they did in "gym."

Ten minutes in the school was more than enough time for me to see what was, or, wasn't, happening. First they called the roll, then they "discussed" what they would play. Then they formed a circle. Since I was a visitor, my child got to start the game. She threw a ball straight up and squeaked "Eleven." The little girl who had that number ran three steps into the circle and caught the ball. She then threw the ball up calling for "Three." Three stepped out of the circle and missed the ball which rolled into a corner. Embarrassed "Three" then consigned the ball to "Ten" and the game continued for the fifteen minutes remaining. Fun it was not; challenging, it was not; physical education, it was not, so I decided my many years of training would stand my children in good stead: I would give them "gym" myself. I had been in the Kosloff Russian Ballet School from the age of four on and off through school. I was varsity in all sports but tennis and had taught dance at Camp Tegawitha the summer before I became a concert dancer with Charles Weidman and Doris Humphrey which was followed by a stint on Broadway. I had plenty of ideas!

"Pick five friends," I told each of my daughters. "We'll meet at the Girl Scout House on Friday at four and we'll exercise." My children had always felt that boys had more fun and *were* more fun, so they invited eight boys and two girls.

Both mothers of the girls called that night to say they didn't want their girls in an exercise class; they'd get muscles. (That kind of ignorance is no worse than another kind going around today—"No pain no gain.") I took the easy way out that time. I assured the mothers that their daughters would not become any more muscular than little ballerinas did, but I changed the name of the game from *exercise class* to *conditioning.* Since no one had any preconceived ideas about *conditioning,* I did just fine. In six weeks I had seventy-five boys and girls running, jumping, leaping, skipping, dancing, tumbling, and delighted . . . for a full hour.

I was a rock climber and my husband and I spent every weekend in the Showangunks, affectionately known as the "Gunks" in New Paltz, New York. They consisted of miles and miles of wonderful sheer cliffs, ideal for climbing practice. At that time only a very small number of climbers knew about the "Gunks" and the group had two leaders, Fritz Wiesener and Hans Kraus. I knew of Dr. Kraus's interest in sports injuries, and one sunny morning as we were sitting on a ledge dangling our legs over five hundred feet of space, I asked him if he had a test I might give my young exercisers. I wanted to know if my "conditioning" was having a good effect on them. He said he had a test, but it had been developed in the Presbyterian Hospital Posture Clinic and it was really for sick children. I could use it, but all healthy children would pass too easily.

I got the test. In the fall, as we tested about 100 children who were new in our school, I discovered to my horror that over 50 percent failed what we came to call the Kraus-Weber Minimum Muscular Fitness Test for Key Posture Muscles (see an outline and explanation of the test on page 81). Named for the two doctors who had devised it, it tested the minimum fitness of the body's key posture muscles. When I called the doctor to tell him the results he didn't believe me; I must have administered the test wrong. But I hadn't; he got the same results, and then asked if I could test a town. Certainly! My friends were on the Rye, New York, school board and they would help me. We started with Rye and then went on to many cities, towns, and even rural villages. I recruited the mothers of the children who had scholarships in my now-burgeoning school and we tested thousands of children. The failure rate came in at 58 percent. For the next two summers, in conjunction with rock-climbing vacations in the Italian Dolomites, the Austrian Tyrol, and Swiss Alps, Dr. Kraus and I tested 3,000 European children. Their failure rate was eight percent.

The Heckler Report says that *"Breaking precedent, the [Heckler] study measured fitness in health-related terms rather than by athletic ability."* They didn't break any precedents; they just didn't do their homework. Using a medically valid test, I had already determined the fitness state of American children as compared with children of three European countries. I was invited to the White House in 1955 to present the findings to President Eisenhower. The president said he was shocked and would certainly do something about the condition of our school children. He formed the President's Council on Youth Fitness which developed, through the administrations of seven presidents, as the President's Council

on Physical Fitness and, of late, as the President's Council on Physical Fitness and Sports.

The events that led up to the meeting with President Eisenhower proved again that it isn't what you know, but who. We had returned from Europe with the horrendous knowledge that while the European children failed our minimum muscular fitness test at 8 percent, we, the richest country in the world, failed at 58 percent. Nor was that the worst of it. We had noticed that children failing more than one of the six tests (which took 90 seconds to administer) seemed to have insufficient physical outlet for the stress under which they lived. Almost no European child failed more than one test, but 32 percent of the Americans failed more than one and some failed them all! Since both the failures and the emotional implications should have been of interest to the medical community, we wrote up the study for medical journals and presented the findings at a medical convention. Nobody turned a hair. It was as if a brand new invention called a "wheel" had been rolled off an Atlantic City pier, sinking at once to the bottom. The media, however, responded quite differently. The wave was slow in starting, but in a matter of months it was rolling along gathering size and momentum; the newly invented wheel floated to the surface.

A young athlete, Jack Kelly, brother of Princess Grace of Monaco, read about our study and showed it to his father, John B. Kelly, one of our elder statesmen. John Kelly met with Dr. Kraus and me at the New York Athletic Club and asked if we would be interested in presenting the results of our study to President Eisenhower. By that time subsequent tests all over the world showed that India's half-starved children had only a 39 percent failure. Guatemala's children, many loaded with intestinal parasites and at least as malnourished as the Indians, failed at 21 percent. Japan's children, just recovering from a terrible war, as were the Austrians and Italians, failed at 15 percent. I felt sure President Eisenhower would want to know that America's children were the weakest in the world.

"I'll be in touch," said Kelly. If you are young . . . if you know something awful is happening . . . if you know what to do about it and have already proved that you can . . . when a person of importance says "I'll be in touch" you hit cloud nine. Our entire study had been done by volunteers, some in exchange for their children's lessons. There were no computers in those days and yet thousands and thousands of cards, each carrying six separate test results, were computed individually, by sex, by age, by school, by town, and by me in the middle of the night. My husband took a dim view of all these goings-on and they were not allowed to interfere with his evenings. So I learned patience. I would wait until he was asleep and then descend to the basement where the day's "take" in test results awaited my hand-done arithmetic. I lived with a sleep deficit for months. The payback to each school was a full report on each child by name plus the correlatives needed to alter the situation. Each school received a chart showing where it stood in comparison to the other schools in the system and, since the classroom teacher makes a tremendous difference when it comes to the comparative fitness of the children, the principal was given a chart with all

the class results. That test done in the fall would have told any intelligent principal what the fitness level of his or her school was and where the real problems, both physical and emotional, were likely to lie.

In Europe Dr. Kraus and I purchased ten dollars' worth of candy to distribute among the tested children in Italy and another bag for Austrians. Later, I made the same investment in Guatemala. In cold, hard cash, other than the layout for the Guatemalan testing which was not connected with a vacation, "The Report that Shocked the President" cost about thirty dollars. I've often wondered what it would have cost had the study been undertaken by a government agency.

So, in a borrowed hat and with a very dry mouth, I headed for the White House to lunch with the president. Not even in my wildest dreams had that ever happened.

In order to catch the attention of the country, since nobody was really interested in either "health" or "fitness," the White House had invited about forty sports "Greats" to attend my presentation. Of all the people there, the only one who was really equipped to understand what I was about to say was the president himself. He had seen American boys in action in two wars and already knew something was amiss. When I told him that American children *entered* school with a 54-percent failure in our minimum test due to the fact that they didn't move around much at home, and that after twelve years of "physical education," they left school with only 2-percent improvement, the muscles in his jaw tightened. After hearing the rest of the report, he said something must be done about it. He meant it and I believed him. Unfortunately, between a president's mouth and executive action lie light years of delay.

What did come of it, and by a long, slow process, was what we have today—an awakened awareness that fitness is important. The various councils and the media have helped make adults aware, but, unfortunately, very little has filtered down to the children. Think: who's jogging? Is it a man or a boy?

At first not too much attention came our way until the physical educators began a marvelous controversy regarding the fitness test: they said it was too hard. We replied that if it was so hard, why did the Europeans pass so easily? It was a gymnastics test, they said, and Americans were games-oriented. That didn't hold water either, because the average six-year-old is not a gymnast, but that age group entered American schools with a 54-percent failure. Finally they decided that the thing to do was invent a test that showed "our" strong points (baseball throw) rather than our weak ones (strength and flexibility). The designers liked the test, but the teachers who had to give it didn't. It took too long and there was too much paper work. However, the children did look better when averages were computed. The trouble was, they still looked pretty bad when compared to children of other nations even when these other nations used the "American" test. When the British girls beat out the American boys, the American physical educators let their new test die.

One interesting sidelight: When we compared the results of public schools versus private schools, the statistics showed that while little children entering both public and private schools had almost the same failure rate (private school entrants were about 4 percent worse off than public school entrants), the results at graduation were very different. While public school children had improved 2 percent in twelve years, private school children had improved 44 percent. Why? The answer is obvious—more sports, more exercise, more real outdoor play.

No matter what the people in charge of public school physical education did or said, they have not been able to make their pupils any fitter. Today they use the test put out by the President's Council on Physical Fitness and Sports. Most students fail it and since "everybody flunks" nobody minds—out loud. Inside is another matter. Even if "everybody flunks," everybody *wants* to pass, and wants to think of himself or herself as "fit." *Fit is it* these days, but if flunking the "President's Fitness Test" is any indication, most of today's kids can consider themselves as "gross."

And, alas, they are our beloved grandchildren.

"As I approve of the youth that has something of the old man in him, so I am no less pleased with an old man that has something of the youth."

Cicero

Of course Cicero was addressing his observations toward men only. This does not detract from his remark, which applies more to women than to men since so many of them outlive men. Put a little more inclusively, one might say that the grown-up whose "inner child" smiles out through bright eyes has more fun and brings more delight to living.

It was war time, the fall of 1943, when I got to know the ladies at the Osborne Home for Retired Gentlewomen. Several of them worked in the sewing circles I had set up for the Red Cross in Harrison, New York. I had never known any "old" people so I had no preconceived ideas about what older people would, could, or should be able to do. If they had any limitations I didn't know about them, and they certainly knew *everything* about sewing. I could count on them too. Many of the younger volunteers at the circle had problems that kept them away from the work. Some had young children who took sick. If the kids brought home a bug their mothers caught it too. Household help was impossible to find and crises were the order of the average family day; but not for my "Old Guard." They never missed—rain, shine, hot, cold, or holidays. We behaved as though the baby clothes and layettes for the war orphans were as important as ammunition and ships. We had a duty to perform in the days when the word was akin to a celestial mandate, but we also had joyful hours and all of us enjoyed both the work and each other.

Twelve years later Harper and Row asked me to write a book about the state of physical fitness in America, about the testing I had done. They asked that the book also provide answers to the problems I had uncovered. The book that Harper finally published was called *Is Your Child Really Fit?* Dr. Hans Kraus wrote the foreword. It came out in 1956 and my friends at the Osborne Home read about it in the local paper. They called and asked me if I'd come and talk to them about it. I

was flattered and delighted. I had my first speaking engagement as an honest-injun' author. The subject was so exciting to me I felt sure everybody in the world would be interested. I thought that until I walked into the auditorium and saw all those beautifully coiffed white heads. "Heavens! They can't possibly have any interest in the fitness of American school children . . . theirs are all grown and flown. Good grief! What shall I talk about?" But I was saved by a habit I had developed over the years. I always try to find out at least something about the people in my audience, and I already knew quite a bit about how these had lived and what their lifelong interests had been. American children might be unfit, but these ladies had led very active childhoods and adult lives. Right then I coined the title of my talk . . . YOU ARE THE LAST FIT AMERICANS. Then I told them why.

A tiny lady in the back stood up and asked if they were too old to exercise. "Certainly not," I said, remembering my elderly grandfather who liked hitchhiking. He'd been a judge and decided to see the world from his feet. Well, the lady asked, if they weren't too old, would I teach a class? I said I'd be glad to, but when the lady doing the asking said she'd call me Tuesday and tell me how many ladies were interested, I breathed a sigh of relief. I *knew* there would be no takers. I was one of those young mothers with two little ones around the house, a very busy and demanding husband, and no help.

Imagine my surprise when she called to tell me she had thirty would-be students. "What shall we wear?" I had a pretty fair idea of what they had stashed away in the trunks at the home and I knew that whatever it was, it wouldn't do. "Don't worry about a thing, I'll take care of it. I'll be there next Tuesday at ten." I went to New York to see my friend Ben Sommers who owned Capezio and asked for whatever he could spare at low cost. He was just changing his line of leotards and tights from wool to nylon, so he said I could have all the wool outfits I needed. I needed thirty.

Can you imagine that first class? Think about it. Those ladies could have been your mothers, aunts, even grand-mothers. None of them had ever gone without a corset, even in a bathing suit. Now they were easing themselves onto the floor in leotards! I had never real-ized in just how many directions the human body could spread. How to be-gin? Actually there was a precedent and I knew all about it. These nice people had only been inactive for a few years. I would have them start back at the beginning. But where *was* the be-ginning? I found the answer to that in my own experience. Hang in, and I'll tell you about it.

I was badly injured in a skiing acci-dent when I was twenty-one. I had been barreling down Vermont's famous rac-ing slope, Suicide Six, when I fell and sat on a rock at about forty miles an hour. My pelvis was fractured in four places, so I was strung up in traction for three months. Traction is now con-sidered old hat except for the setting of bones, since it often causes the very thing it is supposed to relieve: muscle spasm. I suppose I should have consid-ered myself lucky since just prior to my fractures one of the accepted proce-dures for handling pelvic fractures was to hang the whole midsection of the body in a sling. You can imagine what happens inside the pelvis with that kind of treatment! One could hardly manage to function in that position even with a perfectly healthy pelvis. Ten years after my misadventure, people with such injuries were up on crutches in a few days. Keep in mind, medical modalities change, and what sounds like the *dernier cri* this year may well be in the doghouse next.

Years later, when I finally got my comeuppance—the comeuppance we all get when, long after an injury, there is too much stress to be borne—the pain came not from my old fractures, but from the muscles that had been strained and the fibers torn by traction. When I was finally released from trac-tion and before I even got out of bed the doctor assured me that I would always limp, could no longer ski or climb, and shouldn't have children. That's another lesson: never listen to Gloomy Guses. I had been a concert dancer and an ath-lete before the accident and my body had a louder voice than the doctor's. "Come on," it whispered, "you've been busted before. You'll be OK. What does *he* know?!" It turned out he didn't know right from breakfast.

When I was finally allowed to sit in a chair my husband could circle my calf with his thumb and middle finger. The accident hadn't done that; the de-cision to immobilize me had. Today we know that twenty-one days of bed rest can physiologically age a person thirty years. After ninety days I was thin, weak, trembly, and with little strength or balance. I had no stamina and was exhausted just sitting. I was twenty-two, looked sixty-two, and felt ninety-two. Where do you begin the road back when you have aged sixty-odd years in three months? You begin as though you had aged in the accepted fashion over a period of many decades. *You start easy and progress at your own comfortable speed.* My nurse and I had amassed a record library of pop tunes, and as she was straightening the room she put one of them on. You remember it, "The Dipsy Doodle." Quite without any conscious direction from me, my feet started tapping. That was the beginning. In half an hour I had choreographed a foot and leg routine that felt wonderful. I was in a lather and needed a nap. That afternoon I did another routine to "Caravan." That was even better since it brought in my head, neck, shoulders, hands, and upper back. I could hardly wait for the next day. We added another record and another routine each day (you will find the start of those routines on page 288). Had I known then what I know now about "Bed Ballet" I would never have "aged" at all.

There was my precedent for the Osborne class!

Thirty of us sat in a circle wiggling our toes to Leroy Anderson's "Sleigh Ride." I found ways no one had ever dreamed of to use a chair, my "students" found others. By the second week we were standing behind the chairs, in front of the chairs, using them for support part of the time, but just as often in a game rather like "Musical Chairs." Right then I decided to give my "students" the Kraus-Weber

test. Remember, the failure rate for American children was 58 percent, and 44 percent couldn't touch the floor with their finger tips. The Osborne team had no flexibility failures. They didn't do well on sit-ups, and, at first, getting up and down posed some problems, along with a lot of hilarity. But, using the chairs to help until our knee bends (page 238) gave us the needed strength, we managed.

By the third week we were doing all the warm-ups in this book and several of the kneeling and lying exercises. We had made a big dent in the floor progressions and we'd begn to use small equipment. By the eighth week I retested. My seventy-and-up (eighty-six was the oldest and she was the organizer) Osborne ladies had better test results than the Rye High School students—girls *or* boys!

Why were those ladies so fit and why did it take so little time to recapture strength and flexibility? They had built the same basic bodies you have and they did it the same way. They had walked everywhere and had done gardening, housework, and assorted chores all their lives. It really is no big deal to reactivate a body, even one as messed up as mine has been. It's a lot harder to start from scratch without the basics, which is what today's seekers of fitness are having to do.

If you walked to school you have the basic body.

A BACKWARD LOOK

Now you know why you are superior to the under forty crowd. It will be no trick at all to get you into good condition and keep you that way. Come back with me and see why.

Besides walking to and from school four times a day, you played out-of-doors. If you weren't quick enough to get into the house, out of your school clothes, into your play clothes, and out the door before your mother caught you, she sent you to the store. You had a scooter and skates and probably a bike, and there were safe places to ride all three. There weren't so many cars on your streets and trucks didn't roar through your neighborhood.

There weren't any weirdos around when you were kids and ranging the neighborhood. We all got the same order—"Be home by six." The worst thing that could happen was if we came home late. We read books or were read to. We played Parcheesi, checkers, and Old Maid, and we made things—puppet theaters, boats, doll beds, and slingshots. Try to remember the toys you invented that developed both your creativity and manual dexterity. You put on shows in the backyard and a lot of you practiced the piano. Everybody could and did sing. Saturday was all ours to spend, waste, or use, which we usually did outdoors and according to season. When we got a little older we could walk the several miles to the movies. Saturday was the day for serials, cartoons, double features, and travelogues. We watched Brett Hart, Tom Mix, Ramon Navarro, Lillian Gish, Kay Francis, Douglas Fairbanks, and Mary Pickford. Nearly everybody lived happily ever after, and the Hayes Office made sure we saw only things that were fit for kids to see.

Then came the radio. I was about ten when Billy Group made one out of an oatmeal box and some copper wire. It was called a crystal set. My father, a representative for national advertising in newspapers, was offered a chance to get in on the ground floor of radio, but he said it would never out-sell newspaper advertising. Pretty soon the radio meant evening entertainment. Most of us had to get through the dishes fast in order to settle down for "The Lone Ranger," "The Shadow," "The Green Hornet," and "Amateur Hour." There were lots of strange noises, yelling, and shooting, but no blood. Only the villains bit the dust and rape was unheard of. "The Scarlet Letter" was about as "bad" as movies ever got, and my mother took us to New York to see "An American Tragedy." Was she trying to tell us something?

Few of us were latchkey kids. Most children had someone to come home to. We came home to milk and oatmeal cookies or bread and jam. There were no cokes or potato chips. Once in a long while we were allowed to make fudge. If you walked to and from the library instead of spending your dime for the trolley, which cost a nickel each way, you had enough for a hot chocolate with whipped cream and a wafer. When we felt wicked we smoked corn silk and assorted weeds. Nobody had ever heard of pot.

Try to remember what you learned on the way to school besides the occasional four-letter word. Life for our generation was completely sensual, even though our parents never used the word. You luxuriated with the warm sun on your back in spring. You walked through rainstorms and the water ran down your face and into your mouth. It had a sweeter taste than tap water, and while you liked it very much nobody told you that the flavor was actually you. You waded in flooding gutters and broke the first brittle ice panes covering winter puddles. Frost feathers grew on your way and in spring they were replaced by violets. Your sensitive nose picked up the aromas of lilacs, lilies of the valley, roses, and the grapes in the arbor three houses away.

In that faraway time we climbed

rocks and slid down grassy hills. We danced in March winds and rolled in the leaves of autumn. There was a tantalizing smell of leaf smoke that even today will bring you good feelings. You will never forget the blackened potatoes, baked in bonfires. When you thought they were "done" you slit them, salted them, and shoved in a hunk of sooty butter. No baked potato has equaled that since. In winter your first move was to the window to check for the snowfall you'd been expecting for a month. When it finally came it was your job to shovel the walk. You came off the sliding hill to sip hot cocoa and to replace sodden mittens with dry socks over bright red fingers. Remember the smell of wool steaming on the radiator? When you finally gave up because the sun was gone and the hill was blue in the frosty twilight, there was that marvelous aroma of supper cooking. While you waited there was a good chance that someone would sit you on a lap and read you a story or the funnies. Television doesn't have a lap and it doesn't smooth your hair and ask, "And how did it go today?"

A FORWARD LOOK

The twenty-first century is just around the next bend and the generation that will stand where you are now will be very different. It is already different. We are so used to things improving in America that it may take some stretch in your thinking to understand that those coming generations can never be your equal. At the close of the most important building years, birth to six, most of today's children fail a minimum fitness test. Only a few of you would have failed and those could have been quickly redeemed. Today's children have few ungranted wishes. Their taste buds, assaulted by the extremes of flavors, know nothing of sour grass, wild onions, or birch bark. Accustomed to the smooth texture of butter pecan ice cream, they know nothing of stealing chunks of crunchy ice from a wagon moving along the street, its driver pretending not to see the theft. They know nothing of chewing pine resin or the bubbling tar in a summer roadway. For them, if it isn't in a bright wrapper and for sale, it doesn't exist.

Start looking around you, and become aware of what you see. In forty years I haven't seen a bunch of kids running around the block just for the *feel* of it. There are plenty of adults doing it, but when did you last see a kid? Most of children today have never played "hide-n'-seek," "cops and robbers," "this old witch," or "red light." At the hour you were out hunting bugs to glow against your pillow, they are glued to TV. At the age when you got a wild thrill from squeezing into a hiding place with "The One" as you played "Sardines," today's budding lovers are watching somebody on television maneuvering somebody else into bed. Even that is mostly second hand.

Everything that happens to today's young happens too soon. They aren't growing up the way you did, wild and wonderful in the fields of a great, proud, and free country. They are caged, stuffed, and forced. You know, and even they would be able to tell you, what happens to young animals under similar conditions. But that need not continue. One man alone, John Walsh, started an organization, the National Center for Missing and Exploited Children, which focuses on finding lost or stolen children. His little boy, Adam, was kidnapped and murdered and there was no accepted way to alert the country, the public agencies, or even the folks in the next county. Now you see pictures of missing children everywhere, and even children are looking for other children, thanks to John Walsh. One woman alone, Candy Lightner, whose little girl was killed by a hit-and-run driver, in despair over the inability of the law enforcement people to get convictions for drunk drivers, started MADD, Mothers Against Drunk Driving. Candy Lightner and John Walsh felt that something had to be done, and did it. They had no more experience than you or I in changing their world, but that didn't stop them.

AND A WORD OF ADVICE

Find something that really interests you, and put your many talents and energies to work. What could be better than helping America's young people to become fit, to learn about the world that was yours and which you can still find for them? After all, many are your beloved grandchildren.

MYTHS AND HOW TO JUNK THEM

MYTHS NO CHILD SHOULD KNOW AND EVERY ADULT SHOULD FORGET

Beware! There are many myths about growing older. One of the first things to know about these myths is that they are often invented by "experts." I've been around long enough to be very nervous (and sometimes insulted) when I'm called an "expert" because most of those so named aren't expert at all. There are, for example, more fitness "experts" writing books and magazine articles, putting out records and tapes, making appearances and pronouncements, than there are fleas on a prairie dog. You can check your own mind for a list of experts. Just ask yourself how many "good" teachers you have had in a lifetime. The answer will probably be "less than five." Then count the people *called* teachers and compare.

The first thing to do when an "expert" sounds off is say, "Name your source." If you are really interested you can check it, but remember that "sources" are a little bit like "experts"— their statistics are often "creatively" used to prove their own points. In the long run, you will have to use your own experience, powers of observation, and common sense.

Prior to 1958 most of the information gathered on older people was based on those living in homes for the aged, alms houses, charity wards in hospitals, and other such institutions. Those elderly people had three things in common: they were old, they were poor, and they were there. They were in places where the old were grouped together in numbers large enough to give weight to statistics and to present an image. That these people were poor, overworked, malnourished for years, and probably ill didn't seem to make any difference.

Back in 1958 when the "experts" were deciding what those people were like and therefore what *you* are like, the youngest member of our after fifty crowd were busy scrambling for identity and raising a family. The furthest thing from your minds was a group called "The Elderly." Unless one of those "Elders" was a member of your close family and perhaps ill or giving trouble, you never thought of them at all. If any of us thought about them it was as the thin tapering end of life's candle. That within our lifetime the candle would switch directions and we would be the solid, growing, burgeoning end could never have entered anyone's head except perhaps Dr. Butler's. I certainly cannot be numbered among those with that kind of foresight. I hadn't thought about older people since my Osborne Home days, and even then I didn't think of them as a generation, just as a group of my friends. But in 1977 I began to sense the change. The people in Washington were starting to take notice, and what they'd come up with was anybody's guess. I decided to take a look. I discovered that the after fifty crowd is the most fascinating of all the ages and that once you scratch the surface, there's no end of depth. Each

member of our crowd is a world filled with history and adventure. Each is a survivor.

I also discovered that the mythmakers were in full cry and just as stupid as ever. I got madder and madder as I discovered how successful they still were. It was bad enough for the brothers Grimm to stain the minds of little children with nasty old lady witches, all bent and warty, but when the modern counterpart did the same thing to the people they purported to be helping, that got my Irish up and the hunt was on.

They're looking at *us*.

Before we start dissecting and demolishing the myths, let's look at something hopeful. There are some new "modern" sources of information regarding *homo senex*. There are many scholarly groups observing and testing us in our own habitats, rather than in zoos.

They are discovering (surprise, surprise) that their subjects live like other human beings, with dignity and independence. We are a mixed bag. Some are healthy, some have problems. Some work, some have retired. Some are well educated, some have limited education but great native intelligence. Some lost out on sex, some are as interested as ever. Some are busy with projects, friends, travel, grandchildren, and the future. Some have turned themselves over to TV, their doctors, and the obit section of the newspaper. Whatever they are up to or have given up on, they present exactly the same kaleidoscope of personalities, states of health, interests, successes, and failures as any other age group.

Some of our behavior patterns, attitudes, and conditions are merely observed and noted as we pass through observation posts, such as hospitals and nursing homes. Others are covered in universities as members of the older set offer themselves as guinea pigs. Those volunteer subjects check in at stated intervals for physicals and psychological and intelligence testing. Other groups of observers present statistics that are gleaned from the census bureaus, insurance companies, and such unlikely parties as prison officials, fashion editors, and sports organizers. One of the amazing "new" discoveries about us "elders" is that basically we are exactly like everybody else, *but with experience.* Amazing?

At first, tests comparing the intelligence of older and younger people were weighted in favor of youth. The same complaints that are often lodged against intelligence and aptitude tests today would apply to those weighted tests, for (1) comparing apples and oranges, and (2) using language that is comprehensible to one group and incomprehensible to the other. Apples and oranges might represent our grandparents who did not go to college as opposed to the average young person today who does.

Most of our grandparents were denied a college education, even when male. Females were not even considered. The University of Virginia had been conceived by Thomas Jefferson as ideal for young men. It was considered very advanced when in the summer months it lifted its ban on female students and, in the early years of this century, opened its doors to more than a thousand teachers-in-training for the Virginia public schools. The comparison of time alotted to men versus women (never mind course content!) tells you where education was just before World War I. But the whole attitude toward education was different then. The average ambitious young man could make his way quite well in a pioneer country where native intelligence and stamina played a bigger role than four years behind ivied walls. Many a boy started out to make his way while still in his teens; his acquaintance with tests had been limited to arithmetic, spelling, and "composition." This does not mean that our elders couldn't "figure." They could, and they built America with that basic information. "Composition" meant actually being able to marshall thoughts and put them on paper logically, correctly spelled, and in legible (and often beautiful) penmanship. But the kinds of tests that are part of today's young people's education were not a part of theirs.

When the experts, who were more curious than wise, compared the test results of "elders" with those of students still in college (who had been tested regularly since first grade), the results were not really valid. However, valid or not, there are still researchers who accept the test results as signs of the "elders" failing intelligence.

And they're creating myths. About us.

Where should we start? With the myths a lot of you believe? The three that come up most often are senility, poverty, and the nursing home. Everyone seems to be terrified of the first, many are worried about the second, and for some, the conviction that the third is where we all go to die is as solid as the one about there being a hell down there. In fact we aren't too sure that the nursing home and hell aren't one and the same!

MYTH 1
Myth: OLD PEOPLE "GO SENILE,"

LOSE THEIR MINDS, CAN'T RE-
MEMBER ANYTHING, WET THEIR
PANTS, AND DRIBBLE DOWN
THEIR BIBS.

Junking the Myth: *Some* old people
suffer from senile dementia. Some
young and middle-aged people aren't
very stable either. There's been so much
about Alzheimer's disease in the papers
in the last couple of years you'd think
that was the only thing that could happen to us other than stroke, cancer, and
heart attack. Two of my skiing buddies
died of strokes within a year of each
other and they were in their forties. Two
of my young students have cancer right
now and one is just over it. My ex-
husband died of a heart attack at forty-
seven. Death can come at any time. Is
it any surer or less sure because we are
nearer the end or the beginning? My
sister's boy, who died on the Cambodian
border, didn't give much evidence of it.
If you are a man, at birth your risk of
running into Alzheimer's is 1.8 percent.
If you are a woman, 2.3 percent. What
you ought to be worried about is the
hospitalization before you "get away,"
as the Irish so nicely put it. That is a
real threat, and one of our jobs right
now is to lessen the danger of not being
allowed to "get away."

For most of us, senility can be post-
poned for a long time and maybe for
always. We read and hear about horror
stories, but they are like the news: If it's
bad, you'll hear about it; if it's very bad,
you'll hear about it fast; if it's really
awful you'll hear about it every night
for at least a week. Good news is slow
in coming, not because it isn't there,
but because it isn't an attention-getter
and it doesn't sell. So let's look around
and dig up some of the good stuff.

When Irving Berlin was 97, he was
still dressing like a fashion plate and
still had what looked like his own hair
and could have been his own hair for all
I know, but that's hardly important.
Premature alopecia hits both young
and old and has nothing whatever to do
with brains, vitality or virility. Irving
Berlin was still running his music company as well as his household. Lillian
Gish, who is over ninety, was recently
honored by all of Hollywood. She looks
as though she has just stepped out of a
bandbox. Averell Harriman is ninety-
four and I wouldn't want to risk my dollar up against his! George Abbott, the
Broadway producer and playwright,
was writing another play at 96 and may
have finished it by now. Dr. Karl Menninger, whose book *The Human Mind*
got me into trouble in the New York
subway (a lady said, "What's a nice
child like you doing reading a book like
that?), is over 90 and still chairman
of the Menninger Clinic which he
founded. Andrés Segovia, one of the
world's greatest guitarists, was ninety-
two at last count and still had a full
schedule of bookings that takes him
around the world for most of the year.
For every one of those very bright, busy,
with-it people in the public eye, there
are thousands and thousands we don't
know but who are equally bright, busy,
and with it.

Before we go any further I want to
call your attention to what causes a lot
of what passes for senility: prescribed
drug addiction. Doctor number one
prescribes Drug A. Doctor number two,
who has a different specialty, prescribes
Drug B which has an antipathy for
Drug A. Doctor number three, another
specialist, prescribes yet another drug
unfriendly to Drug A. Soon the patient
can't remember which drug was for
which symptom, but for some hard-to-
explain reason, stops none of the drugs

and asks no questions. The use of drugs for more sinister purposes isn't new. There are still instances when they are used by self-seekers in charge of often helpless elderly persons. The intention is to cloud minds that would otherwise be clear and aware. Less venal perhaps, but equally unacceptable, is the use to which "calming" drugs are sometimes put, turning "calm" into *non compos mentis*.

Then there are the over-the-counter drugs which are often the same as drugs A, B, or C, but in smaller doses. However, if you think an OTC drug is completely safe you are not very smart. Overuse of these drugs can cause more problems than they solve. If any drug doesn't get along with what you are already taking, it can spell "Poison," and your reaction can be spelled "Senility." A drug is a drug and you should do everything in your power to stay away from them, which means not *need* them. Every positive study of older people I saw said, "If the person is healthy, he or she should be able to continue to work if that is what is desired, enjoy an active sex life, be independent, and take part in all the wondrous things life has to offer, with the added lift of appreciation." Staying healthy should be our main goal, not searching after a new drug. Health is not to be found in a bottle. The after fifty crowd buys 20 percent of the over-the-counter medications and fills 25 percent of the prescriptions. It will take information, intelligence, and character to withdraw from the habit of a lifetime: *If you hurt . . . take something.* With an understanding of *Myotherapy* and a tailor-made exercise and fitness program you won't have to hurt. Imagine how many medications will be made obsolete, just for

you! Multiply that by the rest of us, and there will be billions to spend on exactly what we would like to have. Also, we'll have enough left over to help those among us who have been less fortunate, and we'll have the healthy energy to seek them out.

Older we are, and still older we will be with any luck, but poverty stricken and senile most of us are not, nor will we be, *unless* we lose or give up our health because of ways of life incompatible with health. . . . *or unless we take to drugs.* How does that work?

As a nation we have been taught by our parents, by our doctors, by our magazines, newspapers, by the radio, TV and by our peers, to "Take something for the cramps," to "take something for that cough," to "take something for the fever," "Something for sadness," "something for nerves," "something for sleep," "something for overweight," "something for arthritis," or "something for aging . . ." and those are only for starters. What we take are chemicals. If we mix any one of them with other drugs or alcohol (another drug) or even some foods, we get a synergistic reaction which can be dangerous to our health. That too is just for starters. That mixing can also be dangerous to our brains and our very lives as many have discovered when their loved ones made that mistake. In order for a drug to be strong enough to "do" anything, it must also be strong enough to cause some unpleasant and unwanted things called side-effects. If they don't seem to "do" anything it is the American way to try two or even three of the same pills or doses. If they "do" the job and render us painless, we may overlook the fact that they are also "doing" something else. A noisy "something else" would be diarrhea or vomiting. A quiet, easily overlooked "something else" might be a slightly dry mouth or skin, cracked lips, dry, thinning hair, brittle nails or ringing in the ears. All of those are called "signs of aging" as well, but *are* they? Before you think "aging," start thinking "drugs." What are you on? Why are you on it? Have you tried not taking it?

Where drugs are concerned don't be your own prescriber even when the drug sounds harmless such as the whole spread of *over-the-counter* medications. Second, *always* know what the drug is *supposed* to do and every possible side effect. Above all, rearrange your thinking about drugs; they are *not* the simple answer.

Another thing that is totally in our hands is what we do with our brains—the ones we're so worried about. We know full well that children left to languish untended, unstimulated, badly fed, and without anyone to talk with, become "retarded." So do adults. A lack of mental stimulation is deadly. Conversely, any faculties that we do use will hold up. That's what Head Start was all about. Researchers found that rats kept in large cages with lots of friends and toys developed very differently from rats deprived of space, friends, or toys. The food could be the same, but still the stimulated rats grew heavier brains and were much more chemically active than their impoverished brothers. Far from diminishing with age, our learning capacities continue to grow, as do our vocabularies and conceptual skills. And we do actually become wiser with time *if* we use those abilities.

Stop worrying about becoming senile. Find things to study; go after old skills and revive them; make friends, go

places, see things, and be discriminating about another dangerous drug—television. While you are sitting, you are not moving or growing. Worry is also unproductive, so don't do that either.

MYTH 2

Myth: OLD PEOPLE ARE POOR, THEY CAN'T WORK ANYMORE. AND THEY HAVE TO LIVE ON SOCIAL SECURITY AND BE SUPPORTED BY THEIR CHILDREN. HOPE I WON'T BE LIKE CHARLIE. HE HARDLY GOT HIS KIDS THROUGH COLLEGE WHEN HE HAD TO START SUPPORTING HIS AGING PARENTS.

Junking the Myth: All this howling about how much older people are going to cost the younger generation! When these same howlers were younger they were screeching about not trusting anyone over thirty. The scary thing is you may even believe all that. There is no question that there are a lot of older people who don't have enough money. In some studies we read that 17 percent of us are worried about money all the time, and in others the number runs as high as 20 percent. Two facts are glaring, and they are facts we will have to address when we get it into our heads that safety can be found in numbers. We have those numbers: Let's look at the 80 percent who are either just OK, OK with enough left over to tie a bow, or very OK.

I didn't think all old people were poor until I began to read about the "elderly" in newspapers back in the seventies. Here in the Massachusetts Berkshires we began to get flyers advertising workshops for "Senior Citizens," "Active People Over Sixty," "Your Elders and

How to Treat Them," and many others. Being a Fitness Institute, we were on many mailing lists. Then I began to get invitations to demonstrate exercises for older people. Harking back to my Osborne Home team, which had ultimately become a demonstration group good enough to go on The Today Show, I began to look into these meetings and workshops. I was horrified. At no time did I hear anyone talk of the well-to-do elderly and their needs, only the poor and theirs. I knew older people who were well off and in some ways more needy of companionship and care than the very poor, who at least had some friends, but that wasn't the message—it was *always* the poor. There are all kinds of hungers, and when we think of them we should think *human* hungers, not just the hungers of those who have few material comforts. It is true that some old people are poor and some are terribly poor, but to stereotype *all* old people as poor, feeble, and vulnerable is a form of discrimination. Anyone who says all old people are poor or even that most old people are poor has never been to Florida in winter or Europe in summer, sailed on a cruise, or sold Cadillacs.

People who are sixty-five and up are said to be "older," and 23 million of them are heads of consumer households. The per capita income for this group is $11,263, considerably higher than the national average. Of the older families 20 percent have an income of $20,000 and three-fourths of them own their own homes, many free and clear. If you realize that for those people rent isn't eating up a high percentage of their income as it does for many younger Americans, then you have a different picture of the "elderly poor."

Of the nation's discretionary income, 55 percent is in the hands of the after fifty crowd who are between fifty-five and sixty-five. That's double what it is for people between the ages of eighteen and thirty-four. There's a vast difference between spending for what you absolutely have to have and what you would simply like to have. (Older Americans spend one dollar in every five spent by the entire nation for home food. Do you remember the home-cooked dinners for which you had to be on time with clean hands? A whopping 88 percent of Americans spend the other four dollars in every five for home food. The rest of the time they eat out.) Last night I counted sixty-two restaurants along fifteen miles of Route One, and that doesn't include the restaurants in towns at either end of that stretch. Most of the restaurants were fast food eateries, and all had full parking lots.

People over sixty-five make up 11.8 percent of the total population, receive 11.9 percent of the personal income, and (back to discretionary income) their kids are through school. Many if not most of these older people have already made the major purchase of a lifetime, a house, and the mortgage is paid off. The major worry and the major expense is a long-term illness. While 23 million of our older brothers and sisters live in consumer households, of which many are the heads, they still pay 30 percent of the $220 billion spent in this nation on personal health care. That's disgraceful in a nation that *could* be full of healthy people of all ages. Our really great advances in medicine came with *prevention*, not pick-me-ups, stick-me-ons, and take-one-every-four-hours. It's time to look into more preventive measures. There are people who "need" to be sick in order to get attention, but they are few and far between. The rest of us need to be well in order to attend to the happiness life has to offer.

The government tells us that their sources prove that older people who are on social security and have other benefits are better off than any other group in the country. They assure us that "myths" about old people eating dog food and freezing to death in Buffalo are either untrue or greatly exaggerated. They *are* true about some old people just as they would be true about some younger people and God forgive all of us, they are true of children as well, but the mythical part is that the statement usually takes in everybody in an age group. Right now the government is painting a rosy picture of us, and there certainly has been an improvement in our overall image in the last years. But you can't get blood out of a stone, and the country is in financial trouble. We should be aware of that and plan for our future by staying in control of our lives. That we can do as long as we have our health and our strength. For most of us, that is within reach.

It is no myth however, that this country, affluent to the point of gross obesity, allows many of its people to suffer abject poverty, ill health, neglect, degradation, and avoidance. We used to think of ourselves as a clean, beggarless country with a chicken in every pot and a bed for every head. Not so. We have the usual social pattern: a group noted for conspicuous consumption of the world's goods; a middle mass struggling to stay afloat in a fluctuating economy; and at the end of the spectrum, the poor, the millions of illiterates, the sick, and the old. At the furthest end are the poor, sick old women who have everything working against them including their pasts, whether those pasts were productive, valued by anyone at all, or simply a lifetime of struggle without reward.

The rewards for having been a diligent housewife and child raiser are in inverse proportion to the amount of time and effort put into the job. The more time spent *in* the home, the less could be spent outside either in part-time work or in developing a network of supporting friends. The fewer the outside contacts, the greater the self-doubt later when the supporting ego has been eroded through death or divorce.

The only job I had held before marriage was that of a concert dancer. A concert dancer is like a concert pianist or a prima ballerina. An entire life and every ounce of strength is put into her work, with about five hours of practice a day. It isn't the kind of job you can drop and then pick up again eighteen years later. During the intervening years I kept house and raised two little girls. I never even learned to type and still use only two fingers . . . but *fast!* I never thought I would have to use my hobbies to support myself and my children. But I did. You should think about your strengths, skills, and talents. Better than that, get a job, go to school, volunteer for all sorts of things. Your talents and deeds probably won't count on a resume, but *you* will know you have the experience. The key is to depend on yourself and no one else. There were all kinds of dire predictions about what would happen to women now that they are sharing the stresses of management (as if there were no stresses in a home with children!). But the heart attack and other stresses disease levels didn't rise; quite the contrary. Women working outside the home have a better health record than those confined to their houses.

Many women who did not have the opportunity to work outside the home are now old, frail, and often both malnourished and ill. However, they don't inspire sympathy. They are not beautiful lost children nor are they the needy young with a future to underwrite. Mostly they are alone, and that means unprotected in a land seething with crime. They are frightened, and fear attracts the worst elements of our society who mug them for the pittance they carry and often injure them badly in the process. As you will learn later in the book, any injury to an older person brings to life damage that was done in past years. That adds pain and weakness to an already burdensome task: getting through each day alive.

There is something else about that group: they are forgotten and ignored. When you have finished this book you will know how to protect yourself and those you love from the perils suffered by so many of our crowd. And when you have that protection, you will owe something to the others. Each of us has a specialty and if we were to toss a little time from each of those specialties into a pot, we would have millions of hours devoted to helping one particular part of the After Fifty Crowd—the ones who need it most. Ask yourself what it is you could do to help . . . and then do it.

MYTH 3
Myth: ALL OLD PEOPLE END UP IN NURSING HOMES . . . THEIR CHILDREN PUT THEM THERE
Junking the Myth: You will be glad,

as I was, to learn that only 5 percent of Americans ever get there. Of those who finally make their way into nursing homes, most are over eighty-five and only half of them have families who could take care of them if they wanted to. Half of them stay only a matter of months while they recover from an illness or accident. And most get out alive. If you are worried about dying in a nursing home, know that 70 percent of us die in the houses we were in at age sixty-five. As for being socked away by uncaring relatives, that certainly happens sometimes—to helpless people of any age. I was six when I was placed in an orphanage, and no one took the trouble to look past the front parlor to see what went on where the potted palms ended.

I had a revealing experience with younger "put away" women when I set up an exercise program in the back wards of a state psychiatric hospital in New Jersey. There they sat in the day room, hats on, purses in laps, day after day, and they hadn't said a word for years. A friend of mine who worked as an occupational therapist wangled permission to use the day room, and we did an Osborne Home job on them. We set the chairs in a circle, recruited a couple of "joiners" to get the ball rolling, and started to do chair exercises to Leroy Anderson's music, which was hard to ignore. Pretty soon one woman started to follow with one hand, purse clutched firmly in the other. About the third day one zombie, who hadn't spoken a word for years, turned to her neighbor and said, "They made my neck hurt." Her neighbor neighed back, "Your neck! You should feel my back!" But they didn't stop. In a few months they were talking up a storm, left the wards to exercise on the lawn, wore exercise clothes, and were *alive*. Rage had kept them silent, as it did some of the orphanage children. *Why were we locked up?* That's what our silence asked. But there are worse things.

That there is child abuse, woman abuse, and abuse of older people is no myth. At least 4 percent of our after fifty crowd are abused every year, and if the truth were known the nearly one million who report it or are discovered are just the tip of the iceberg. Who does that sort of thing? Usually a son or a daughter, but not always. I had an experience in a hospital once that soured me on the healing profession. An elderly woman had fallen on the ice and broken her hip. Her hip was pinned, and sometime around ten at night she was brought down from the recovery room and put into the bed next to mine. She was still out of it, but seemed to be sleeping quietly. Early in the morning a nurse came in to check her and uttered the universal "Shit!" called for at moments of anger or frustration. The mostly unconscious lady had urinated in her bed. Would you believe, the nurse called for assistance, woke up the miscreant, and in the most vulgar language I'd heard in a while (and I've heard plenty) bawled her out, picked her up as roughly as possible, changed her bed as though she were a totally healthy gymnast, dropped her poor little moaning self back on the mattress, and stormed out. Later, when I told a doctor about it over the phone he said, "And I bet I know just who they are." "They" are still there and I'll bet nothing was ever said to that nurse.

Abuse happens to people who are disabled, dependent, and without access to help. That lack of access may be self-imposed. Women who have taken some kind of guff for a lifetime often don't find either reason or strength to change. They don't even complain; they just endure. What's behind most of it? Alcohol, drugs, stress, anger, ego ... and frustration. Avoiding possible future abuse is one very good reason for forming a network of friends who will protect you and whom you will protect. No one should accept, "Sorry, she can't see you today" more than once or twice. Few black eyes happen by running into doors at midnight, at least not more than once. Set up a home care and hospital protection group. Start now to plan and if you can, plan now for where you want to live later. Friends are essential and you can't form friendships while sitting in front of the TV set. Join things. There are some of us who aren't natural joiners either, but everyone can learn.

Senility, poverty, warehousing in nursing homes—those are the three areas most people bring up when questioned about the fears of the older generation. But there are secondary worries, too.

MYTH 4
Myth: POOR OLD THINGS; TOO BAD THEY NEVER HAD ANY EDUCATION. WE DON'T HIRE THEM AT OUR PLACE AFTER THEY HIT FORTY-FIVE; UNRELIABLE YOU KNOW, AND THEY DON'T HAVE ANY OFFICE SKILLS.

Junking the Myth: "Them" is us. So let's look at the facts: Just how well or poorly educated are we?

Of today's over-ninety-year-olds, 20 percent were immigrants right off the farms or the fishing boats and had less than eight years of education. This does not really impress me, as my own formal education adds up to considerably less than that. Those people came to this strange country, learned a new language and new ways, and, in many cases, built personal fortunes. All of them contributed to the building of an almost-new nation. Today, if one of those ninety year olds has occasion to hire one of today's college graduates, he may well have to send that college graduate to remedial classes to learn how to read and write a simple business letter. Older Americans are often far better educated than the younger generation. And what about the eighty percent who got better than eighth grade educations?

Roughly 35 percent of the senior members of the after fifty crowd finished high school, but only 7 percent got through four years of college. Because college graduates were such a rare breed, Americans, like Europeans, attached far more importance to a college education than the results deserved. A close check on the men who made the largest fortunes in America reveals more ruthless tenacity than classroom experience. However, the trend was upward mobility and parents were determined that things should be better and easier for their children. College seemed to guarantee a white-collar job. But a college education today isn't what it once was; standards are lower. Possibly because of this, a degree guarantees nothing more than a ticket in. Once past the door, ability comes into the picture. What seems to be lacking in education, both physical and mental, are the basics. American students are very short on basics of any kind.

For the most part, older people have the basics. The elderly proprietor of a hole-in-the-wall grocery in Barbados can tot up a column of figures and give you an accurate accounting before the American college-graduated tourist can get his calculator out of his pocket.

A new wind is blowing in American educational circles: the after fifty crowd is going back to school. That strikes a chord in my heart because when I was thirty, had had my children and was flush enough to go to school I applied to a famous college in New York, Sarah Lawrence, where I was told I was too old. (At least they didn't tell me what Father O'Sullivan told me when he refused my request for the job as altar boy, but then Sarah Lawrence was a girl's school at the time.) Today, forty years later, my application would be taken seriously, and I'd be welcome. The opportunity to improve, to open new doors and fulfill dreams put on ice during the family-raising years is available to people of all educational levels and all age levels. As time passes and the "youth creep" (that appearance of looking, acting, and feeling younger than you are chronologically) burgeons, more and more of us will be involved in multiple careers. The careers we enter after fifty will be very different from those we fell into or were pushed into when we were younger. *These new careers will be ones we really choose.* We are already preparing. "But *how?*"

There are a number of ways to get back into education and one is to write the Adult Education Association of the USA. This association is made up of a large cross section of people who are in the education field. They can provide answers to specific questions and tell you where to turn for your individual needs in your own community. Write to

The Adult Education Association of the USA, 810 18th St. NW, Washington, DC 20006.

You may want to get started right now, but going outside the home may be difficult. That brings us to home study, at least for starters. The National Home Study Council would be helpful. Its address is 1601 18th St. NW, Washington, DC 20009. The council can give you a free directory of accredited courses and institutions. That sort of guarantee assures you of

- A competent faculty
- Educationally sound, up-to-date courses
- Careful screening of students for admission
- Satisfactory educational services
- Demonstrable student success and satisfaction
- Truthful advertising of courses
- Financial ability to deliver high-quality educational services

Perhaps you have a summer or part of a summer free and would like to try getting your educational feet wet a week at a time. An Elderhostel program might be a good start in the right direction. Elderhostel consists of on-campus courses for older persons at low cost. I have a friend who has taught Elderhostel courses for several years and finds the students wonderfully aware and interested. If you have ever taught the other kind of student, the one who can't imagine why he or she is *there*, you know what a bonus such a group would be to the teacher and to the other students. Elderhostels don't give credit, but that's not what you are there for; you want to find out what really interests you. A week's investment of time isn't all that earth shaking. The instructors don't give any outside assignments, so that means lots of free time to meet other people and enjoy them. Elderhostels provide campus accommodation, housing, and meals, as well as use of all other facilities. There is no cost for the courses if you are sixty-five or older. Depending on financial factors, those under sixty-five may be charged tuition. For information, contact Elderhostel, 80 Boylston St., Boston, MA 02116.

Don't waste another day. Check out one of the above organizations, or drop in at your nearest college or write the one nearest your heart, and ask what they have to offer. The ecnomic situation has taken a lot of the arrogance out of colleges. As government support drops away they are going to need you and your tuition more than ever. Foundations that give colleges financial support ask how many living, breathing students a college has—not how old they are. If you are there, you count. If you get a runaround, write to the president of the college and complain. Type your letter and make it succinct. I get hundreds of letters a week, and when I'm on the air the mail can run into thousands. I get tired when I get long letters and am apt to put them aside "until I have time" which can take forever. It's also tiring to read careless handwriting. Make your complaint short, clear, and neat. Arthur Godfrey told me he could get 500 complimentary letters about a show and three nasty ones. He answered the three because they challenged him. The college president will feel challenged too; he's catching it because an underling didn't do the job he or she was hired to do. That's *annoying*. Two letters from two different people doubles the urgency and five cannot be ignored. The after fifty crowd should be reminded that there is both safety and power in numbers.

One of the facts that have surfaced regarding education and the after fifty crowd is that education enhances our chances for living longer. Better education, better job. Better job, more money and benefits. More of those mean better nutrition, medical and dental care, housing, and recreation. The latter assures physical outlets for emotional stress. Better and more positive statistics on this will be forthcoming after the beneficiaries of the G.I. Bill get into their eighties. If there are more over-eighties than teenagers today, what will it be like in twenty years?

MYTH 5

Myth: YOU CAN'T TEACH AN OLD DOG NEW TRICKS.

Junking the Myth: Some aspects of intelligence continue to grow as long as we are healthy. The real key that affects both young and old is interest. People learn if they want to and when it's no chore. I took forever to learn even a modicum of French and no time at all to do well in both German and Italian because I fell in love with men who spoke those languages. Leaving the studies on aging done in almshouses, nursing homes, and hospitals behind, let's see where we really stand. And let's understand that those biased studies have led to tragic consequences. Many people now dealing with older Americans feel that countless intellectually vigorous lives may have atrophied due to the erroneous results of "studies" done in the past. Believing that you are "through" very often brings on the con-

dition of mental deterioration just as believing that physical activity is not possible, makes it impossible. The expectation of both mental and physical decline is a self-fulfilling prophecy.

We have become very interesting to researchers for a number of reasons, only one of which is our growing numbers. Granted, the fact that there are so many of us leads to the possibility of many problems. It is to be hoped that the various researchers are also thinking of answers to the questions they are so busy raising.

Our friend Dr. Robert Butler, who was the founding director of the National Council on Aging and is now the head of the geriatric medicine program at Mt. Sinai Hospital in New York, says, "The belief that if you live long enough you will become senile is just wrong. Senility is a sign of disease, not a part of the normal aging process." There is other good news: it is also thought that declines in intelligence can be reversed in some instances and that pronouncements about the loss of brain cells as people age are dead wrong. Not only have the researchers come to the conclusion that those reports about inevitable loss were in error, they even feel that for those of us who remain emotionally and physically healthy, some of the most important forms of intellectual growth can continue well into our eighties. It is my opinion that as health improves with painless exercise, eighties can stretch to nineties and beyond.

Warner Schaie, an eminent researcher on aging, did the kind of continuing study that makes sense. His was one of the first studies to show how various mental capacities change as people age. Begun in Seattle in the mid-fifties, the study now has over 3,000 participants, some retested every 7 years for a period of 21 years. Some subjects have been followed well into their eighties. Dr. Schaie, writing in *Longitudinal Studies of Psychological Development* (Guilford Press), reports that on average, declines in mental abilities such as fluency and spatial relations have little practical significance until the mid-seventies or eighties, and other mental capacities decline very little or not at all and can be reversed with tutoring. Other mental capacities decline very little or not at all and can even improve with years. He feels that the use-it-or-lose-it principle applies not only to the physical, but to intellectual performance as well.

A propos of comparing apples and oranges, or young college students with older subjects, Dr. Jerry Avorn of the Division on Aging at Harvard Medical School was very critical of the "scientific" literature. For one thing, most college students are free of major illness while the same cannot be said of oldsters. In addition, there is a second hidden bias: the medication given oldsters to "control" their various diseases such as diabetes, high blood pressure, heart disease, etc. You have already read about what drugs can do, so you know that the bias is not only hidden, but considerable.

THREE TYPES OF INTELLIGENCE

Three aspects of intelligence come under scrutiny here. One is called *crystallized intelligence* and is a key mental capacity that continues to increase during the lives of healthy people. It denotes a person's ability to use an accumulated body of general information to make judgments and solve problems. This type of intelligence is what you need at a town meeting where no issue is black or white, merely shades of gray. Dr. John Horn, a psychologist at the University of Denver who has done the main research on crystallized intelligence, says that it continues to increase throughout life, although in old age the increments become smaller.

As for the intelligence that may be lost, Dr. Jerry Avorn says, "The deficits found in the healthy aged are in a minor range and not at all clinically impairing. At worst they are a nuisance, like not being able to remember phone numbers well." I'd settle for that any day. From as far back as I can remember I can't recall names when I need them. I also have a terrible block when it comes to introductions. I've even been known to "lose" my sister's name . . . and I was probably thirty or forty!

The increase in crystallized intelligence occurs despite the simultaneous decline in another form of mental capacity, *fluid intelligence*. This form involves seeing and using abstract relationships, such as when playing chess. Happily, as Martha Storandt, a psychologist at Washington University in St. Louis, says, we learn to compensate for the decline. We can still learn what we want to learn; it just takes a little longer. I find that what takes me longer to learn also seems to stay with me longer.

A third aspect—one that should be of interest to all of us—is what is called *world knowledge*. That is the information people acquire in both their formal education and day-to-day experience. This sort of knowledge ranges from the name of the general in charge on D-Day to how to get the car started on a cold day. The total score of that information increases with age through the seventies and the oldest group tested had better recall of facts than did people in their twenties. And we have many more facts to recall!

HOW TO KEEP GROWING MENTALLY

Researchers have turned up some key factors that might allow us to maintain our mental capabilities. For one, we must stay socially involved. Those older people who withdraw from life socially are not long for this world when it comes to "living." Do you remember Barbra Streisand's song, "People Who Need People Are the Luckiest People in the World"? Well, everybody does need people. The ones who *know* they need people and *do* something to provide themselves with people are the really lucky people.

Another helpful factor is staying mentally active. Well-educated people who continue their intellectual interests can actually continue to increase their verbal intelligence into their old age. There's a story about Oliver Wendell Holmes, Jr., who was a member of the Supreme Court. When he was unable to attend due to frailty, President Roosevelt felt he ought to pay a call on him. When he heard no sound coming from Holmes's office, he entered quietly, thinking he might be napping. Not at all. He was reading a book in Greek. When the president asked him what he was doing, Justice Holmes told him, "I'm improving my mind." I use language and crossword puzzles similarly. I "play" at German, Russian, Greek, French, Spanish, and Latin. I'm no good at any of them, but I love all of them. It's fun to practice in any of

them, to try to remember that the word *bread* has a different name in each language and yet many words are related. At least I'll never go hungry!

Dr. John Horn, says "The ability to bring to mind and entertain many different facets of information improves in many people over the years . . . they can often say the same thing in five different ways."

Having a flexible personality is considered another plus. People who are able to tolerate ambiguity and enjoy new experiences in middle age usually maintain mental alertness through old age. I could always count on my mother-in-law to say, "Sure, we ought to be able to knock fun out of that," no matter what I suggested we do. When she was ninety she still had a mind like a steel trap and the laughter of a young, delighted girl. I never knew any young person who could match her, even when she was very old.

One of the real "scaries" is the idea that the brain degenerates all at once as well as over a period of time. There was and still is a claim that every drink destroys thousands of brain cells. Woe to the martini drinker! This little gem must have been put about by somebody in the WCTU because when Marion Diamond, a neuroanatomist at the University of California at Berkeley, tried to find its origins, she could find no trace of such a study. Her own work is one of the few studies ever done that assesses cell loss rates as the brain ages. She discovered that while there certainly is some cell loss, the greatest decrease is early in life. Subsequent losses are not significant even late in life. Recent studies state that "the healthy aged brain is as active and efficient as the healthy young brain."

What seems to matter most is what you have done all through life—the experiences you have had, the adjustments you have made, and the knowledge you have garnered.

Yes, there are all sorts of studies going on concerning our brains and us. There's no question that there has been mental deterioration in about 5 percent of the over sixty-five-years-olds, but if 50 percent of the hospital beds in the country are taken up by mental patients, we must ask what other age groups are similarly affected. It is also true that one in four of the eighty-five-and-older people will deteriorate, but you have to ask how many of those were handicapped by the work laws, or by illness. How many were driven out of this world by drugs, and how many gave up thinking because there was nothing to do, no place to go, and nothing much to think about? The stimulation that is essential for rats and children is also essential for us. We need to share our thoughts; they are more important than you think. Whoever you are, what you have to offer is needed even if you (especially you) may not know at this moment what that something is.

Ninety percent of us show no memory loss, so why zero in on the 10 percent who do? I'll settle for an increase in insight even if I do forget my own telephone number. I don't call myself, anyway.

Just to make my "use it or lose it" point stronger, here's a brief list of people who made major accomplishments happen in their later years.

- *Benjamin Franklin* shared in the design of the Declaration of Independence at the age of seventy.

- *Douglas MacArthur* came out of retirement at age sixty-one to lead the Allied Forces to victory in the Pacific in World War II. He then commanded the United Nations forces in Korea at the age of seventy.

- *Frank Lloyd Wright* did some of his best work in his eighties and designed the Guggenheim Museum when he was close to ninety.

- *Winston Churchill* not only saw Great Britain through a terrible war when he was in his sixties, but he stayed on as prime minister until he was eighty-one. Then he tried a very different lifestyle and wrote *A History of the English Speaking People* when he was eighty-two.

- *Konrad Adenauer* was seventy-three when he became chancellor of West Germany, and he led that country out of one of the worst defeats in the history of the world, staying with it until the age of eighty-seven. He was known affectionately and correctly as Der Alte, "The Old One," but there was no denigration attached to the name.

- *Giuseppe Verdi* wrote the "Ave Maria" when he was seventy-six.

- *Pablo Casals* played the cello and conducted until he was almost ninety-six.

- *Grandma Moses* started to paint when she was seventy-seven, and continued to produce until she was over one hundred years old.

- *Cornelius Vanderbilt* managed a financial empire until he was eighty.

- *Johann Goethe* completed "Faust" shortly before he died at eighty-three.

- *Mohandas Gandhi* was assassinated at the age of seventy-nine, but not before he led India out of bondage.

- *Martha Graham* continues to inspire the modern dance world at the age of ninety.
- *Arthur Rubinstein* was still playing magnificent piano until he was eighty.
- *Oliver Wendell Holmes* was still a Supreme Court judge at the age of ninety-one.
- *Mother Teresa*, at the age of 75, continues to supervise the operation of schools, hospitals, orphanages, and food centers in more than twenty-five countries.
- *Coco Chanel* remained one of the most imitated of designers until her death at the age of eighty-seven.
- *Golda Meir* was prime minister of Israel in her seventies.
- *Bertrand Russell* continued to be a leading philosopher when he entered prison as a radical protesting nuclear arms at the age of eighty-nine.
- *Arthur Fiedler* was still conducting his famous Boston Pops in his eighties.

People who continue with interests of all kinds tend to increase skills all through their lives. Those who can, do. Those who can't, make myths! So make a list of what interests you. Don't hold yourself back with self-limiting ideas of your abilities. A long time ago I was given a slip of paper carrying a Latin motto. I was supposed to copy the beautiful handwriting of Madame Loyola and thus, with the phrase written a hundred times, improve my own which was undisciplined, poorly directed, and smudgy. I guess my writing improved;

it's very different now, but better than that, I made the motto my own and have lived by it.

Ad astra per aspera.

Literally it means "To reach the stars—through difficulty." Colloquially I'd translate it as "The sky's the limit." God knows there have been difficulties in my life, but there have also been stars—I have lived with both. Decide on the star you want and head for it. Keep in mind that what interests *you* most will be easiest for *you* to conquer.

MYTH 6

Myth: THE DATE FOR AN END TO SEX IS SET SOMEWHERE BETWEEN FIFTY AND SIXTY. OLD PEOPLE ARE JUST NOT INTERESTED IN MAKING LOVE, IT'S ALL OVER FOR THEM.

Junking the Myth: People who are warm, loving, appreciatively sensual, and who have enjoyed sex in their earlier years don't give up such joys because of a date on a calendar.

My mother-in-law had a way of saying very revealing things about herself that today I would view as cries for help. "Sex," she announced archly, "drives half the world crazy" (she meant me) "and bores the other half to death" (referring to herself and most of her contemporaries, who were fifty-five and up). Since half of the statement that pointed to me was unquestionably true, I assumed she knew what she was saying about "older" people. Then I went skiing and learned differently.

I was sitting in a ski train headed for Vermont and there were four of us in the group. I was on the aisle, riding backward, and across from me was an "older" couple. "Older," to most people, means fifteen years senior to the person using the designation. I was approaching thirty-five. The couple was holding hands and staring out the window. Suddenly he turned and looked into her face. His look was filled with such love, such desire, such incredible yearning, I felt I had blundered into a forbidden garden. I wanted to turn away, but I couldn't. I knew I was seeing something not meant for me, perhaps never meant for me. The longing I lived with, the one I had tried to explain to my mother-in-law, rose up in me and overflowed in tears. How do you explain sudden tears to three merry skiers? You don't; you go to the ladies' room.

I pondered my own aloneness all that weekend. Sunday evening after I had risked my neck a dozen times racing down the mountain, pursued by my loneliness, and had endured endless slow rides on the lift, one of my three skiing companions joined me for the Ski Patrol sweep. We stood there in the sudden silence that follows the last ride up. The trails were already flattening in the twilight and we could see the lights of the town below shimmering like fiery gems. "Is it so bad?" he said. "Yes," was all I could muster, but for a wonder, I was no longer alone. Something magical had happened; someone understood. Years later my friend told me that we are all lonely stars in a huge dark firmament and that the best we can expect is to be able to see each other. If we can signal a simple message of friendship and encouragement, we are doing well. He reminded me that we are born alone and in essence we live and die alone. Our comfort comes from reaching out across the dark abyss and saying, "I am here." That's what happened on the train. It never occurred to me to wonder if those two older people slept together. Of course they did! Nothing, I thought, could be as wonderful as the love those two people felt for each other . . . then I realized, with a shock, that those two in-love people were *old!*

My mother-in-law really did find sex boring, and like many another disappointed person, she turned into a mythmaker. There were others, of course, just as there have been for you. At the convent Reverend Mother Whoever told us sex was sinful. We called her "Shredded Wheat," and she lived up to every crackly, dry, wispy, unsalted, unsugared stick of it. Mythmakers talk about the end of our sex drive, having never been satisfied themselves. The sex killers are as right as their brother and sister mythmakers who claim we are all poverty stricken, all ill and feeble, all meant to end our days in nursing homes and will undoubtedly have big ears, big noses and shrivelled everything else.

There are some facts of life that are facts and are useful. One is that healthy men can go on making love happily and satisfyingly for all concerned and there isn't a cutoff date. Many (more than you might suspect) have an impotence problem and while it used to be thought that most of it was "all in your head Mac . . .", more and more it is recognized as having physiological causes. The first question we ask a patient with that complaint is, "What was your sport when you were a teenager, as a young man, and what is it now?" If the sport involved running on cement (or for women complaining of spastic pelvic muscles, dancing on a similar surface); if there was constant foot pounding as in basketball, or body pounding as in football; or if there was an injury to the groin or coccyx, or menstrual cramps or jaw pain, we think first of muscle spasm. All your parts are hitched together, and ever since birth you have been hurting one muscle or another just getting through each adventure each day. In the chapter on Myotherapy you will learn about trigger points, little irritable spots that get into muscles when they are damaged in any way, from a cut with a kitchen knife to a fall down the stairs to small, but repetitive movements like those employed in using a typewriter. Those invisible points have the power to throw those once injured muscles into spasm, which can range from mild (your hands are cold from poor circulation caused by muscles) to extremely painful (your back is "out"). Their power doesn't stop there either; they can refer pain to adjacent or distant places. Damaging leg muscles by running or jumping on cement doesn't merely cause shin splints, calf pain, sore knees, tendinitis, or what your grandchildren call "growing pains." Those same painful, spasmed muscles tie into the pelvis as well as their other terminals, the feet, ankles, and knees. The pelvis houses the sex organs and if the pelvic floor is influenced into spasm, things that should work . . . don't.

Heading still farther north in the body . . . if the abdominals, groin, and seat muscles are in spasm, they can refer pain to the upper back, chest, neck, and head. If someone comes to a Myotherapist with TMJD, or jaw pain, we check immediately for the original trouble in the groin and the seat. If pelvic pain, impotence, or spasticity in the vaginal area is the complaint, we would look first to the legs and feet. The good news is that when the causes of sexual

dysfunction are muscular, they can usually be fixed—with myotherapy.

Until fairly recently women almost always married men older than themselves. Since men die an average of eight years earlier than their mates, if they start out even, there can be a long, lonely time for many women. Men, on the other hand, have always married women younger than themselves and when they are either widowed or divorced they usually take on someone *much* younger than themselves. The field is weighted, so to speak. There is a lot to be said for marrying a younger person if it brings youthful enthusiasm, new interests, satisfying sex, and health. I love to watch the turned-down mouths of mythmakers when that drops on their plate, but they turn down even more when the opposite happens and an older woman marries a younger man.

When I was fifty-one, a man I found thoroughly enjoyable asked me to marry him. It was tempting for many reasons, but I refused. He was sixteen years younger than I and in my most logical manner I said, "My dear, dear friend, it's great now but imagine what it will be like when I am seventy! You will be fifty-four!" We parted, friends. A year ago I met him again. A lot had happened to both of us, to be sure, but while I looked to be in my fifties, he could have been close to seventy. Think what we had missed because of mythmakers! *Now* she tells me!

Recently on the Donahue show there was a program on a group of such marriages. "How could you have done it?" was written on almost every face in the audience. They should take a trip to Florida and watch healthy, sprightly, attractive, well-groomed, well-dressed, active, and perfectly capable women driving and leading very aged men around as if they were children. Those women aren't ready for the heap. They are caught in the net of life. The myth-makers, however, see them as equal couples. Stop thinking of years when it comes to sex and start thinking of lov-ing. Sex is a short, sharp bark of a word. Sensuality and loving are long, caress-ing, and euphonious.

Women are capable of enjoying sex as long as they have a partner who in-terests them. If a woman with a satis-fying partner runs into trouble that could be labeled sexual, there are prob-ably physical reasons. Think Myother-apy first, and if that isn't the answer you may want to investigate estrogen therapy. I am not recommending it, but medical researchers are learning more and more about hormones and estrogen in particular, since it plays a part in treatment for osteoporosis.

The nice thing about sex and the after fifty crowd is that there are a lot of us, and most of us are very loving and content. More of us are "living to-gether," much to the amazement and some discomfort of our children, not to mention the same to our parents who wish they could have done it too. The main keys to the sex part of loving and sensuality are health, energy, and phys-ical attraction which does *not* have an age tag.

DON'T BE AFRAID TO LET GO
In "the olden days" people stayed to-gether until death did them part, never noticing that death of love, desire, hap-piness, and loyalty had crept into their beds and wreaked the kind of havoc that suffers no survivors. Today the younger members of the after fifty

crowd are keeping up with still younger people when it comes to divorce, and more and more often we are seeing di-vorces between people married for twenty-five and thirty years. Certainly it's heartbreaking, but so is a lot of other stuff in today's world. As every-thing moves faster and faster we can't get things under control and again luck plays a part. Who were you when you married? Who were you ten years later? Who are you now? Birth, marriage, and death are three major undertakings for which we have no preparation. So, in-stead of tearing out your hair and pounding your head on the wall think about it this way for a moment.

If it's over—the marriage, the affair, the interest or whatever—don't blame your lack of arousal, or ability to arouse, on your age. You will ultimately do whatever you think is right—part, endure, or sublimate—but at least understand what has happened. A fire that has burned out cannot be rekin-dled from ashes. Sometimes there are unburned timbers that can be made to live again, but that is going to take time, effort, care, consideration, and above all, patience. At no time does it mean the repetition of old habits. Per-haps taking a long vacation during which you rebuild yourself is in order. If you can, go away somewhere for a while. If you can't, move your mind over to a place where it can rest and then go to work on your body.

Misery loves company and unloved, unloving, unsatisfied, and unsatisfying mythmakers are counting on you to share their loss. Don't do it. Go out and make the most of your life.

The next myths all run together and remind me of my little relative who ran screaming out of the bathroom. When he was finally quiet enough to be understood he sobbed, "There are a million centipedes in the tub." "How many, dear?" asked his patient mother. "Well, two anyway."

MYTH 7

Myth: THEY'RE ALL CRAZY. THEY'RE ALL UGLY. THEY'RE SICK ALL THE TIME.

Junking the myth: The after fifty crowd is much less likely to develop emotional disorders than are young people between the ages of twenty-five and forty-five, and for a lot of reasons. The stable survive. Olders aren't one whit more neurotic than younger ones nor are they any more subject to depression except as it is related to drug addiction. That kind of depression should usually be labeled "iatrogenic." Older people see doctors more often than younger people do, and the treatment suggested is all too often a drug.

As a society, we were so carried away by our truly great medical discoveries that we began to think of medicine as an exact science instead of as an art. As medications became more sophisticated, the growing pharmaceutical houses tried to fill in the gaps left in the doctor's education which really didn't assign much time to pharmacology. They trained "detail" men to let doctors know about new medications. Today no busy doctor could possibly keep up with what's on the market without those fellows who visit them regularly, leaving samples in their wake. As the pharmaceutical industry became larger and more important to the practice of medicine and their products proliferated it became big, then bigger and now very big business. It made good sense to spend millions on research to keep up with or ahead of rival companies, and that investment was followed by millions more for advertising. Logic: Pharmaceutical houses sell medicine and whom do they use as their middle man? Your doctor. Who goes to the doctor more often than anyone else? The after fifty crowd. Who takes the most medicine? The after fifty crowd. Warning: Being "stoned" at twenty-five is accepted by society as a passing phase. For the older person the word "passing" is accepted as terminal. For our crowd "stoned" translates to "crazy."

FACTS ABOUT UGLY

It's true, some people get ugly as they age. Some weren't all that attractive when they were young either. It is also true that the very, very old are wrinkled and have spots, but try to remember what life has been like for the very old. They have already lived between eighty-five and one hundred years and they began life when it was neither easy nor safe. The ninety-year-olds were already fifteen before the first tractor clanked down a furrow, and since this country was primarily agricultural many of them were overworked farmers. They were well into adulthood before one of the worst scourges, tuberculosis, was vanquished. They were almost thirty before insulin began to save diabetics. They were forty before sulpha came to the rescue against everpresent and often lethal bacteria. How many bugs had they already fought without help?

Today's very old were too old before the Pill came to prevent millions of babies from aging them too fast. Childbearing is hard, physical work and it takes years to get over each pregnancy. Raising a family in those days was even harder physical work and for many it went on and on, multiplying as it went. Paying the bills was also hard, physical work. Yet despite all of these difficulties, more and more people are making it to eighty-five, ninety, and one hundred.

You will be old in a different time. You have escaped the grinding toil of today's very old. We've had automobiles, vacuum cleaners, and washing machines for a long time now. We also have permanent waves, hair stylists, and clothes that can *do* something for both men and women. We know how to change bodies as you will see in the section on self-image (see page 72). It's how you sit, stand, and move that counts. It's your vitality, your energy level. Calling again on "famous people," since we all know them:

Claudette Colbert is over eighty and Gloria Steinem is well into the after fifty crowd. So are Dan Rather and Barbara Walters as are Angie Dickinson, Cicely Tyson, Sophia Loren, and Shirley MacLaine. Lena Horne, Lauren Bacall, and Dinah Shore are past sixty, and Phyllis Diller, who becomes more beautiful with each "lift," is over sixty-seven. Mary Martin is over seventy and her son, Larry Hagman, is in the after fifty crowd, as are a goodly number of very current male stars.

Tomorrow's "old, old" will look younger, act younger and *be* younger and they won't need to worry about looking ugly. They and you and I will know how to prevent it . . . starting now.

FACTS ABOUT SICK

Everybody can get sick, especially when we are tired or stressed. Older persons do have some problems as does every other age group, but 75 percent of the difficulties attributed to "oldsters," and often accepted by them as well, are due to the attitudes imposed on them by the American public. Only 25 percent of the difficulties are actually due to aging, and that includes illnesses we suffer. Only 10 percent of us are confined in any serious way, and a check with the VA hospitals might tell you that the young men who returned from Vietnam have had to put up with some of that confinement at age twenty.

Actually, older people have far fewer acute diseases than do younger ones and when they do catch a bug they recover faster. They do have more chronic diseases from wear and tear, but these don't seem to interfere with daily living, and once you learn to banish pain, they will interfere even less. Most diseases that attack Americans today are invited. They are the result of a lifestyle that is very unhealthy indeed. As a result of that lifestyle, about three-fourths of us don't reach our full life span. We can change that, of course, but to do so three things are necessary: knowledge, self-discipline, and a reason to use that discipline. Perhaps the last should come first. We are all born with the will to live and the love of pleasure and satisfaction. If life stresses us too much, that will to live becomes dulled. If nothing we do turns out the way we want it to, we forget the pleasure of satisfaction. We are also born needing people. We need to interact, we need to share, we need to be near. Lacking those things we grow careless, and even if we knew the answers to health we would not use self-discipline; we might just not see the reason for it. Which comes first, the chicken or the egg? Do we go for health or happiness first? We go for health, freedom from pain, and the energy to go out and round up the rest.

MYTH 8
Myth: THE OLD AREN'T SOCIALLY ACCEPTABLE: THEY WET THEMSELVES.

Junking the Myth: That's called incontinence in the old and "pants wetting" or bed-wetting in the young. For women who have had children and for those who find they have "leaked" after a cough, sneeze, or good hard serve in tennis, it is called embarrassing. There is usually more than is at first apparent in all four. The bed- and pants-wetting stage used to be called "willfulness." In the orphanage when I began my bedwetting stage I was made to lie in it foodless all the next day. It was for my own, good of course, but I did not improve. I was very willful.

At the other end of life about one person in sixty-five suffers with incontinence and most of them are women. What would common sense tell you about that ratio? First, you would have to ask yourself what was the difference between the sexes. Every little girl with a brother could tell you what the Germans say best—"Was bruder hat ist mehr practisch"—from the first minute she saw him piddle in the bushes while she had to dash for the house. But in addition to that difference, women produce babies. What does labor do to the floor of the pelvis which houses both useful and pleasure-giving apparatus? It stretches, strains, and often wounds.

In the chapter on Myotherapy you will learn that whenever a muscle is damaged a situation is set up which can come back to haunt you years later.

Childbirth sets women up for incontinence, hemorrhoids, and sundry aches they would never connect with anything so remote as a child's birth twenty to fifty years before. Damage to the pelvic floor can cause back pain, what seems to be a spastic colon, or kidney pain. It can cause constipation, aching legs, and menstrual cramps. Weakness is another result of old injury and weakness interferes with sex. You don't have to be a woman to have pain, weakness, or problems with sex; it just helps! You will find surcease for the whole weary litany in Myotherapy and exercise. Both will improve the sex lives people think their elders don't have. There is also a series of preventive exercises for incontinence. You want to be in control . . . always.

Speaking of control. In nursing homes 50 percent of the residents are incontinent as of right now. Virtually no effort is being made to help most of them. Diapering is not helping, and the elderly person will be lucky if he or she isn't catheterized. Drugs interfere with control as do stress, illness, fatigue, and confusion (which are often drug-caused). You might look into that if you have occasion to visit elderly relatives.

So build up the muscles of the pelvic floor. Continence won't be the only bonus!

Now you know what *isn't* true; we've junked the myths. We're *not* senile, poor, and warehoused, nor are we stupid, sexless, crazy, ugly, sick, or socially unacceptable. Whoopee!

Exposing myths is fun and it's very useful as well. Every one you blast with the bright light of common sense is one less pitfall waiting for your own foot. We are all in a way historians. We write the history of our own times and sometimes we are able to influence it; we certainly have a duty towards it. A French historian, Jules Michelet, who died back in 1874 (the year before my father was born), said: "The historian's first duties are sacrifice and the mocking of false gods. They are his indispensable instruments for establishing truth." Gladly should we sacrifice old, worn-out, erroneous myths and delightedly should we mock the myth-makers.

Now, let's get on to some truths.

THE CROSSROADS OF CHANGE

Now you know who your "enemies" are, the ones you must be fit enough to combat and to overcome: the mythmakers. It's time to look at the positive aspects of twentieth-century life, so read on and learn the real *facts*—facts that will make you both safe and dangerous: safe in a healthy self, and dangerous to the mythmakers of the world.

Here are some of the good things that have happened in this country, the events that have helped make your generation and mine The Last Fit Americans. I've fit them into events and memories of my own life, to show how these "special happenings" have touched me.

FORTY-THREE SPECIAL HAPPENINGS

It's time for you to start writing in the margins. Don't let your mother's voice (or the librarian's) haunt you. They said, "Books are your friends, never deface them." Indeed, they are your friends—and you should talk to them as only you can do. Write in the margins, laugh there, expostulate, even weep your despair to them. There have been many years when I had no one to talk to but books. I started reading "Over the Top" by a man named Empey, when I was nine. I read it ten times, and each time I read it I had more to tell it.

If I could find that book today it would be a book about me, for me to read. That book was my friend.

Back to those major changes—all forty-three of them.

1. The first major changes came when our grandparents were living their lives as we are living ours right now. The first medical wonders were about to burst on a world of pestilence. One of these wonders was the development of anesthesia. Ether had been around since 1540, but like a lot of other things that are "around," people didn't know how to use it. My hitchhiking grandfather didn't trust the stuff. He'd been a criminal lawyer and then a judge, and he didn't trust much of anything. During his time on the bench he'd sent a lot of men to prison and two of them eventually got out. They waylaid him on his way home at dusk and put two bullets into him. One bullet entered his chest just above his heart, ending up somewhere near his armpit. The other lodged in his liver. When he finally got to the operating room, my grandfather refused the alcohol and ether that were offered him. My grandmother had died of alcoholism, and he wouldn't touch a drop even as an anesthetic. He'd take his operations cold, not even a glass of brandy. He survived the ordeals of being shot and left to die by the road, the long wait for help while stanching his wounds with his handkerchief and a piece torn from his shirttail, and being strapped to a table as the surgeon cut through flesh and sinews and probed his open chest and abdomen, grappled with chunks of lead, tied off arteries, and poured antiseptics into open wounds before putting in drains and sewing him up. He survived, but the shocks changed him

from a cold, judgmental, powerful politician to a gentle old soul who loved to hitchhike around town. He also spilled on his shirt front and forgot his address. The change wasn't all for the best.

Ether probably could have prevented my grandfather's deterioration, but it was then used as a popular intoxicant, which was where the old gentleman got hung up. In fact, ether was the cocktail of its day. Folks would gather round and inhale it to get what we'd call "high." One day, a doctor who was trying to talk a patient into a necessary tumor operation discovered the real value of ether. He had run out of whiskey and laudanum, the pain deadeners of choice, but did have some ether on hand for parties. On the off chance that it would work he gave the patient a couple of whiffs. The patient went out like the proverbial light and the operation was a painless success. Then, as often happens with incredible discoveries, ether as an anesthetic was forgotten.

Four years later, a dentist by the name of Morton used ether in front of an audience, and his fortune was made. The power of an audience and the press must never be underestimated. Three years after that a Scottish physician introduced chloroform. Make a list of all the operations you have had and see how many you would have survived or even undergone without the help of anesthesia.

2. That same year a brilliant and heroic doctor by the name of Ignatz Semmelweiss changed something else for us: he washed his hands before examining young women in labor. He found that the disease rate dropped dramatically, and he tried to influence

his colleagues to do the same. This was especially important for those coming directly from the morgue, where they had been working on women who had died of a disease. However, there were problems. For one thing, people didn't wash very much in those days; but there was something much more important to consider: doctors were known by the patina of blood and pus on the lapels of their frock coats, which they only took off at bed time. The patina increased with time and the constant wiping of bloody hands as doctors worked with patients or corpses. If hands were washed, where would the distinguishing patina come from? Forget it, Ignatz! They ignored his hand-washing advice and, indirectly, they killed him. This is not unusual in history when someone, ahead of his time, demands change.

3. How many of you have ever had a fracture? A fellow by the name of Dr. Mathysen saw how many arms and legs healed badly, leaving limps and impaired function. He sought something better than two splints and inadequate bindings and came up with bandages impregnated with plaster. So simple and so helpful! Dr. Mathysen has given many of you straight, well-functioning limbs, which can certainly make a difference in the quality of life.

4. One year after Mathysen made his discovery, Alexander Wood used a kind of hypodermic syringe for subcutaneous injections. Prior to that time the only occasion a syringe was used was to squirt holy water into a uterus at a dying baby to assure its entry into heaven. Think a minute of the injections you have had in your lifetime, what they were for, and how you might have gotten along without them. That they may be over-used today is not the fault of the modality, but rather the practitioner. The syringe is merely the modality; what's injected is something else again. This is the first time in this book, but not the last, that you will be reminded that you *must* know what medications you are getting, why you are getting them, and what their side effects are. If a syringe is used, please know where it was before it was aimed at you. Syringes, like dirty hands, carry diseases. Thanks to Alexander Wood they also prevent them.

5. A year after Wood's discovery, a singing teacher who was curious about the causes of some of his students' difficulties invented the laryngoscope. Imagine—the first peek into a functioning throat made without causing a wound was taken by a singing teacher. There is something else exciting, up ahead, for singers: another singing teacher, using Myotherapy, has been able to improve tone, breath control, and skill.

6. Cocaine was the next "discovery." The conquistadores found the Peruvian and Bolivian Indians chewing and sucking on wads of coca leaves smeared with ashes. This mixture was said to make a hard life bearable. No one is quite sure how it traveled north of the border, but from 1800 to 1900 cocaine was "in." It was laced into almost everything—chewing gum, cigarettes, soda, tea, nose spray, patent medicine, and wine. The real explosion came when a Corsican named Angelo Mariani concocted Coca Wine. Everybody loved it, including Thomas Edison, President McKinley, Freud, Sarah Bernhardt, John Philip Sousa, and Pope Leo XIII. One hundred percent pure cocaine was sold in drugstores without prescription and thought to be as harmless as a lot of the over-the-counter drugs we pur-

chase without a qualm today (and may turn away from in horror in years to come).

Today cocaine is back as middle America's drug of choice, with three differences: it's illegal, which makes it much more expensive; its purity is a thing of the past; and God knows what's added to it. That means it can be deadly . . . fast.

7. Five years after Mathysen's plaster cast, the chemist Louis Pasteur made a big change in our lives with the development of pasteurization. Actually, he wasn't looking for a cure or preventive for disease, he was trying to save the French wine industry which was in trouble because "something" was turning the wine bitter. That "something" turned out to be a nasty little entity now called a germ. Heat destroyed the germs in wine and in milk. Germy wine may have been bitter, but germy milk was deadly.

8. The very next year Baron Joseph Lister used carbolic acid on an open wound, and antiseptic surgery was born. Go over your operations again and count your blessings, then give thanks to someone else we have taken for granted.

9. The year my father was born Albert Bilroth discovered two of our most virulent enemies, streptococci and staphylococci. Unfortunately for two of my father's young cousins who died because of one of them, it was quite some time before doctors knew how to use that information.

10. The father of those two boys hadn't recovered from that terrible blow when anthrax got into his cattle. A German bacteriologist had already discovered the anthrax bacterium, but again, knowing only part of the story isn't enough and my distant relative's

herd was decimated. Pasteur had been given encouragement by the discovery, and went to work and found the desperately needed vaccine.

11. Parasites were another "ugly" floating around the world. The damage they did was usually blamed on sin, witches and devils, miasma, night air, and unsanitary conditions. The margins of my books all contain references to my father's sharpshooting escapades, Teddy Roosevelt, the Panama Canal, and boys dying in heat and stink. My father, who was a volunteer orderly during the Spanish-American War, washed the young soldiers' awful sores and was caught by President McKinley one day standing on his head in a basin of water. Why? Soldiers in those days had absolutely nothing to divert them; no books, no radio, no TV, only a scrubby, gangly teenager with a funny crooked smile who would do just about anything to elicit a smile or a glint of humor from glazed eyes, even wear costumes and stand on his head. The president, against all the rules, was visiting the "pesthole," as the smallpox area was called, and walked into one of the tents just in time to see the very end of a minstrel show made up of one actor. It wasn't much as entertainment goes, but it was the best they had, and if the president had come a few seconds later he would have seen the pajama-clad youth playing a mandolin in that unique position. In any case, my father's career as an entertainer was cut short by malaria which never really left him. That's why I have no trouble remembering Charles Louis Alphonse Laveran, the French pathologist who discovered the malarial parasite.

12. Pasteur never rested on his laurels and probably rarely rested at all. He came up with a vaccine for chicken

cholera, and vaccines displaced a number of witches and devils. Arthur Nicolaier developed a vaccine for tetanus, the disease that had most of the mothers of the world frantic every time a young one stepped on a nail.

13.   We are coming closer to "our" time as doctors were able to replace laudanum (tincture of opium) with the non-habit-forming painkiller phenacetin. At just about the same time, the Japanese bacteriologist Shiga discovered the dysentery bacillus which had carried off babies, oldsters, and millions of soldiers.

14.   For a while things quieted down on the "Remarkable Cure" front until one happy day when a German bacteriologist developed salvarsan, the cure for syphilis.

15.   My father had already survived diphtheria as a little boy before Emil von Behring discovered its antitoxin, but the dread disease claimed my mother's little brother and two of his classmates in one week. I wasn't quite here in 1913 when Bela Schick developed the diphtheria immunity test. Do you remember baring your arm for that test in grammar school when we stood in long lines to get "jections?" We made a lot of fuss over those and some of our mothers came to school wearing red and furious faces. They had probably never seen a child slowly choking to death as a false membrane grew over the inside of its nose and throat. If you are a graveyard buff as I am, you will remember having seen the old markers for whole families of little kids, two, three, four, and five years old who had all died within days of each other. It isn't surprising if you know that those germs lurk in noses and throats and one uncovered sneeze could infect every

susceptible person in the room. Those were the days when every sneeze should have been followed by "God protect us all."

How old were you and what were you doing in 1926? I was twelve, living in Mount Vernon, New York, and planning to become either a veterinarian or a surgeon. I'd already had considerable experience as the former, but felt that the latter was more something-or-other. "Prestigious" wasn't in my usable vocabulary yet, though I knew what it meant. I was then on my second trip through the dictionary which I would never have found fun it we'd had TV.

16.   George Minot had started to treat pernicious anemia with liver abstract when I was twelve. My mother decided that if liver extract was good for anemia, liver must be too. We had it twice a week until she forgot about it. Now they use Vitamin B$_{12}$, but back then the word "vitamin" wasn't known. Now you can't go to a drugstore without falling over a display of vitamins in a two-for-one sale.

In 1929 the Depression hit. If you are fifty now, you couldn't have cared less: you weren't here yet. If you are now fifty-five your mother was probably having a fit. You were on the way and how were they going to handle the Depression and a baby too? If you are sixty you didn't know much about what was going on, even if you were poor. Almost everybody else was in the same boat. But if you are now seventy, the economic climate upset your dating something fierce. There we were, just us and the radio. Nobody had the money to go out or the clothes to go out in. If I accepted a date it had to be an evening date or a horseback riding date in the park. I did have evening clothes left over from better times, and those styles don't change so fast. If I didn't grow anymore, my riding habit would last forever. My school clothes (one brown wool skirt and two white blouses) couldn't have gone anywhere.

For the most part we were fit and healthy. There wasn't much junk food around yet. National advertising was still limited to Bon Ami, Dutch Cleanser, Campbell's Soup, and Nabisco. Most of us didn't smoke, in spite of the little guy yelling Philip Morris on the radio, and almost none of us drank anything alcoholic. Ginger ale was the party standby. Whether we liked it or not, our way of life was on our side. And the scientists still struggled, often underfunded, underfed, and certainly undersung.

17.   In those years of despair, Christian Eijkman, a Dutch hygienist and pathologist, received the Nobel Prize for his discovery of Vitamin B_1. The Nobel Prize does a lot more than recognize an important person; it publicly recognizes an important discovery. If Nobel had been around when Semmelweiss lived, doctors might have washed their hands sooner ... *you* would have insisted on it. I can remember my mother bustling about in our bathroom before the doctor came to visit one of us. She laid out a clean hand towel, a new piece of soap (which she threw away afterwards), and a bottle of alcohol. Her cheery, "Everything's ready for you in the bathroom, Doctor," signaled to us, and I guess to him, that whatever germs were on his hands were about to be killed dead!

Back to Vitamin B_1. Why should it make such a difference in your life, especially now? Because if you are deficient in B_1 (or niacin, which has been synthesized into thiamine chloride), you will exhibit several symptoms that ignorant people call "aging." Thiamine is needed to change carbohydrates into energy, and if you were to ask your doctor what most people complain of when they come for a check up, you'd learn that it is fatigue. Ask yourself right now, "How often do I say 'God, but I'm *tired.*'" Lack of thiamine also causes irritability and sensitivity to noise. Sometimes that noise is caused by people you love and all too often by the little people you love. There's worse: you can become a nervous wreck, and forgetful to boot. A lot of unpleasantness attributed to "aging" is really caused by poor diet. One of your after fifty resolutions should be to find a good course in nutrition.

18.   Right after B_1 became news, blood grouping was recognized. Considering the war clouds gathering over Europe, it was just in time. If there is one essential (other than ammunition) in wartime, it's blood. Now, soldiers and civilians could be assured of getting the right type blood.

19.   A year later came Vitamin A, responsible for bone growth and tooth structure. Two items the after fifty crowd should always keep in mind are teeth and bones. False teeth are white and shiny, but your own are better suited to your face. If you are a woman, start preventive treatment against osteoporosis *now*. Actually, you should have been informed about that danger when you were in high school, where your beloved granddaughter will soon be, but the information is just now available. We are told to drink milk, take extra calcium, and exercise. There are some suggestions regarding estrogen, but that is a matter for discussion

between a woman and her doctor. Learn more about osteoporosis, then tell your granddaughter and her friends. They may not listen to parents, but they often do listen to grandparents, especially grandparents who know what they are talking about.

Another thing Vitamin A does is fight infection and there's plenty of that around, especially if for one reason or another you are shipped off to a hospital. While hospitals are a long time away from the filth of the Hotel de Dieu in Paris, their shiny cleanliness is only comfort-deep. Chances are that you may go in with one infection and leave with another that you got there. I went into one of America's top hospitals to get my first hip replaced. I came away with a new hip . . . and hepatitis.

20. In 1932 there wasn't a lot going on besides despair. I had left boarding school and we had moved into one of those resident hotels New York was famous for. The Depression was in full force, and at an age when today's teenagers are taking part-time and weekend jobs, there was absolutely nothing available. I went to a wonderful high school up on 120th Street, Horace Mann School for Girls. At night I took courses at Columbia University on 116th Street. In between I spent every available hour up at The College of Physicians and Surgeons learning to cut up cadavers (after hours) and watching operations (illegally). All but two of the boys I went out with were interns. That year, while I was assisting some of those interns with bugs I had no business being around, Dr. Fritz Mietsch quietly gave us sulphanilamide. It wouldn't have been an answer had any of those bugs gotten into a hangnail, but it was the forerunner of a drug that

had always been needed. The need would soon be crucial, as the elite of the world tried to blow each other to bits.

In 1933 I graduated from Horace Mann, which was quite an accomplishment considering my study habits, my home life, and what I wanted to do with my life. Having been told for several years that I wasn't college material, I didn't feel too badly when there was no money to send me there and no counseling to suggest anything else. My mother had been wringing her hands for a long time. "What are we going to *do* with her? What will she become?" Today there are athletic scholarships for girls; then there was nothing. I divided my days between the Grand Central School of Art, journalism and psychology courses at Columbia, and the Humphrey-Weidman School of Dance, the rival of Martha Graham. I decided to cover all bets and see what life offered. It offered the theater, and I became first a concert dancer and then started to appear on Broadway. Heaven! I was young, I was successful . . . and I was in love.

21. With no help from me, riboflavin, or Vitamin B_2, was discovered. It is the vitamin needed for good eye function. The last time I went to the eye doctor he wanted to know what my diet was; I told him it was like Pritikin's, but with lapses. Then he wanted to know what my exercise regimen was and I told him "Some *every* day." Then I wanted to know why he wanted to know. "Because your eyes haven't changed a bit in five years. You must be doing something right and I'd like to try it." I told him about riboflavin which also helps in the promotion of oxygen. If you don't have enough of that you can develop cracks in the corners

THE CROSSROADS OF CHANGE 49

of your mouth, a sore tongue, or scaly skin around nose and ears. Light can bother your eyes. That's not age fellows, that's a vitamin deficiency.

22. The male hormone androsterone was isolated in 1934, and the first sulfa drug, prontospol, was used in the treatment of strep infections. Strep throats need no longer lead to rheumatic hearts. There now was help if you were wise enough to see the doctor.

Between the discovery of streptococci and the ability to defeat it there had been a lapse of fifty-one years, over half a century. Think of your forebears who fell to those septic sore throats, scarlet fever, septicemia (blood poisoning), puerperal fever, and several kinds of pneumonia. Do you remember when Calvin Coolidge's son developed septicemia from a blister on his heel . . . and died?

In 1936 I succumbed to love, married, and went to Europe on my honeymoon. It was to have been a wonderful time, but we started off in Essen, Germany, where my husband had many aunts, uncles, and cousins. I sensed danger almost immediately and have always been amazed at friends who attended the Olympics in Germany that year and didn't catch a whiff of the underlying horror. Germany was loaded with malevolence. I'd been there in the summer of '29, and sensed something bad then too, but it had been different—despair and hopelessness, but not evil. As a teenager I had met a lot of European youngsters and people in their early twenties. They had no plans for the future and were fond of saying, "Oh, you are American, you would never understand."

By 1938 a lot was going on, but it was ignored by most of the world when it wasn't ridiculed. To anyone with a Jewish connection though, it was anything but ridiculous. My father-in-law's home was one of the American stations on the underground that funneled many of Germany's great scientists into this country. Some stayed only a few days and were hustled on to other stations. Some, like Professor Richard Courant, came with his whole family and stayed for weeks or months.

23. Vitamin B_6, Pyridoxine, was isolated in 1938, and I got pregnant. The latter made the bigger impression on me. For one thing, I didn't know what was the matter with me. My return from my six-week honeymoon in Europe had signaled a whole new life.

After the Depression when my parents had lost everything, and I mean *everything*, it was hard going. When my future husband and I were dating and courting I was forced to fake a lot. Evening clothes and riding habit, shorts and sweaters I had. Day clothes, suits, and dresses I had not. I would leave school on Friday at 116th Street and take the subway to Van Cortlandt Park, where my future father-in-law's chauffeur would pick me up. I would change for dinner and look pretty good. The next morning I would be up by seven and my soon-to-be father-in-law and I would ride for three or four hours. Styles of riding habit don't change, and since it pleased him to have me ride side saddle, I borrowed my mother-in-law-to-be's skirt. It was too big, but that made it fun. We always got back too late to change for lunch.

Afternoons if the weather was good, we played tennis. I owned shorts and had my school sneakers. My terror, however, had to do with the maids: they always wanted to unpack my bag. I had to beat them to it or they'd find out that the inside of the bag was ratty, my pajamas were fit for a child, and I didn't own a toilet case. My only makeup was a Tangee lipstick purchased at the five-and-ten, where I also bought my underpants. I didn't own a bra (neither needed nor wanted one), or a petticoat (ditto), or a second pair of stockings, or a bathrobe. This state of affairs went on until I graduated from high school, went to all those schools in New York while my fiancé was at Dartmouth, and went on the stage [and finally made some money which mostly went to the dentist]. Just as things got better, I got married.

My new life was based on a wealthy, highly cultured, German-Jewish style of living. I had a lot to learn. For several months, until we found a little apartment in New York, I lived in the family house in Harrison, New York. My background hadn't prepared me for what I now faced. Every room had fabulous paintings, and I didn't know one of the painters. I bought *Lust for Life* and learned about Van Gogh. I "played" the piano, sort of, but that didn't prepare me for the Philharmonic every Thursday and Beethoven's nine symphonies and Artur Schnabel. I loved theater, but "Mourning Becomes Electra"? Concert dance was out! Earning money was out! My old crowd was out! Lots of things were out.

While the world changed, I did too. I learned to adapt. The only thing I could fall back on was drawing which I did with a vengeance . . . that and study. My father-in-law plied me with books that would help me to understand him, and he found me to be a good student. I really was interested. My mother-in-law became my model. I tried, oh how

I tried. When she was away I became the hostess. Go over the menus, arrange flowers, call in the grocery lists, preside at meals . . . ye gods! Was this life?! Then she offered me the huge playroom and hall as mural space. At last! Something to do. When those walls were finished, a hospital asked me to paint murals with the same Mexican children motif in the children's wing. Then another door closed: I had my first baby. "Bonnie has a family to raise," and that was that. It would be ten long years before I found the key that unlocked the door, and when I found it I walked out and never returned. I took heart and fled out into the sunshine.

But in 1938 I was sitting on a ladder painting murals and feeling sick all the time. Was it the paint? It must be the paint. It wasn't the paint. My mother-in-law returned from New York through the teeth of that famous hurricane (a hurricane, a tornado, an earthquake—nothing stopped her. I admired her tremendously). "You look sick," was her opening line after being missed by two falling trees, but just barely. "I feel sick; it must be the paint." "Have you considered being pregnant?" I certainly had not. It was not on my schedule. But I was.

24. In 1939 the RH factor in human blood was discovered at the same time I was delivering Petie by Caesarean section. A long-ago ski accident had started (but only started) to collect its wages. The RH factor meant nothing to me in 1939, but a great deal to Petie when she had her own babies twenty-odd years later.

The year 1939 was terrible. Germany had decided to pay the world back for the Versailles Treaty—with interest. Ships were sunk, planes shot down, and countries overrun. "Civilians" ceased to exist for the most part, though there were still islands of safety here and there. That's another plus for the after fifty Americans—they were still civilians. For today's children there is no place to hide, not even in their heads.

25. In 1940 the older sister of one of the Girl Scouts in my senior troop came home with her baby to live in her parent's house. She hadn't wanted to, but like so many young widows in those days, she had never learned how to support herself, let alone a child. Her husband, four days past his twenty-fifth birthday, had died of pneumonia the week before. Only a few months later, Howard Flory developed penicillin as a practical antibiotic. I could only think of nine-year-old Noreen Ailles, my very gentle friend. She had died in a diabetic coma just before insulin was discovered in the twenties.

So many of us awaken after an operation to see a little bottle of antibiotic riding on the IV. If we are aware at all—which may take some time if we know or care about antibiotics and never if we don't—we are grateful for that IV. It's a more comfortable way of getting an antibiotic than being injected several times a day in the seat! What we don't think about are the complications that our parents faced when they lay in similar hospitals undergoing similar operations. Their chances of post-surgical complications were many times what ours are today.

26. During the thirties a friend of mine, Robert Oppenheimer, had been away in Norway studying something I couldn't visualize: heavy water. It was top secret and not to be discussed, although he was an oft-time visitor. We never knew where he was when he

wasn't in New York. Now we know that in 1941 he headed up something called the Manhattan Project in Los Alamos, New Mexico. What he and his associates were working on out there would change everything for us forever.

You and I can put the atomic bomb into some sort of perspective because we have known both the best and the worst of the twentieth century. We had a chance at real childhood, real youth, both the good and the bad. Whatever else our childhood was, it was real and we had it. We made our way through courtship and we had our kids. Today's younglings can only look in one direction—forward. And what they see, or *think* they see, is often devastating. Physically their world is no-support, and mentally it's no-man's-land.

Do you remember when the long lazy days of summer took forever to pass? Fall was kind of slow, too, even though there were Halloween, Thanksgiving, and Christmas holidays to speed things up a little. But oh, between Christmas and Easter! There just seemed to be a *lot* of time. Then everything began to move faster and it wasn't just because we grew up and grew older: it was a fact.

27. In 1927 my sister and I had stayed up all night praying for "Slim Lindbergh," that he might get to his destination safely. My mother was convinced that our prayers alone would keep him in the air, and we behaved accordingly. He made Europe in an incredible 33½ hours, and my mother kept comparing his time with our ancestors' crossings from Ireland. In 1941 the ferry command was crossing in 8½ hours, and that same year similar speeding planes bombed Pearl Harbor. Where were you that day and what

were you doing? What did that awful news mean to you?

Today, people under forty-five hardly remember that war. It was ours. We each had a part in it. Some of you fought in it, some of you were caught in its most horrible aspects, concentration camps. Some of you did war work on the home front, and others fought to get through the days and nights and news, waiting for word. Europe was totally submerged in the murder and any illusions that might have survived its bloody history were burned, blown, and blotted out. America, winning as expected, hung onto its naiveté a while longer, but somewhere between our war and now, things have changed. There probably always was rot somewhere, but between World War II and today someone kicked over the fallen log to expose the decay underneath. Where we as children smelled autumn leaves burning, were given aspirin for sniffles, and married the kid next door, today's children smell pot burning, sniff cocaine for depression, and maybe they will marry her or him . . . but then again, maybe not . . . and does it really matter? That is the crux of the difference—*does it really matter . . . does anything?* It is only one short step to "*Nothing really matters.*" We were very lucky. Things did matter and they mattered very much, especially while we were growing up. People mattered and love mattered. Our parents mattered and so did our children and our friends . . . they still do. Let's keep it that way.

28. In 1942 Fermi split the atom. Do you remember? I can remember that we were mildly impressed. It was a little like most people's attitude toward the discovery of sulfanilamide: "Ummmmm, and what's for dinner?"

They would not have been so complacent had they known its future value and threat to life and limb, nor would we have been could we have visualized the results of another discovery made that year—the computer.

29. In 1943 my best excuse for escaping school—tuberculosis—was made obsolete. Waksman found streptomycin, and tuberculosis became a disease of the past, like the Black Death. My friend Gwen had tuberculosis and we were free of school because of it, but my cousin Helen had it and died of it in Saranac.

Streptomycin interferes with the growth of microbes, including those that cause typhoid fever (which my father had after the war), dysentery, undulant fever, gangrene, and even infections of the urinary tract. Infections of the urinary tract, ever had one? Here's something to think about, talk to your doctor about, and warn your family about. One of the best ways to get a urinary infection is to allow yourself to be catheterized. Indeed, there are forever-lasting infections that can *only* be contracted through catheterization (which is very often done for the convenience of somebody else). About 500,000 people die every year as a result of catheterization during or following operations they underwent in order that they might live long and well. Catheters are sometimes essential but very often they are used "routinely." That is a word that should wear the Surgeon General's warning "*May be injurious to your health.*"

If you are taken to a hospital and a nurse comes at you with a catheter to be used "routinely," rear up in bed and say, "Call my doctor," the person you have already discussed this with. Be an aware and well-informed, even if difficult, patient. You'll live longer and with more comfort. It is no secret that doctors are the worst patients in the world, and for good reason: they know about "routines" and "procedures." Beware of that word, too!

By 1945 the Atomic Age had begun, though most of us were unaware of what it would mean to us. To our military it meant we had beaten the Germans in the race to produce the ultimate weapon. To the Japanese it meant horror past imagining. To Robert Oppenheimer it meant that the evil genie had been let out of the bottle and there was no way between heaven and hell that it could be gotten back in again . . . ever.

Where were you in 1945? What were you doing? What were you planning? What were you worrying about? If you are now forty-five, you were part of those who can be considered the last fit Americans, but your ranks are thin. You may have been waiting for Daddy to come home from the war. If you are somewhere between sixty and seventy you may have been Daddy, or perhaps mother or the girl back home who waited. For most of us life stood still while the war swirled around us, but in 1945 it all began to move again. Two years later an American plane flew at supersonic speeds.

30.   In 1946 a fellow rock climber, Bill Shockley, invented the transistor for Bell Lab. He probably should have stopped while he was ahead and not gotten involved with sperm banks. But then, when you have a mind that operates light years ahead of the next fellow's, you are apt to jump the gun.

31.   In the same year aureomycetin and chloromycetin were discovered.

They both affect Rocky Mountain spotted fever, various types of typhus, and viral pneumonia. Chloromycetin affects bacterial dysentery and also does a number on typhoid. However—and here's a big "however" because it is a sign of pollution, which we hadn't had to worry about before—aureomycetin has gotten itself a bad name. We have been feeding it to poultry and hogs to speed their growth. It gets into the human system through the food chain and one day, when one of us might need its help, it will no longer work for us. That now goes for a lot of medication which is prescribed with the "guarantee" of the huge pharmaceutical houses. The trouble is, when they pull a drug that has caused illness and death off the shelves, what good is the guarantee? It is good policy to take all drugs with extreme care and avoid the newest ones until they have been proven over many tests and the test of time.

32.   The Kinsey Report on *Sexual Behavior in the Human Male* shocked a lot of Americans out of their socks. Some folks found it hard to believe that "The All-American Male" did all those things. *That was our generation they were claiming to be so shocked about.* I knew, and yes, you know, they did all those things, but we (females) thought they kept mum about it and they (males) didn't think anyone knew! When the sky didn't fall in and nobody was excommunicated, people began to wonder why there had been so much secrecy before. The closet door opened a wee crack and a gremlin peeked out.

33.   Cortisone was next and it's like fire. It's great if you use it wisely, under control, and for things that need fire. Cortisone really did look like a miracle drug to match some of the earlier

breakthroughs, and when it's the right drug used with discrimination and care, it does seem a touch miraculous. As the drug-of-the-week, it's a bust. That's the trouble with many discoveries. There's no way to prove them except on people. Rats simply won't do: the information they give is often inaccurate, especially when drugs to be used on older people are tested on young rats. Their metabolism is different. Even the metabolisms of people are not the same. Don't be all that happy or boastful to friends when you are told you are getting the latest discovery, the newest thing. All that means is that what's been tried didn't work and now you are a human guinea pig. You are being "observed" to see what the drug or treatment will do to you. It might be just the ticket, but on the other hand your hair could fall out, you could lose your sight, or you could come under the heading "once was." If it's a last ditch try to save your life, that's different. Then it's no holds barred and let's hope for the best. But to get rid of pain . . . no way. Stick with aspirin until you learn how to use myotherapy. And if you do use aspirin, remember it's an anticoagulant and may cause bruises.

Cortisone was discovered by Philip Hench and was hailed as the answer to "arthritis." It is also used for "bursitis," the name often given to shoulder pain. Read up on both in the section on problems (pages 153–166).

34.   In 1949 neomycin, yet another antibiotic, was introduced. A U.S. Air Force jet flew the Atlantic in 3 hours and 46 minutes. The U.S. launched a missile that landed 250 miles away, and while we didn't think much about it, we lost our protective moats, the Atlantic

and Pacific Oceans. I was too busy to notice. I had my exercise school in Westchester, and was busy using the minimum fitness test on anyone who would stand still. I knew American school children were in terrible shape, but our school had developed a program that could bring the failure rate down to 4 percent in weeks.

Think back, what were you worried about in 1950? What kind of emotional stress were you under? What about your family, what state were they in? I had a growing business, two little girls, my husband had had a nervous breakdown, my marriage was having one too . . . and I had a backache. Could you handle all your problems then, and if you couldn't, what was offered to you?

35.   We were told a whole new world was about to open for us and on the other side we would find happiness, serenity . . . and Miltown. Yes, Miltown, a meprobamate, was the answer. I didn't hear about it because I didn't have a doctor, and if I had I would never have thought of going to him for my "nerves." The only doctor I knew was a rock climber, and when I said I was worried he said, "Come climb 'sixes' with me and you'll forget all about it." He was right. I climbed 'sixes' at least two days a week every week and spent the rest of the time teaching exercise to happy, stimulating music. My troubles didn't go away, but I grew emotionally taller and was able to carry my troubles better. That is a very important aid you will be able to use very soon: if you are physically active, especially out-of-doors, you will be able to make your heart ache less. But that's not what happened to those who listened to the siren song of "nerve medicine." They took the drugs and got hooked on them.

They sold today (however bad) which is reality, for tomorrows that never came. Try to keep that in mind. *You really only have today.* Make that TODAY in capital letters. Yesterday is gone, and good or bad, there's nothing to be done about it, so don't live there. You can think about tomorrow, but all any of us have is today. Do the best you can with it and try to knock a little fun out of each one. Even bad days have a purpose, though it's hard to recognize it when you are in the middle of it. Keep in mind that tranquilizers steal today and often render you incapable of using tomorrow. By the way, tranquilizers often masquerade as "muscle relaxants." Believe me, you won't need them when you have finished this book. There's a much better way to get muscles to relax, and it won't do weird things to your sex life!

In 1951 J. Andre Thomas invented the heart-lung machine, making heart operations possible in a country beset not only by a very high rate of death from heart attack, but by the fear of heart attack. This fear was to lead to the jogging craze which is now beginning to find many of its champions dying on the track or roads while running for example, Jack Kelly, Jr., the young man responsible for getting my fitness study to President Eisenhower, dropped dead while running near his home at age 56. His brother-in-law died seven hours later doing the same thing.

There were other changes approaching, changes that we could never have envisioned in our wildest imaginings. One of them was the sexual revolution which was already in the works, but we had not really recognized it yet.

36. In 1952 the contraceptive pill, phosphorated hesperidin, was produced. It was to be hoped that in a liberate country it would lead to fewer gruesome deaths by illegal abortion and even fewer children who could not be supported. It led to a lot more than that.

37. The year after the Pill came Kinsey's second shocker, *Sexual Behavior in the Human Female.* Had my mother been alive it would have done 'er in. She had spent many hours telling us "No," warning us about sex and morals, and here was a book that made her out to be totally ignorant (which I doubted) or lying in her teeth (which I had started to suspect when I was twelve). That same year a rocket flew much farther than the one that had been so highly advertised at 250 miles. The new one flew 1,600 miles which should have sounded a warning. If we can send one that-a-way, *they* could probably send one this-a-way. My husband, who smoked three packs a day, didn't listen to the warnings that had begun appearing about smoking and lung cancer and heart problems.

38. One of the last big developments came in 1954. Jonas Salk developed a POLIO vaccine and mothers everywhere breathed easier. I was just wrapping up the testing on school children, had collaborated on a couple of medical papers, and had gone to Reno for a divorce.

Since the fitness tests we had given in the states and in Europe were medically valid tests, it seemed only right that the papers should be written for medical journals and presented before bodies of medical people. Neither caused the slightest stir. There was a good reason for that: doctors are not like other people. Only a very few of them ever go out for baseball, football, or basketball, as insurance men do.

Doctors like sports such as tennis, canoeing, hiking, back packing, and climbing. Since there is nothing to attract them to sports in the American school system, they grow up cheated of things physical. Later, when children are brought to their offices they don't *think* physical. Unless the child is grossly obese, has a fever or spots, it's a healthy child.

So when a report comes in stating that American children are unfit, what does that mean to doctors? Nothing. Some researcher with a grant has been counting the white whiskers and the black whiskers on rabbits again. They know all about such studies; the woods are full of them. Had it not been for Mrs. Eddie Eagan, wife of the boxing commissioner, no one might ever have heard. She told a friend at the *New York Daily Mirror.* Our study had taken years of work and worry and it almost got lost, but not quite. One article led to another and, as you know, I was invited to the White House to give my report.

Life is a funny business. Had I tried directly to reach the president—who *runs* the United States—with my really horrifying information, I could never have done it. But imagine this chain of events. Among the articles sparked by our study was one in *The Winged Foot,* the magazine of the New York Athletic Club. John Kelly, Jr., a champion sculler, read the article and remembered that his father, the wealthy Philadelphia contractor and champion sculler in his own right, had had the assignment during World War II to check out the fitness of American children. That had been a frustrating assignment for Kelly in a frustrating time. Where would he start—with physical educators? They were convinced that what they were doing was right and would have shown him baseball scores. With the doctors? They would have shown him records of vaccinations. In addition, he was underfunded. What he did have was the knowledge that compared to his healthy, athletic children John Jr. and Grace, (who later became Princess Grace of Monaco) other kids looked less healthy and couldn't perform very well physically. Now he realized someone had done his research for him and the proof was a telephone call away. He called and made a lunch date with Dr. Kraus and me. He wanted to know all about the testing: who, how, where, when, and the results. All the results. Then he flew back to Washington, and the next link in the chain came into play.

Some time before, Senator James H. Duff had been governor of Pennsylvania, John B. Kelly's state, and had worked to reduce the pollution of the Schuylkill River. That led to the revival of rowing on the river and to a friendship between the two men. As soon as he got back to Washington, Mr. Kelly called the senator and told him what we had not only uncovered, but had proven beyond a doubt. The senator was both shocked and upset and went immediately to President Eisenhower saying, "Here we are, only a few generations from the frontier, and one of the most serious problems facing us now is the physical deterioration of our youth." Thereupon they decided on the upcoming White House Sports Luncheon where we would launch the report. It was held in July, 1955—more than thirty years ago.

Among the guests were Vice President Richard Nixon who later opened one of the annual meetings of the President's Advisory Council on Youth Fitness with the most sensible comments I ever heard expressed from that august body: "Let's not scatter our shots, let's make this physical fitness, and let's not overlook girls." Now that may have been because he had daughters, but I rather think he knew who should be able to do a good fitness job on American children if given the tools and the training: the young mothers of America. Unfortunately, nobody was listening.

Sports Illustrated covered the luncheon and reported that on hand was probably the greatest array of sports stars ever gathered together in one place. Thirty had been invited . . . Earl Blaik, Bob Cousy, Max Elbin, Eddie Erdelatz, Jack Fleck, Ford Frick, Isaac Grainger, Hank Greenberg, Ralph Gugliemi, Jack Kelly Sr., Jack Kelly Jr., Jack Kramer, Sammy Lee, Willie Mays, Lloyd Mangrum, Harry Moffit, Archie Moore, Billy Joe Patton, Barbara Romack, Bill Russell, Wes Santee, Norbert Schemansky, Tony Trabert, Gene Tunney, Mal Whitfield, Kenneth Wilson and William Woodward Jr. among them.

I was scared spitless, as we say when we have just climbed a "six." I remember very little except that on my right was Ford Frick and on my left Dr. Hans Kraus who had designed a test for sick children and caught a nation of them. The president was sitting right across from me listening to Archie Moore. Suddenly there came the awful summons. Mr. Kelly was saying, ". . . and now, Mr. President, Mrs. Hirschland will give you the report." I was still Mrs. Hirschland in those days and didn't even have a self-image. I was also very timid. The president grinned. Do you

remember that grin? It went from ear to ear and I went into my act. "If you will just pretend you are lying on the table here in front of me, Mr. President, I'll talk you through the test so you will know exactly what we are talking about. Put your hands behind your neck and I'll hold your feet down." I went through it step by step. "Americans fail at 58 percent and Europeans at 8 percent." He understood and said, "This is really shocking." Our study became known as *"The Report that Shocked the President."* Dr. Kraus then gave a report about what happens when people are unfit. The first problem he addressed was back pain, one of the conditions that the minimum fitness test can predict. How many of you have back pain? How many of your friends or colleagues? The answer is somewhere around 60 percent for you, but it will be around 85 percent for your children and almost 100 percent for your grandchildren.

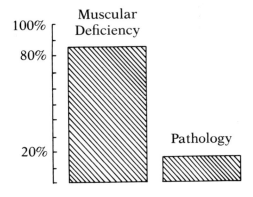

Figure 1. *Low Back Pain*

We had coined a word for the conditions suffered as a result of inactivity. It is HYPOKINETIC DISEASE and there are a lot of them.

The first study Dr. Kraus quoted in his report was one done at New York's Presbyterian Hospital. Thousands of people with clinical back pain (requiring the attention of a doctor) were examined. They were given a whole battery of tests, including blood and urine tests, blood pressure, gynecological exams, and psychological screening. Subjects were also given the minimum muscular fitness test you will give yourself in the next chapter. Over 80 percent of the "back achers" flunked nothing but the muscle test. When they were given exercises to recondition their muscles, they not only passed the test, they were free of pain. That was the end of the pain for the ones who could be induced to keep up with their exercises. Others, less disciplined, were soon back at their doctors' offices. Retested, they flunked. Reexercised, they were made strong, flexible, and pain free again. It was like turning the tap water off and on. Of course, some never learn.

The results of the study proved (again) that there is a level of muscular fitness below which you cannot go without getting into trouble. When we had been in Austria and wanted to test, the head of the National Health Department had asked us why. We quoted the results of the Presbyterian Hospital tests and we predicted that children who had failed the test would one day have back pain. While the failure rate in America was 58 percent, the rate of back pain in adults was 60 percent. "Then our children will fail at 10 percent because that is the rate of adult back pain in Austria," he predicted.

They failed at 9.5 percent! How does that make you feel when I tell you that children in our country enter school today at between 85 and 100 percent? Of course, in the same breath I can tell you that that can be prevented. And you can do it.

Probably the only statistics that really interested everyone at the White House on the day of my report were the ones on heart attacks. We were still living in a time when doctors would say to a perfectly healthy young man, "Quit shoveling snow; next time it may not be your back. You want to have a heart attack?" The president had not yet had his famous coronary which would change that attitude completely. When Dr. Kraus said people who did heavy work had half as many heart attacks as those who were engaged in light work, the athletes looked smug, though they needn't have. Their hearts may have been better while they were doing the

Average annual mortality rate per million men aged 45–64

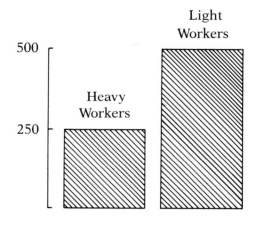

Figure 2. *Coronary Heart Disease*

"heavy work" required of competing athletes, but athletes are forced to stop the really heavy workouts rather early in life and, unfortunately, the conditioning doesn't hold.

The executives in the room leaned forward. Nobody, athlete or executive, would do anything about the news that day or for many years, but they did think about their closest friends and think, "Poor George, we'll miss him."

The president understood the next statistics better than anyone else in the room: they had to do with draft rejections. Of the 3.7 million young men under the age of 26 who had been examined by the armed forces for the draft, 1.7 million were rejected as physically unfit for fighting. That was over 40 percent.

That was our generation at its best and those were just the males. You can imagine what the females were like, if not then at least a few years after childbirth. Now hang those figures up against what the young people of today would produce!

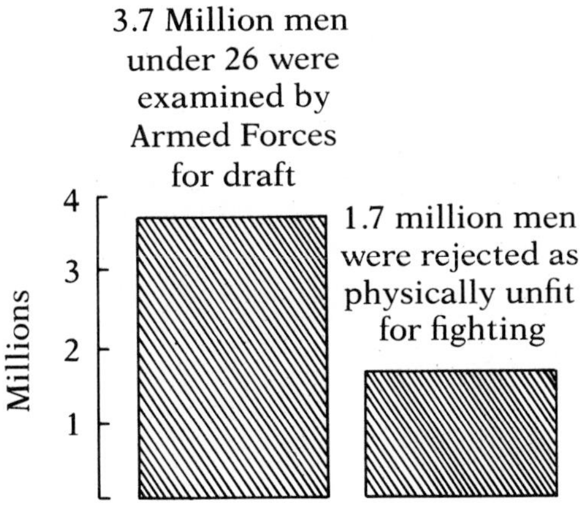

The decay had already begun. In spite of better housing, better food, better general conditions, more money, in fact more of everything, our people were beginning the descent which usually accompanies the march of civilizations.

We touched on another interesting facet of fitness but I don't think we were understood, as there were neither psychiatrists nor psychologists present (the only people, as a group, who would have understood the connection between a person's physical condition and his or her mental outlook and behavior). Our crème de la crème, West Point cadets, had these statistics to offer. All incoming plebes were given tough physical fitness tests. The young men who fell into the lowest 7 percent had roughly 12 percent of the discharges from the Point with psychiatric endorsement. The top 7 percent had no psychiatric discharges at all.

The level of fitness runs parallel to emotional difficulties. That point isn't hard to make when West Pointers are being used as examples; they can be tested and observed for four years. But those same observations apply when looking at men and women in ordinary lives: the more fit, the more emotionally stable. The less fit, the less chance or base for stability. There are many reasons—Stamina, opportunities for the physical release of stress, a satisfying self-image, continued successes, self-confidence, attention to nutrition and many other facets. These qualities start early in life and last late. It doesn't matter where you are in the scheme of life, physical fitness will make a huge

3.7 Million men under 26 were examined by Armed Forces for draft

1.7 million men were rejected as physically unfit for fighting

Figure 3. *Draft Rejections*

West Point cadets discharged with psychiatric endorsement

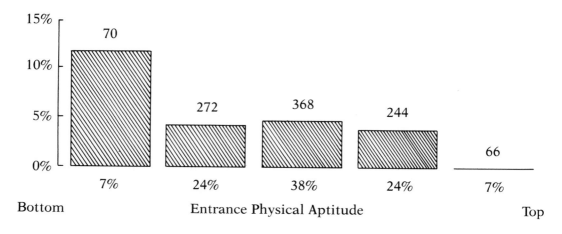

Figure 4. *Psychiatric*

difference to your emotional make-up. NO MATTER WHAT CONDITION YOU ARE IN AT THIS MOMENT, YOU CAN MAKE IT BETTER.

The last message we gave to the president, to the athletes, and, we hoped, to America was that the majority of the Americans in our generation had become sedentary. We said that the physically active showed better adaptability to stress, less neuromuscular and emotional tension, and less fatigue. Active people age later and their weight tends to remain stable, both in comparison to their own weight in earlier years and in comparison to others who, due to sedentary living, gain.

And then we all went home. The athletes had had a nice lunch, been lionized by the press, and hadn't heard a word. The president appointed a committee to investigate and act upon the matter, but he was soon engrossed in his own personal problem: his heart attack. Two groups heard, however; the first was the YMCA, who decided they could use this "new" condition to push their programs. They began to build family Y's, tested thousands, and bore out nationally what had been proven primarily in the East. The other group, the physical educators, fought us tooth and nail, and stiletto. Once they had turned away from real physical education, the type we had adopted from Europe and the British Isles, and once they had adopted "play" as their curriculum, they couldn't admit to a lessening of fitness levels without admitting a mistake in direction. All of us know how hard it is to admit error, and for some it is not possible. For some of the people directing physical education it was totally impossible.

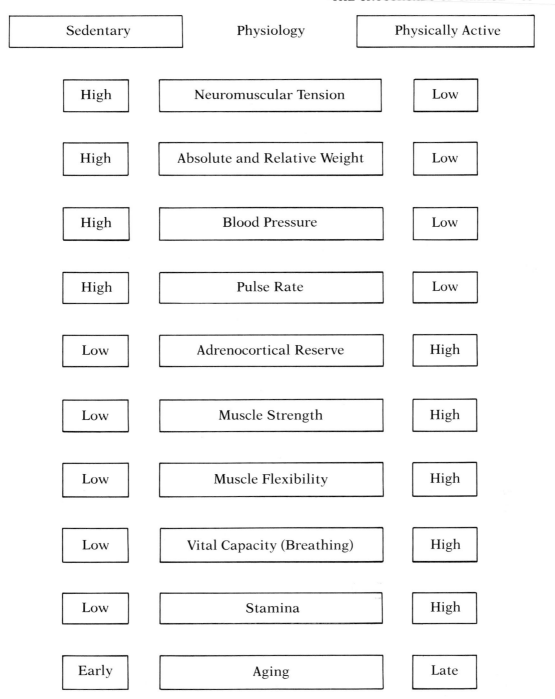

Figure 5. *Sedentary Living vs. Physically Active*

AN ENCOURAGING WORD

Now let's get back to you: You can be reclaimed. Many of you lead sedentary lives and are primarily spectator sports people. Those of you who are active have certain advantages which the rest of you are entitled to and can have, starting right now. What's in it for us?

- Active people age much later. Why not wait till you're ninety to look and feel ninety?
- Active people show better resistance to stress; this adaptability can help them avoid drugs and prevent alcoholism with its consequent decay.
- The active do not tend to put on weight and their blood pressure is lower. That means avoidance of the drugs that put a damper on sex.
- Due to exercise, active people are stronger and more flexible.
- They have greater breathing capacity which means more oxygen throughout the entire body.
- Their pulse rate is slower denoting better heart action and less strain on a crucial organ.
- They have less neuro-muscular and emotional tension and are rarely tired.

A lot of us would settle for that last one alone, or would place it first on the list!

All in all, it makes sense to improve our physical, mental and emotional states, especially since we have such a good basis for all three. Keep in mind that there is a war going on between the After Fifty Crowd and the Mythmakers. We are the largest "minority group" in the country and of all the groups suffering discrimination, we have the best chance to combat it, for ourselves and for others to come. We are the generation that believes in helping others. We were trained to help and we can and must do it again. In order to do it, however, we must begin with ourselves, and to begin with us we need to know where we are right now.

In the next chapters you will find out a lot about yourself. Some of it will annoy you but some of it will please. Take the pleases and run with them; the annoys will be left behind.

39. President Eisenhower's committee on fitness became known as The President's Council on Youth Fitness and was given a Citizen's Advisory Committee on which I served for three years. However, those of you who have served on large committees know how effective either you or they can be. I resigned. I had to be where I could really do some good.

40. *Sports Illustrated* took up the banner of fitness and reported what was happening around the country—and what was not. I soon began writing an exercise column for SI, the first to appear in an American magazine. Many of you tell me you cut those columns out, used them, and saved them.

41. Television caught on to exercise for a very interesting reason: I wore fashionable exercise clothes in my column layouts. A man who read the magazine told his wife, who was in charge of Arlene Francis's wardrobe for The Home Show, that the producers ought to do a show on "fitness fashions." They in turn called me in, we did a show, and I became a regular. When The Home

Show finished its run I moved over to The Today Show. On TV a different hour is a different audience and a different audience is a different dimension. Dave Garroway was king of the TV world back then and we had a ball. If he could get down on the floor, everybody could. And so I opened the door for a multimillion-dollar industry in health, exercise, and diet books. I also opened the door for the greatest mass of junk ever to hit the American public. The minute the advertising media smelled money in the fitness field anything could happen . . . and did.

Beginning in 1956 I began producing books and records on exercise for all ages and shapes—babies, young children, teenagers, executives, women.

42. Exercise, once considered beyond the pale, had been accepted. There would be many false starts and dead ends, not to mention damaged muscles, but the word at least had some sort of meaning and, to many, attraction. Doctors came to recommend it, schools to claim they taught it, clubs, spas, and assorted emporia to make money on it.

In 1965 I began first to walk down a long and lonely road which would bring me to Myotherapy, the last of the five influences to make you the last fit Americans. The circumstances under which I began that trek are important because they apply to everyone who has any kind of chronic pain. I was under terrible emotional stress and had been for many years. Now, although I was unaware of it, I was breaking down physically. While I was teaching a five-day workshop in the Berkshires with everything against me—inadequate facilities, cold, damp weather, and no staff—I pulled a muscle in my right

thigh which proceeded to worsen until the last day when it "went" altogether and my knee would not support me. Most people think "knee injuries" are in the knee; most of them are not.

That was the beginning. I continued all summer lecturing, teaching, doing The Bonnie Prudden Show from Canada, and trying in every way I knew to make fitness palatable to the public. I turned no job down and the stress never let up. It never entered my mind that those spasmed thigh muscles were pulling my right leg short.

I fought the deterioration and the agony for five stress-filled years and finally had my ailing hip replaced. Most people who have that kind of trouble think that the problem lies solely in the hip. Some of it does, but be sure to check the thigh, calf, and hip muscles, and the stress level. Above all, check the stress.

By 1975 my stress level carried me to the brink of suicide. As I look back on those terrible years I think the only reason I'm still here is because I am supposed to be. I hadn't finished, so to speak. Four months later I found myotherapy.

43. Myotherapy came as a result of an injury sustained by a young woman of twenty-one who didn't have the sense to learn to ski before taking on a steep hill. Her search for pain relief covered thirty-seven years, most of the modalities short of back surgery, and most of the medications not even short of Indocin, a drug given for arthritis with more side effects than a fall down a mountain. What Myotherapy is, you will learn in the next chapters. You will learn how to use it for yourself and your dear ones, including those beloved grandchildren who will need it tomor-

row if they don't need it already. What it can do, you will learn right now.

- It can make you painless and stronger.
- It will open the way to exercise that can do all the things we told the president.

You've heard our nation's fitness story—and mine. Now let's write yours.

PART TWO
GETTING BETTER AND BETTER

TAKING STOCK

Taking a good, long look at yourself is interesting because you always learn something about the person who should be the most important human being in your life . . . yourself. When you are comfortable with that person, you are a joy to everyone around you. One of the things you learn is what you really think of yourself. Once you have that information you should ask yourself where it came from. You will use it either for or against yourself for a lifetime.

For years I thought I was a "bad" kid. I got that idea from my mother, and my father did nothing to counteract it. On the other hand, he promised me he'd take me hunting "when I got sense." He never did. I was sure I wasn't bright or talented. I got *those* negatives from the nuns when I was at the orphanage, though how they could be so sure when I was so little I never figured out. I was "hopeless" at math. Miss Okerstrom at P.S. 9 told me that "fact." I was not very attractive, but I certainly was "healthy." All my mother's friends had said so when viewing my sister and me in the same eyefull. I was also an "urchin," a "rag-tag," a "vandal," and a "misfit," all various appellations applied by adults to a child who was trying to decide what to be.

At Marymount when I was a teenager—that time of life when you are sure you are a mess and not worth saving—the girls used to play a game called "The Book." Like the confessions wrung out of the Communist cadres it was supposed to make you thoroughly aware of your shortcomings and appropriately humble. One charmer would be the keeper of the book (I never got the job and today I wonder if I would have played). The Keeper would call up one of my classmates and whisper so no one else could hear, "Give this book to the girl with the worst figure." That was for starters and it was all down hill from there. The book would be handed to A who may or may not have had a bad figure, but was or was not a friend of the Giver. No mention was made of why she had been given the book. She then went with it to the whispering Keeper and was told to pass it along to the one with the most pimples, was the most conceited, told the biggest whoppers, or something equally degrading. This would go on for about fifteen minutes; then, each girl would be told why she had been so honored. "I gave Helen the book because she has bad breath," was usually pronounced with both superiority and finality. It was sick time and presided over by Madame Cecelia who thought it was "character building."

I got all the downers at one time or another and sometimes several in a single evening. In that class I was the misfit. I had skipped most of elementary school and junior high, a lot of it taking care of my mother who was an alcoholic (which was why I'd been stashed in the orphanage). My mother, in an effort to give me the educational grounding she knew I'd missed, put me back two years when I went to boarding school. I had probably read well past the required reading for the second year of college, and since my mother had no use for the Catholic Index of proscribed books, my reading had included books and subjects my teachers had never heard of. Did that kind of information and pattern of thinking endear me to my classmates? You can bet it didn't! By the time I got out of there after two years of "shaming," I couldn't walk straight through Grand Central Station but had to slink around the edges where no one could see me. I was nineteen before I could be made to understand that the young man on the phone wanted to talk to me and not my sister. I was married and the mother of two children before a wonderful man made me feel that I was an attractive woman. *Are you sure that what you think about yourself is the truth?* If it's nice, keep it. If it isn't, let's get rid of it, all of it.

LOOK YOURSELF OVER

We are about to make a checklist that will help you learn about yourself and change what you want to change. It will also help you keep track of these changes and encourage you to persevere. You will grow younger in body, mind, and heart with each passing week . . . and you will know it.

The first things to check are physical, because they are fairly easy to spot.

HOW TALL ARE YOU?

You want to know your exact height because of the myth that "all older people shrink and shrivel." It is true that eventually we will become shorter. Some of the fluid in the discs between the vertebrae disappears and the cushions are less padded. What causes the real (and preventable) shortening, however, is muscle spasm, even the kind you can't feel. If you can feel spasm in the form of back and neck pain, it is happening faster than need be and must be stopped. The back muscles are doing a tightening act and compacting you. I have seen people who have had polio, back pain, or torticollis get off a Myotherapy table and find that they have "grown" an inch or more in a single hour. Did their bones grow? Certainly not; those bones were taken out of the crushing clasp of once injured muscles which later went into increasing spasm. You will shorten some day, but when? If you clear your muscles of spasm and give them daily release through the right kind of exercise, the shortening process will happen much later in your life.

HOW MUCH DO YOU WEIGH?

You want to know your weight for several reasons. Overweight gets to your self-image and bothers you. It interferes with self-discipline (ahhhh, why bother, I don't eat much anyway and look at me?!). You are not in any danger of anorexia or bulimia, both diseases of the young, but overweight is also a disease and far easier to correct. It entails knowing what to eat, when, and with whom. You can (should) scrap all those magazine diets and enroll instead at a good college with a course in dietetics. You don't need a certificate, just information on how to properly feed yourself and your family in a world of fast-food factories reeking of rancid fat. Make copies of the Eat Sheet (page 78) and use it faithfully. If you are in the market for weight loss put three of your charts together: Weight Chart (page 76), Measurement Chart (page 77), and Eat Sheet. In a couple of weeks one (or more) of several things will have happened.

- *You have lost inches, but not weight.* That means you are tightening your body, improving tone, putting on muscle, and dropping fat. You are right on target.
- *You have lost weight but not inches.* Fat is leaving, but you are not yet working hard enough to do much about tone. You are still on target, but a less ambitious target. It's fine; keep on with it.
- *You have lost neither weight nor inches.* Ask yourself how you feel. If you feel more alive and less stiff, you are still on target. Keep going. At the end of a week if nothing has changed, make a decision. You have to shake yourself up and there are just two possibilities: eat less or exercise more. Don't try to do both at the same time or you will lose track of yourself. Make an intelligent choice, not an emotional one. Perhaps until you are in better shape it would be easier to eat less. Look over your Eat Sheets, note your patterns, and choose one item you could live without. It could be dessert or it could be bread. Decide, and stick with your decision.

If you'd rather increase your exercise regimen, either add repetitions or use weight bags (page 367) with your warm-ups (page 229). You might decide to make two trips upstairs for every necessary trip. If one week of change doesn't make a difference repeat it for another and then—but only then—take one more item off your menu. Eat less *or* increase the exercise. By then the latter will be easy. As soon as you can, turn your feet toward hilly country in your daily walks.

There are expensive ways to find out if you are "obese" (hateful word!). You could go to a sports medicine center and get into a tank of water. This will show how much of you is fat and how much ought to be. These centers are famous for tests and infamous for programs. The inexpensive way, which is just as good if not better, is to go into your bedroom, take off your clothes . . . and look! If you feel like saying "Ummmmmm, yummy," stay as sweet, handsome, feminine, masculine, whatever, as you are. If your reaction is "Agggggggggh!" you are probably right. So let's get after it.

FORM FOLLOWS FUNCTION is a fact. Whatever tasks your body is called upon to execute often, will determine the form it takes, how it feels and looks, and what pain you will ultimately have. If your daily occupation is that of CPA, or bookkeeper, hematologist, surgeon, secretary, or computer programmer the function of your chest muscles will be to contract in order to bring your arms forward. Gravity will pull your head down and your abdominals will be slack. On the opposite side of your body the antagonist muscles in the back of your neck, shoulders, and upper back will be constantly on the stretch. Any sitting job will foreshorten the hamstrings at the backs of your legs and the groin muscles in front. What form can your body take from that sort of function? Eventually you will be round backed, forward leaning, neck straining, potbellied, soft bottomed, in short, physically inadequate. If you are forty you will look fifty, at fifty, sixty, etc. Not good.

Now, suppose you are aware of the problems entailed in your job or the job you retired from. In the first instance you can prevent disaster and in the second, correct it. And both with the same

system. Check with the list of occupations which are accompanied by the needed muscle work (see page 171), the necessary exercise, and the fun "x-x"— which stands for "extra exercise" (see page 278). These are outside the calesthenics program you will set up and are easy, pleasant ways to build exercise into your life. Your choice does not lie with whether to exercise or not but rather, which exercises must be done and which ones give you the most pleasure. A full exercise program plus a balanced diet will lead to a firmer, trimmer, healthier body, with—an added attraction—the right weight for *you*.

HOW IS YOUR POSTURE?

For your Posture Quiz you may need an unbiased assistant. You can see a round back in the mirror and you can usually hear echoes of "Stand up straight dear, you'll be old before your time." A sway back, too, is easy to recognize (you think your bottom sticks out). If you've had scoliosis since junior high (when the condition usually becomes apparent), nobody needs to tell you, but a flat back in which your back doesn't nip in at the waist, is often overlooked. You will also need some help with forward lean which makes you look like you are always heading into a wind. It means that the groin muscles have shortened and are pulling the upper torso downward. It puts a terrible strain on your lower back which you can feel, if only as fatigue. Your friend needs to walk with you and take note when you are not trying to stand straight. A forward head is also hard to self-spot. If your upper back has rounded, so has your spine. When your posture is well balanced your head sits neatly on your shoulders and your eyes look straight ahead. In a round back the head tips forward as the upper spine does and all you can see is the ground in front of you. You handle that by lifting your chin, bringing it not only up, but forward. This puts strain on every face, head, neck, chest, and upper back muscle. Not good at all. What's more, you look like a turtle.

HOW IS YOUR HEART?

You may want to know what your heart action is, since the slower it beats the better it's doing. Once a month you can check with the Step Test (see page 79), but it isn't essential. Don't get sucked into an exercise "stress test." They are just money-makers and are inaccurate, giving both false positive and false negative results. Your doctor can give you an accurate report as to what your heart is doing in a matter of a few minutes without charging you for a test that can tell you you are sick when you are healthy as a horse, or well when you are not.

HOW IS YOUR VITAL CAPACITY?

As your lungs enlarge you have better vital capacity. Your lungs determine how much oxygen you will have available and that determines almost everything else. An inexpensive way to find out your vital capacity is by using a tape measure. Of course there are expensive ways (there are *always* expensive ways), but let's spend the money on something more fun than a spirometer. Here's a simple test:

Measure your chest empty and then full. Run a tape measure around your chest right across the nipples. Exhale every bit of air you can and measure the size of your chest. Then inhale as

fully as you can and take that chest measurement. The difference in inches between empty and full is called your vital capacity. As your body improves and you exercise more, you will find your chest expanding. The increased oxygen in the improved lungs will add to your feelings of zest, well-being, and control.

HOW MUCH STRESS IS IN YOUR LIFE?

Stress is the bottom line. It starts when the first contraction of the womb grabs us like a giant fist and forces us, ready or not, into the world. It never goes away. It is hard to see why people today are going in for "rebirthing": it cannot have been anything but painful and terrifying the first time. Pain and terror both cause stress. So do worry and injury, anger and illness, frustration and despair. And while only a few of the poets have labeled love as a disease, it is one, and it causes all kinds of stress— even when it's perfect.

Thirty-odd years ago the Canadian doctor Hans Selye noticed that no matter what diseases his patients had, they all exhibited similar symptoms: they were listless, felt terrible, and didn't care if school kept or not. His rats behaved the same way, and when he opened them up he found the same things wrong with many of their organs: it didn't matter what disease he had inflicted on them or what injury he had done them, even to drowning them in icy water. Their adrenals had shrunk and they had developed little ulcers, for example. In time, Selye named the collection of symptoms G.A.S. or General Adaptation Syndrome.

What Selye had noted in rats and then applied to humans was the ability to adapt to stress for a time. This echoed what Walter B. Cannon referred to as homeostasis in *Wisdom of the Body*. But when normal stasis is disrupted and requires enormous amounts of energy to maintain, the body begins to break down. Young people and young rats were behaving like sick, tired, old people and rats. Uninterrupted stress and resulting exhaustion eventually cause death. In modern man and woman, stress is the pervasive killer.

Think about the stress in your life this way: Jack and Jill go after a pail of water, but no sooner have they filled the pail and arranged it between them for easy transportation than they see smoke on the horizon in the direction of their house. Jill shouts, "Ohmigod, I left the beans on the stove; bring the water, Jack, we may need it if the house is on fire . . ." and races off to rescue the beans and perhaps the house as well. Jack (you) is now forced to carry the weight alone and without balance. He bends as far away from the heavy pail of precious water as he can and hastens down the hill and across the fields. His body has adapted to the load, but in no way is he balanced. He is caught in a stressful situation. The load is terribly heavy and adapt as he will, he is tiring fast. Adaptation has its limits but he—like so many of us—dares not stop, nor can he lighten his load. Eventually the strain will be too much and something will give in Jack's (read "your") body. It will be called "sickness."

Later you will learn that chronic pain does not exist without stress and that chronic pain is your warning that your stress level has risen beyond the body's ability to adapt. Exhaustion is not far off.

We are all stressed to some degree every day of our lives. If you question your friends you will find that their "arthritis" pain started during or fairly soon after a time of great stress. We all live with germs, but disease hits only when we have used up our strength and our resistance to stress. Our General Adaptation ability is running low, we are close to exhaustion. Have you ever noticed how often, when two people work incredibly hard to amass enough money to retire to ease and comfort, one of them is apt to sicken and die less than a year later? That is the stress of overwork. Cancer often occurs several months after a loved one dies: that is the stress of loss.

Sadness is a stressor, loneliness is a stressor, anger is a stressor. Overwork, jealousy, overeating, drinking too much, and drugs are stressors. How many of the above can you control? Had Jill checked the stove before she left the house the beans would not have burned. Had the two of them kept a rainbarrel full of water under the eaves they could have run home together to handle the fire. Had Jill realized that the exhaustion would cause Jack to have a heart attack she could have said, "To hell with the house, let 'er burn, you are more important."

What were their errors of commission and omission?

1. They didn't plan very well.

2. They didn't take sensible precautions, and

3. Their priorities were wrong. They didn't think ahead to what might, could, and did happen. Jack was more important than the house. *And so are you.*

HOW IS YOUR SELF-IMAGE?
Sit down and write a book report on your life as you see it right now and in the past. The title you confer on your

opus will tell you a lot. I've written volumes that could only be labeled "Gaslight," "Hatter's Castle," "The Seventh Level of Hell," and "Whatever Happened to Bonnie Prudden." Those titles would no longer apply (thank heavens), but even in the last year I wrote one entitled "What Did I Do to Deserve This?"

After you've settled on a title, give the author a name. Each of us has many aliases in a lifetime and sometimes "Gorgeous" fits. But there are other times when "Dumkopf" is more apt. Sometimes I was Niobe, Atlas, or Hercules in the Augean stables. I've even felt like P. T. Barnum from time to time. It's also fun to give friends and relatives aliases as you watch them mentally write their book reports (which everybody does all the time). If you want a quick start on a book report, get out the family album and turn to any page containing a snap of you. It will all come quickly to mind—title, author, chapter headings, and ending.

Now, give a brief synopsis of your life as though it were being lived by a character in a book. Describe your character as you now see yourself—your surroundings, hopes, fears, anxieties, all the stresses as if you were viewing them from a distance. Put in the supporting characters as you see them and their contributions to the plot and then step back and read what you have written. Then write a conclusion. Remember, writers can make everything turn out the way they want and choose optimums. When you have examined your story you will find very valid ways to make your life turn out right. Don't think of what might happen; start concentrating on the ending you have chosen. You're the one who's living it—and deciding it.

When people give us advice we have two self-protective words which guarantee the status quo: "Yes, but . . ." When you, the author, are writing your book you will be surprised to discover that you don't use "Yes, but . . ." You can find ways to do what has to be done because, unlike Jack and Jill, you have already sorted out your priorities. Your unbiased advice is better than anyone else's because you know the whole story to date and have decided on the finish. Writers don't feel denigrated when their characters make damn fools of themselves, take wrong turns, or waste time, friends, or money. They are not dismayed when one of their characters gets into trouble; they just get them out again! Scrap any ideas of writing a tragedy. Put the positive ending on paper and then hide it in the bottom drawer for six months. The next step is to change yourself physically so you can make the happy ending come true.

Your self-image is how you see yourself . . . your *self*, all of you, not merely how you look, but what you are. It can change in one night if you have spent that night being well loved. A different kind of change occurs when you meet an old "friend" who opens the conversation with, "My God! What happened to you, you look awful! Are you all right?" If you were, you aren't anymore! My own self image has changed so often I feel like a crowd. Self-images are built brick by brick by what people say, what happens to you day after day, but most of all by what you say to yourself. Your subconscious has no discrimination at all. What it hears it accepts and it might as well be true. Then the poor thing tries to live up to it. That's often what makes bad kids, weird teenagers, dishonest adults, and ugly old people.

I've made some important discoveries in the last ten years. First, I never was an ugly duckling, as I thought for so long. I never was stupid and incapable of adding or subtracting. I never was conceited. I was sure of some things and a leader. I wasn't any more selfish than the next guy and had surprising (for me) spurts of generosity. I'm not a social inept; I just hate parties and find them dull. Notice what all those qualities are and imagine where they came from. Those are all things teenagers worry about. I was stuck with them for years. Criticism starts early and is foisted on us by unthinking parents, disinterested teachers, and less-thinking contemporaries. The garbage can last a long time and should be bagged and thrown out. None of yours is true, either. Get rid of it.

Now to the body and what we lay on it.

DO YOU LIKE YOUR BODY?

I thought I was fat. I wasn't; my little sister just grew past me and was tall and slender. I hated being short. I wasn't; I was merely shorter than my sister. I thought I had a pug nose. They could have called it "turned up," or perhaps "retroussé," but no, I had a "pug" nose. My sister, of course, had a classic one. They could have called it "long," but no, it was "classic." Do you see the game I'm playing? Well, start playing yours. What did you think of your body? What do you think of it now? What would you like to keep as is? What would you like to have back again? What don't you like?

- You don't like eye glasses? What's wrong with contacts? They get better and cheaper every year.
- You don't like gray hair? That's what beauty salons are for. Choose the color that suits your face right now (and you certainly don't have to be female for that any more). If some is missing, fix it. I did a TV show not long ago with two men wearing "rugs." They didn't have to take them off at night and they could even swim with them.
- You loathe your double chin? Well, first get your whole body in shape. Get rid of all the excess weight and then find a first-class plastic surgeon and have a necklift or a facelift or both. Sometimes a job hangs on a facelift and it's no longer something done in secret, either for women or for men. Brains don't deteriorate, but bosses discriminate.
- You don't like your bust line? Lose weight and look again. It may be OK. If not, have it made smaller, larger, or balanced.

Your opinion of yourself is more important than anyone else's opinion of you. It can mean the difference between liking and disliking yourself which will influence your success or failure. At this late date—and fifty plus *is* late when it comes to enjoying the person you are—you want to have everything on your side. So do whatever it takes. Expensive, you say? Sure it is, but so were your braces when you were ten. If you don't do it now . . . then when?

MAKE YOUR GAME PLAN

Now we are about to get down to business—the "doing" part of the book and your new beginnings. Get yourself a notebook. There's nothing like a new notebook when you start back to school. In a sense you are starting school—your own school. You went to somebody else's school before and the motivation may not have been of the highest order. This is *your* school. *You* set the guidelines and goals and every last one of them applies to you and is of interest to you. Make your charts, keep your notes. Study.

- What's different this week from last?
- What can you do this month that you couldn't do a year ago?
- What new thing have you taken up and how are you progressing? Even sore muscles can be a change for the better so long as they are only mildly sore.

Now begins the action, your action. If you obey the rules you will be a very different person a year from now and it won't take anything but consistency, dogged determination, plain stubbornness . . . and what you will come to recognize as secret joy.

YOUR WEIGHT
Make some copies of the weight chart on the next page and paste one on your bathroom wall. Each new chart will last three weeks. Enter the date of your first weigh-in in the top-left square and your poundage about three squares from the top. That will allow for a pound or two in the wrong direction at the start. Buy a good scale, not one of those little ones that require you to squat to see and weigh more or less depending on where you stand. You want the truth. *Weigh in every day.* And write your weight in the box below (or above!) and to the right of the previous day's weight. Don't think "I've got to lose fifty pounds! That's impossible!" You're right, it is. Tell your subconscious you only want to lose ten. Now

say to your subconscious, "If I lose half a pound a week and this chart will last three weeks, I'll need seven charts. By the end of the first chart I'll be a pound and a half less." You've made your point. You were heard. You know that's possible. Now do it. If you happen to do a little better, pat yourself on the back, but don't think past ten. When you get there it will be time enough to think about another ten.

YOUR MEASUREMENTS
There are two ways to measure—every week on the same day, or every day. Every day is tedious, but when I am working very hard to get in shape, I do it. It's gratifying to see the inches come off even if the scale doesn't offer encouragement due to muscle increase. Again, make some copies of this chart and put one on your bathroom wall. Always measure carefully. A quarter of an inch difference is a lot, on the end of your nose or around your wrist.

Arm measurements: Measure your arms half way between armpit and elbow. Be sure your muscles are relaxed.

Chest-bust: Measure across nipples.

Midriff: Measure at the widest point of the chest.

Waist: Measure at the belt line.

Abdomen: Measure just below the navel at the most protuberant point. Be sure to keep the tape measure on a straight line. Check the mirror.

Hips 1: Measure a few inches below the abdominal measurement where the hips are widest when viewed from the front. Be sure not to include the abdominal bulge. Keep the tape horizontal.

Hips 2: Measure the fullest part of the hips a few inches lower than Hips 1.

Right thigh: Measure the top of the thigh at its fullest point a little below the groin.

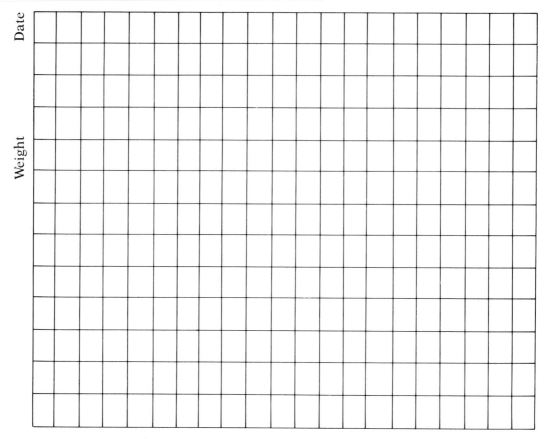

Figure 6. *Weight Chart*

Right knee: Measure just above the knee. If your legs have really lost shape, add another knee measurement just below the knee. When the legs have been cleared of restricting spasm by Myotherapy any swelling should be reduced.

Right calf: Measure the calf at its fullest with the muscle fully relaxed.

Right ankle: Measure just above the ankle bone. Check for reduction after Myotherapy to the legs and use "Im-

mediate Mobilization" on page 166. Do the same with the left leg. Write your measurements in black and compare the results with the day (or week) before, writing losses in red and gains (I hope not, but it always happens) in black. That way you will see at a glance where your program is having its best effect and where it is lagging.

YOUR DIET

List *everything* you eat, including the

Date						
R. arm						
L. arm						
Chest-bust						
Midriff						
Waist						
Abdominals						
Hips 1						
Hips 2						
R. thigh						
R. knee						
R. calf						
R. ankle						
L. thigh						
L. knee						
L. calf						
L. ankle						

Figure 7. *Measurements*

snack you sneak at your desk, the peanut (each one) you have with your cocktail, *and* the cocktail (in ounces!). When you list something like eggs, steak, chicken, or fish, write down the manner of its preparation. Poached, broiled, or boiled are fatless. Fried is another matter. Later, when your weight is stubborn and you are looking for something to give up, it might help to switch from one way of cooking to another. Fat is what most of us do *not* need. There is a difference between veal cutlets lightly sautéed and Veal Oscar with a thick cream sauce. There is even a difference between Shredded Wheat and my favorite cereal, Raisin Bran. The former is totally free of both sugar and salt and the latter is 28 percent sugar and Lord only knows how much salt!

When I contacted Dr. Jean Mayer, the famous Harvard nutritionist, about one of the more famous breakfast foods he said, "Well, it doesn't keep my rats

	Sun.	Mon.	Tues.	Wed.	Thurs.	Fri.	Sat.
Breakfast							
Break							
Lunch							
Cocktails							
Dinner							
Evening							
Snacks							

Figure 8. *The Eat Sheet*

alive." You shouldn't think of staying alive on our typical breakfast cereals. Their very preparation robs them of nutrients. My father-in-law always loved bran which he ate for its fiber and one other reason: "I like it." Learn to like things that, though they may not add to your health, at least take nothing away. Most cereals (according to what we see on TV) are carriers for milk and fruit. Like my father-in-law (and maybe because of him) I use breakfast cereal for fiber and get my nutrition from a well-balanced diet the rest of the day.

Get a food scale if you are going to do it right. A "helping" of beef stew could fill the top of a double boiler. How *much* of a helping are you helping yourself to? Too much "good" food isn't too much better than the same with junk food. Weigh your helpings.

Learn what *not* to eat. Homogenized milk has trapped fat. Sodas contain phosphates that contribute to osteoporosis. Commercial baked goods are mostly empty calories and boxed stuff is loaded with additives to prolong shelf life. If the bugs (who are usually smart about food, with the exception of sugar) won't eat it, why would you? That's the fun part about nutrition. Get good books and learn about what you are eating and what you are not eating and why. The enormous food companies have much in common with the enormous pharmaceutical houses . . . they are in business, and you are the consumer, not their responsibility. Who is responsible for you, then? *You* are— now and tomorrow.

YOUR HEART ACTION

Lie down comfortably for ten minutes. Don't get up for anything, just lie there. Then take your pulse. The easiest way is to lay the tips of your fingers on your larynx or voice box. Then, if you are using your right hand, lift your fingers off the larynx and slide them about an inch to the right into the soft tissues of

Date	Rest	Standing	Action	After 1 min.	After 5 min.

Figure 9. *Heart Action Test*

your neck, to rest on the pulsing artery. There is also a pulse in your thumb which might confuse things, so don't use it; use your fingers.

Count your heartbeat for a full minute. Enter your resting pulse under *Rest*.

Stand up and take your pulse again, but this time for only fifteen seconds. Multiply that beat by four and enter it under *Standing*.

Next you want to know how your heart behaves when put under a little pressure. In the course of one minute you should be able to step up onto a stair with one foot, bring the other up next to it, step back down with the first foot and bring the second back down, about thirty times. If you are in very poor shape or just recovering from an illness or accident, be satisfied with fifteen times in half a minute. To get the right cadence, count yourself through it. On the count of *one*, step up. On the word "*and*," bring the other foot up. On the count of *two*, step back down with the first foot, and on the word "*and*," step down with the second foot. When you have finished, take your pulse immediately for one full minute and enter the results under *Action*. The minute required to take your pulse will have provided one minute of rest, so as soon as you have entered the rate under *Action*, take your pulse again, this time for fifteen seconds and multiplied by four. Enter the result under *After one minute*. Sit down for five minutes and take your pulse once more, using the fifteen-second multiplied-by-four count.

OXYGEN DEBT

When you are very active, you burn oxygen at a much faster rate than can be replaced in the body right then and there. No matter how fast you breathe while the action is going on, you can't replace all the oxygen you are using because your body can't absorb it fast enough. You go into what is called oxygen debt. Since you have already used up all the oxygen you had free in your body, you borrow from your own tissues with the tacit understanding that you will "pay it back" with a lot of fast panting when the action has been terminated. It's like setting out on a trip and suddenly running out of money. You wire home to your brother, who lends you what you need until a time when you can find work, earn the money, and pay it back.

Naturally, if you are in good shape, you will be able to pay your debt quickly and efficiently. The debt itself won't be so great because, since your circulation, lungs, and heart are good, you would have more free oxygen available at the start. As the months pass and you stick to your exercise program, you will be improving your heart action, lung capacity, and circulation. You will soon find that your heart returns to normal faster than it did at the start. In time, your starting pulse will be slower. You will have improved your heart action along with your general level of fitness.

YOUR VITAL CAPACITY

In addition to improving heart action, your lung capacity will also pick up. The better your lungs behave, the better you will feel. More oxygen is available for your body and therefore you can accomplish more with far less fatigue. Like everything else lungs improve or deteriorate according to use. Riding in the car, even with the windows open, doesn't do much for your lungs. Climbing five flights of stairs, even with the windows closed, will. If you've had unpleasant surprises lately when you had to dash to catch a bus or take the stairs two at a time, it is not due to age. It is due to disuse.

Put a tape measure around your chest at its widest point and exhale every last ounce of air. Measure your chest. Then inhale fully and measure again. Note the difference in the tape. Some children in our testing had as little as one-half inch expansion. Singers and mountaineers may go as high as five or six inches. What's yours?

THE KRAUS-WEBER TEST FOR MINIMUM MUSCULAR FITNESS

This is the test you've heard so much about—the one so many of our children fail. It tests your key posture muscles: the back, abdominals, and hip flexors known as the psoas. The test will tell you if these muscles are weak or inflexible.

Date							
A +							
A −							
P							
UB							
LB							
BHF							
Substitution							
Leading elbow							
Arch							

Figure 10. *Kraus–Weber Test (K–W)*

HOW TO TAKE THE TEST

A+ (Abdominals plus psoas)

- Lie supine with feet held down and hands clasped behind head. Roll *slowly* up to a full sitting position.
- If you can do that, even with struggle, you pass. Give yourself a check next to A+ in the box above. If there was a struggle add a small c which stands for "with difficulty." (Whenever you have a small c after a test you must realize that an injury or an illness will move you into danger of failure, and you will need to do the correctives as part of your regular program.) If you can't sit up, you fail. Give yourself a zero and check with the correctives immediately (see page 87).
- If you found it necessary to sit up with a jerky motion or with a straight rather than rounded back, you pass, but you are substituting. That means the back muscles are weak and other muscles, not designed for the job, are taking over. Enter a check in the smaller box

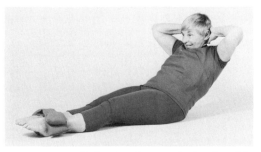

next to *Substitution* and check with the correctives.
- If, when doing either the sit-up or roll-down, you found one or the other of your elbows leading, there is uneven muscle function in your torso. Enter R or L in the box next to *Leading elbow*. Then, when you have hunted for the trigger points (you'll learn about those in the chapter on Myotherapy) which might be contributing to weakness on one side or the other, do the suggested roll-downs described in the correctives, but with the opposite elbow leading.

A- (Abdominals minus psoas)

- Lie supine but with knees bent, feet held down, and hands clasped behind head. Roll up slowly to the full sitting position.
- Mark a check for pass, add a c for "with difficulty," and a zero if you failed. The same substitution or leading elbow may occur. Be sure to note them in the smaller box and check with the correctives. One thing more: if either test causes muscle pain *anywhere*, check with

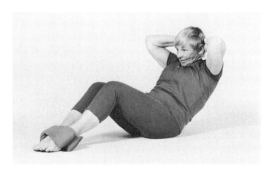

the pain list at the end of the section on Myotherapy.

P (Psoas)

- Lie supine with hands behind head and raise both legs to a point about eight inches above the supporting surface. Hold for a slow count of ten.
- If, as you lie there (especially as you lift your legs), a very high arch appears in the small of your back, enter a check in the box next to *Arch*. It indicates a tendency to swayback. You will need to do the

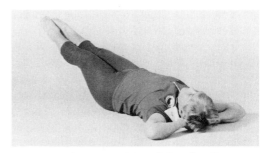

exercises suggested in the Posture section (page 90).

UB (Upper back)

- Lie prone over pillow with feet held down and hands clasped behind your head. Raise the upper body high enough so that your chest can clear the floor or table.
- Your build will affect the amount of weight needed to hold the upper body in the air: the longer the torso, the more weight.
- Hold the lift for a slow count of ten.
- Enter a check next to UB in the large box; add c if it was difficult (not the number while you were counting to ten and your chest touched down). Myotherapy to

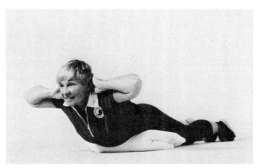

your back will improve your score and ability to hold your position; even a second or two longer is progress. Check the correctives (page 87).

LB (Lower back)

- Lie prone over pillow, upper back held down. Raise both legs and hold for ten.
- Score as in UB and check with correctives. If either test causes any real pain (as opposed to the stiffness accompanying disuse) see the Pain List in the Myotherapy chapter (page 153).

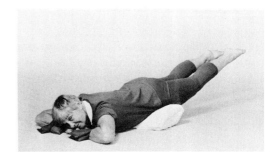

BHF (Back and hamstring flexibility)

- Stand with feet together and knees held straight. Bend forward from the hips and try to touch the floor with your finger tips. Hold for three seconds.
- If the floor is touched and held for three seconds, enter T for touch next to BHF in the larger box. If your fingers cannot touch, enter the number of inches between floor and fingers as minus inches. If you pass, but do so with difficulty (one day of "bed rest," an injury, or a stint of sitting will cause failure; don't be satisfied with a mere

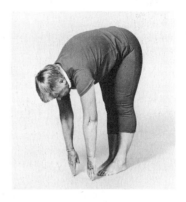

touch). If you fail anything, see correctives (page 89). Next, see Prudden Supplement test.

THE PRUDDEN SUPPLEMENT TEST FOR OPTIMUM PERFORMANCE

We in the after fifty crowd must always remember that human beings use about 10 percent of their potential brain power and probably less than 5 percent of their physical potential *at any age.* That means that only our Olympic athletes step out of the dustbin and reach for the stars physically as do our Einsteins and Oppenheimers mentally. In America today the physical graph compared to that of Europeans is particularly disheartening since we don't really "peak" anywhere along the line. We are in need of rehabilitation when we start school and we go down from there. The after fifty crowd, however, has the basics and we can go up from here no matter where "here" is. This book has been the reclaiming of me. I had allowed so much deterioration (claiming I was too busy, etc.) that I knew the climb back up was going to take all my willpower. But I made it

and you will too. What you *had* to do you always managed to do. I *had* to be in shape to show some of you it could be done.

The Prudden Supplement test was designed for those who passed the minimum fitness test and for you as soon as you do pass. Use it and know that there is no way to flunk. You compete only against yourself and there aren't even any norms. If you can't do a single push-up or pull-up . . . if your broad jump is two feet . . . that's where you are today. One sit-up and a mere floor touch gets you into the game. When I began, one push-up was a groaner. I tell you that because it's so easy to dismiss someone who has a reputation for being able to out-do most people. "Oh you! Of course you can do those things, you've done them all your life. . . ." That gives a lot of folks the excuse not to try. As a rock climber, I can tell you that when you are lost on a terrible face and you can't find a way to either go on or turn back, the sight of a piton, gleaming in a crack above you is like the hand of God at your back. It means that another human, just like you, has been this way and could get through. It says that there is a way and that you are on the right track. It says that someone

had what it took and challenges you to do no less. So let us meet on the summit one day and as we coil our ropes we will tell each other how hard and wonderful it was and how pleased we are that the mountain allowed us to stand on its rugged shoulder and look down at the way we have come.

Date	Push-up	Sit-up	Chin-up	Broad jump	Flex.

Figure 11. *P–S for Optimum Performance*

TEST 1: PUSH-UPS
Lie prone on the floor, legs together, toes curled under, and hands flat on the floor just outside your shoulders. Keeping your body stiff as a board, push up into a full arm extension. (If you can, great.)

Count it as one; lower *slowly* to the floor. So you will always start from scratch, touch your hands in back. Now try for two. Do as many full push-ups as you can without sagging.

Enter your score and promise to do half that number every day as "homework."

CORRECTIVE FOR PUSH-UPS
You can't do a single push-up? Fine; you can only get better. Here's a wonderful

bit of information. If you do a let-down, slowly, starting at the top of the push-up position, you will improve four times as fast as you would doing push-ups. That is because the muscle is working against the resistance of gravity while lengthening rather than contracting as it does when you push up. Try to take five seconds to go down and do five a day. They need not be done all at one time.

TEST 2: SIT-UPS
You already know you can do at least a sit-up. Do that. The next step can be done one of two ways. The more exact way is to use the set of weight bags suggested on page 322. Do the second sit-up holding one pound behind your neck

and then roll slowly down. On the third sit-up hold two pounds, on the fourth three, until you can no longer sit up. Enter your poundage. To improve, do 5 a day carrying half your best poundage.

The other way is to use repetitions. Never exceed ten if you want to avoid injuring your coccyx, which can lead to nasty complications involving the pelvic floor. If you can sit up ten times easily, then check your library. Choose a book that weighs close to a pound and do the same number. If you survive, next day repeat the test with a bigger book until you find one heavy enough to stop you. Then do five daily with the next lightest.

TEST 3: CHIN-UPS
You are going to need a chinning bar, so see the section on Self Center (page 321) and put one in your bedroom door. Hang at full length (which for most of us means bending our knees so our feet clear the floor).

With palms facing your face (curl) try to pull up until your chin clears the bar. Then let yourself *slowly* down taking ten seconds to touch down.

Next, grasp the bar with your palms facing away (reverse curl) and again bring your chin to the bar and let down slowly. Do half of the best score every day with palms facing each way.

"Ha! I can't even hold onto the bar, my arthritis hurts so bad I can't lift a pot off the stove, I haven't been able to comb my hair for a month, and you want a chin-up!!!?" No, I don't. I want you to use Myotherapy until you are as painless as I now am for the first time since 1965. Then I want you to test yourself and enter a zero if that's what you can do. Then get with the Weight section and go to work. Put a box next to the door and step up so your chin is above the bar and let yourself slowly down every time you go through the door. At first you'll descend in two seconds flat. In a week you'll hold for three. You can only get better from then on. If anything hurts . . . fix it. You'll know how.

TEST 4: BROAD JUMP
Put a piece of tape on the floor and stand behind it with toes on the tape and feet together. Jump both feet forward as far as you can. If you manage six inches that's a start. Enter it on your chart. It's better than no inches. Then mark half of your jump with a second piece of tape and never go that way without jumping that small space. Three inches isn't going to be anything but easy, but it will set up a habit and you will be constantly testing and improving. Leave the original score on the floor so you can be pleased with yourself (or have a guilty conscience).

TEST 5: FLEXIBILITY PLUS
You have already tested your flexibility and found you could touch the floor with your finger tips. Now you want more. Stand on a box or stair and see how much farther your finger tips can reach past the stand surface. List your score as "plus inches." As your flexibility improves with the flexibility exercises and Myotherapy you will go farther and farther down.

Test once a month.

CORRECTIVES

#1 Abdominals

Sit on the floor with knees slightly bent and feet held down. Drop your head down, round your back, and stretch your arms out in front. Holding that rounded position, roll slowly down, trying to touch each "button" of your spine to the floor as you go.

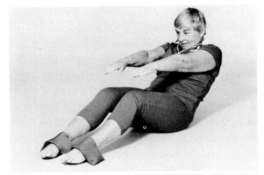

Sit up any old way you can, and repeat. Do five *slow* roll-downs several times a day and as soon as you feel comfortable with it, cross your arms in front of your chest and do them that way. After a short time with the harder version, try to sit up with arms outstretched. When you can do that do the roll-downs and sit-ups with arms across your chest several times each day. Fairly soon there will be a difference in your measurements at the abdominal level.

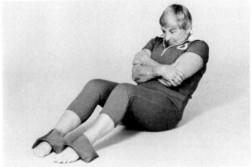

When you can roll down and sit up with your arms crossed in front, start rolling down with your hands behind your neck and sitting up with arms across chest. Soon enough you will be able to pass the test by sitting up with your hands behind your neck. At that point start doing the roll-downs with a light weight in your hands—a book, a one-pound weight bag, or a can of soup. As you improve, increase the weight.

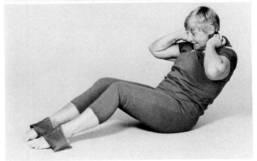

#2 Psoas

The psoas is very important to back and leg function. It attaches to the spine near the waist and also to the top of the thigh bone. When people used to do sit-ups with straight legs, this muscle was forced to pull on the spine which led to a lot of back pain, especially in soldiers after basic training and boy athletes. Girl athletes didn't get much rough training; most female back pain came from doing nothing.

Follow these directions exactly, step by step:

Lie supine with knees bent above the torso. Be sure your spine is tight to the floor. Extend both legs overhead so that the torso and legs form a right angle. Return the legs to the bent-knee-rest position. From the "rest" position, extend the legs again, but a little closer to the floor, *while being sure the spine is still down (no arch).* Retract to the "rest" position.

Extend and retract, each time a little lower, until you find you can't keep your spine tight to the floor. At that point you have gone too far. Extend the legs at the last level when you were sure your back was down, and do two to five, depending on your strength.

Do five extensions daily, always trying to get them a little nearer the floor *while still keeping your back flat on the floor.* In time you will be able to do this with weights.

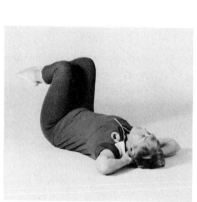 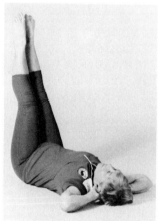 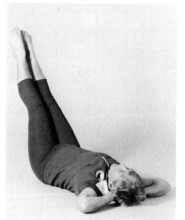

#3 Upper Back

Lie prone (face down) and raise first the left arm and then the right. Alternate sides, being careful to keep your chest on the floor.

• Do not roll from side to side for greater lift. You want to strengthen the upper back and stretch the pectorals. More lift will come after you have done Myotherapy to your chest and groin. Later, do the same exercise using weight bags.

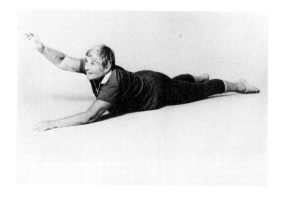

#4 Lower Back

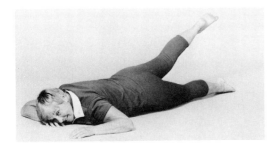

Lie prone and lift first one straight leg and then the other, from the hip. Alternate legs for a count of eight. Start with one set and add as you improve.

#5 Flexibility of Back and Hamstrings

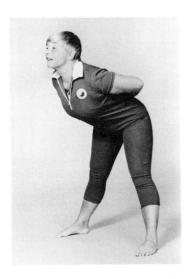

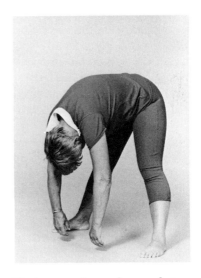

Stand with feet apart and hands clasped behind back. Lean forward from the hips while keeping the back level and the head up. Bounce gently and rhythmically downward eight times. Then drop the arms and upper body downward and bounce again for eight counts.

This makes up a set. Do three sets when you do your daily work on correctives, but also try to remember to do these gentle bounces often during the day, especially if your work entails sit-

ting. Sitting, and any form of stress (including concentration), causes muscles to shorten. Keeping muscles limber and well oiled is like building a breakwater so the seas of time can't carry off the harbor and all the boats in it.

If you failed any *one* of the minimum tests, you have less than the minimum strength and flexibility required for daily living, *it doesn't matter which of the tests you failed.* If you fail any part of the test you are in line for future backache, and if you already have back pain from time to time, the failed test tells you where the trouble lies. You owe your nice body protection and the best protection you can afford it, no matter what your age or condition, is what you've learned on these last few pages.

IMPROVE YOUR POSTURE

Your posture is a dead giveaway; it tells all there is to know about you. You have several kinds of posture:

1. There's lying posture. You probably didn't know you had one, but how you lie when you are supposed to be relaxed tells an educated eye that you probably aren't really relaxed and which of your muscles are tense.

2. Sitting would come next, and that one tells a lot about your state of mind. If you are bored you sit one way; annoyed, angry, frustrated, interested, excited, or terrified, other ways. If you are fresh and rested you have a totally different sitting posture from the one your exhausted body falls into. You have different sitting postures for different activities, different chairs, and different situations. Imagine how versatile your body must be!

3. Standing is something else again. Impatience, interest, fun, exhaustion, and anger are all obvious from the way you stand.

4. The most revealing posture of all is the way you move. That starts to form right after birth and probably a long time before. One of my children floats on cloud eleven one minute and is digging tunnels to China the next. She was doing that before she was born. Beethoven's Ninth Symphony sent her into a dervish and sent my program flying across the aisle at the Philharmonic. My other child kept odd hours, moved to an endless canter, and giggled a lot which tickled. She is still a night person, only gets off her horse to eat and sleep . . . and giggles a lot. She tickles still. My mother told me I spent most of my time in her womb kicking. I am kicking still. I don't think we really change from the time we begin, and posture is the signature at the bottom of the page. Think about your children and what they were like as babies—what their postures were, how they sat when entranced or bored, how they stood as they waited or watched, how they ran when approaching with joy or fleeing in fear—all will tell you what they are doing now in much subtler ways.

Posture is affected by injury, and there is no such thing as a once-was injury. Every injury leaves a scar and every scar collects something you will learn about shortly: a trigger point. Trigger points boss muscles around and make them shorten. Shortened muscles are like tightened rigging on a sailboat: pull hard enough on one side of the mast without equal pull to the other and eventually you will get a bent mast. Every woman who has ever had a baby has muscles that can eventually pull her into the posture affected by Hansel's witch. Ask any little kid in first grade to be that witch in a play and she will lean forward from the groin (where babies come from), put one hand on an imaginary cane and the other on the back pain that has come from groin pull. That's an accurate picture of a witch who has had baby witches!

Injuries cause bodies to substitute, to use muscles never designed for the job. That leads to imbalance and overwork. Sports cause injuries that are not recognized at the time, and much later, when the shortened "rope" pulls, the *mast* (or knee) will be treated—the rope ignored. That guarantees failure of whatever treatment is offered. Typical is the football player whose quadriceps or thigh muscles have been damaged. When he (and fifty others just like him) runs in place, bringing knees as high as possible, he runs with his knees apart as though he had been badly fitted for a tin jock. Later, his knees will "go bad." When he walks on the beach it's as though something very uncomfortable has been inserted; he leaves footprints three inches apart. Walking on two parted rails gives him a ponderous waddle which is damaging to his self-image. For no legitimate reason it makes him look "stoopid."

Sometimes a baby will lie in a crib and look at you with head tilted just a little to one side. He looks as interested as the dickens. Later, he'll look at a girl the same way and she'll think the same thing. Eventually the tilt will turn into wry neck or torticollis and hurt like hell. It was damage, not interest, all the time. After I had my first hip replaced and limped for a long time, but was totally free of pain, I discovered a signal. I was surrounded by people I really didn't like, but one in particular caused me enormous stress. Suddenly I would find myself limping. It became my body's advice to my mind to get out now, before you say something you'll regret. When I finally handled the situation I never limped again.

KNOWING YOURSELF

To people who have never had to read one, a road map can be incomprehensible. Anyone who has never had to navigate a ship or a plane would have difficulty with charts of both sea and heavens. There is no need for most of us to know the latter two and nothing vitally pressing about a road map either. But we all need to know about our bodies. All through this book you will find maps of yourself. On the maps are certain markers. They indicate trouble spots just as maps of our shores point out reefs, sandbars, and currents. You *need* to know where to find the hidden reef causing your backache. You *must* understand that your round back isn't due to heredity, but to a hidden "cable" in your chest.

In order to obtain this understanding and information, look at the maps as though they were pictures of *you*, because they are. Your posture improvement depends on understanding why you do certain exercises because if you don't, you probably won't do them. You must learn how to look for improvement because if you don't see it and understand why it has happened, you won't continue.

The following table of posture problems gives the names of the problems as we all know them. In this book there are some tests you can take to chart progress. They are listed right after the problem. Then comes the map so you can locate the problem as well as the suggested myotherapy which will change it. You need to do the Myotherapy only about once or twice a week, but the Myotherapy exercises should be done every day. The exercises that will help, other than the specific ones that go with the Myotherapy, are next in line. Finally, there are Extra Exercises. They are not musts, but if they were compared to our dinner habits, they would be paté, caviar, a really good vanilla ice cream, or a liqueur. They are fun and bring variety.

Go over the following conditions carefully, enlisting the observations of others where necessary, and then check with the chart on posture corrections at the end of the chapter.

Nobody has *all* these problems, but you need to know which ones you do have so you can begin now to improve, take away unnecessary stress, move better, be less tired and more able to pursue the things you want from life . . . perhaps for the first time.

Check out your family for their posture problems, too!

Date								
Abdominal Protrusion								
Back, Flat								
Back, Round								
Back, Scoliosis								
Back, Sway								
Chest Flexibility								
Cringe								
Flat Feet								
Forward Head								
Groin Pull								
Head Tilt/Turn								
Heel Flexibility								
Limp								
Mince								
Pigeon Toes								
Shoulder Flexibility								
Spread Legs								
Toe Out								
Toe Walk								
Uneven "Buttons"								
Uneven Shoulders								

Figure 12. *Posture Checklist*

Abdominal Protrusion

If your abdomen sticks out there is probably too much in it (besides what ought to be there), namely, fat. Do the recommended exercises and watch your Eat Sheet.

Back, Flat

Fewer people know when they have flat back, but it is a cause of back pain all the same and clothes don't look their best when hung on one. The lumbar curve is less than normal or the opposite of swayback. Enter yours on your chart and do the prescribed exercises.

Back, Round (Kyphosis)

Round back often starts in children when they suffer from anxiety. They try to behave like turtles, pulling their heads in and shoulders up to ward off danger. In adults, the same posture can come with a job over a desk. If osteoporosis has not been warded off, it can round backs, and a "dowager's hump" appears. Look at all the older people you know and see how many cause you to stand up straighter because they stand so badly. Prevent it. Check improvement with the measurements entered on the Posture Checklist for chest flexibility, and the Posture Correction List.

Back, Scoliosis (Curvature)

It's bad enough to have one that is causing your backache, but lately I have seen any number of women who either don't have a curvature or who have one so slight as to be negligible, who have been told that they have se-vere scoliosis and what they need is a course of "adjustments" or they'll turn into hunchbacks. Scare tactics cost the customer a lot. Don't tell me, "But the insurance covers it." Does it cover your time? Of course, if you've nothing else to do I suppose it's as good as going for a manicure, with one difference. "Adjustments" in the wrong hands, like surgery in the wrong hands, *cause* trouble. Scoliosis begins to show at around the age of eleven, but Myotherapy applied early seems to reverse the trend. For most of you, the back "sets" at about the age seventeen. While there is little we can do to change the conformation of the back at this late stage, we can stop the aches and pains. Have your back checked by standing with feet apart. Lean slowly downward letting your head and arms hang loose. Your friend stands behind you and watches the horizontal line of your back as you descend. If one part rises, you have scoliosis. If it remains flat, you don't and your backache, if you have one, is coming from somewhere else.

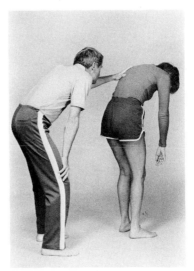

Figure 13.

Back Sway (Lordosis)

Swayback, or lordosis, is an abnormal curve of the lumbar or lower spine which often accompanies ballet lessons, as unformed bodies try to conform to the turn-out or fifth position of the feet. It also goes with the thumb-in-mouth-pigeon-toed-head-down-Daddy's-Little-Girl stance, which looks absolutely ghastly on a thirty-year-old woman. But some women don't even know they have it. Swayback can give you back pain, but it also involves the upper back, neck, jaw, and groin, and can cause turned out feet as the body tries to substitute. Most people know if they have it. If you do, check yourself into the chart and start with the suggested program.

Chest Flexibility

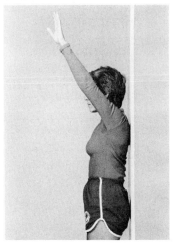

Figure 14.

Stand in a doorway with your heels up against the frame. Press your seat and shoulders back to touch the frame as well. Lift your arm and try to bring the back of one wrist to touch the frame, and then the other.

• Measure the distance from your right and then left wrist to the frame and enter the score in the box as T (for touch) or in minus inches. Check for Myotherapy and the exercises that will stretch those muscles.

Cringe

Everyone knows what a cringing posture is and almost no one would connect it with themselves, mostly because it is intermittent. It comes on with loud noise, quarreling voices, doors slamming, and the sound of automobiles running into one another. Obviously it is a protective measure and doesn't become part of a posture *unless* there have been many occasions to cringe. Ask yourself: were there? Is my grandson's cringing posture due to something other than asthma? No matter the cause, if you cringe too often, muscles foreshorten. Stretch them.

Flat Feet

Flat feet can't be given arches but they can be given strength and freed from pain.

Forward Head

This condition is a continuation, or result, of round back. Ask your friend to check your neck and head when you're walking. See the correctives.

Groin Pull

Groin pulls come with living. Sports cause injury to the back, abdominal, groin, and leg muscles; sedentary jobs injure groins and they can be damaged through childbirth. Groin pulls cause all kinds of problems from aches, jaw pain, mock angina, down to simple bellyache. Ask someone to watch you walk and if you lean forward, you should do the recommended Myotherapy and exercise for this condition.

Head Tilt/Turn

This is invariably caused by muscle spasm and the sooner addressed the better the chances of recovery. Sometimes someone who has a hearing difficulty will develop the habit of tilting or turning. Eye problems will do it too, but the usual is a past injury such as whiplash. Myotherapy should take care of it.

Heel Flexibility

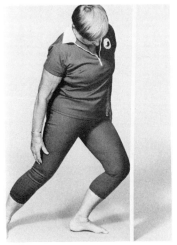

Figure 15.

Tight heel cords are often the problem of little children who walk on tiptoe whenever their shoes are off. Women can cause shortened heel cords by wearing high heeled shoes all the time. Athletes can cause them by running on cement or overworking the legs.

To measure your improvement, stand facing a wall and place the toes of the right foot about three inches from the wall. Bend the right knee and try to touch the wall with your heel stuck tight to the floor. If you can't, then move the toes nearer the wall. If it's easy, move the toes further out. When you reach the point where your knee can just touch, note it on your chart. Measure from toe to wall and then do the other foot. Myotherapy and the exercises will be found at the end of the chapter and, yes, you probably need both. The causes of foot pain and night cramps are usually found in the limiting calf muscles.

Limp

If you are limping because you hurt, go after the pain. If you are limping because your leg is short, go after the trigger points that are causing weakness. If you are limping (as I was) from habit and stress, do the recommended exercises and start all floor progressions backwards.

Mince

A mince is a shortened gait that signifies tight groin and leg muscles and the potential for both leg spasms and back pain. There are many causes for tight hamstrings in the backs of legs; sitting is one of them. Sitting, coupled with old sports injuries, can provide a most unmasculine mince. It's no more attractive in a woman. Today's woman does not want to signal dependence or frightened inferiority. A mincing gait gives that impression. Stretch those leg muscles and when you walk in the house, take longer steps than usual. If you catch yourself taking shortened steps. . . . stretch.

Pigeon Toes

You may have one turned-in foot, or two. The leg muscles pulling the feet in are in spasm and need release.

Shoulder Flexibility

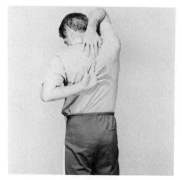

Figure 16.

Testing for this condition requires the help of a friend if you want to be exact. But even alone, knowing if you do or don't have flexibility is easy. Push your right hand down your back as far as possible, and with your left hand try to touch the fingers of both hands together. If you touch, that's good. If there is space, you miss by that much. Then shove the left hand down and the right up. The exercises and the appropriate Myotherapy are listed at the end of the chapter.

Spread Legs

If you walk with a waddle (surely someone has told you) it's because of muscle spasms in the muscles from waist to ankle on the outsides of your legs. Those muscles also help make sciatica worse. Because it helps to copy, think Clark Gable and Ava Gardner. They had the kind of walks you want and can have. Meanwhile, do Myotherapy and exercises.

Toe Out

This often accompanies scoliosis, but can also come along on its own. It usu-

Figure 17. POSTURE PROBLEMS . . . CORRECTIONS

Condition	Test	Map Figure #	Myotherapy
ABDOMINAL PROTRUSION	None	None	None
BACK, FLAT	Same as SWAY BACK		

ally signals spasms in the muscles on the outsides of the legs and poor leg musculature because the legs didn't ever "track" properly. That meant muscles that were in spasm could not be properly trained in childhood. Get rid of the spasm. You will be surprised at your increased stamina and pleasure in walking.

Toe Walk

If you walked on your toes as a small child, and you were a girl, you were considered "dainty" and not handicapped, which you were and are. If you were a boy and you managed to make a team, you had awful "growing pains" as your spasmed calf muscles and even those in the backs of your upper legs fought valiantly to make you a member of the team while fighting themselves and each other. One of our Olympic skiers had absolutely no forward lean (*vorlager*) at all. If he had, his skill and courage might have won him a gold.

His coach never noticed his problem, nor did I know the answer when I saw it in 1956. But it is here now, so you use it.

Uneven "Buttons"

This condition won't show up in a medical book, but it means a torso that leans to one side when the person is sitting. Dr. Janet Travell discovered it in me when my back and hip were in extreme spasm. The long line of small brass buttons from the neck to waist on the front of my dress curved out to the right. When I sat up straight one of my two "sitting bones" left the chair. When I sat back on both, my buttons curved. If you don't make contact with the chair when you sit up straight, you will need to do a Myotherapy search. In the meantime, slide a copy of the Reader's Digest (or reasonable facsimile) under the side that floats free and you'll be a lot less tired.

Myotherapy Exercise	Exercise #	Extra Exercise #
None	1, 2, 27, 32, 33, 39, 44, 47, 50, 52	Chair exercises 133 through 136
7, 8, 10	3, 4, 27, 33, 46, 83	Limbering series 109 rope 185

Condition	Test	Map Figure #	Myotherapy
BACK, ROUND	14	21, 40, 45	24, 32, 41, 46
BACK, SCOLIOSIS	13	21	22, 23, 42
BACK, SWAY	None	21, 25	22, 23, 26, 27, 28
CHEST FLEXIBILITY		(See ROUND BACK)	
CRINGE		(See ROUND BACK)	
FLAT FEET	None	51	Do Myotherapy to the entire leg and especially to the outside of the lower leg (anterior tibialis) along the lower leg bone
FORWARD HEAD	None	21, 40, 45	24, 32, 41, 46
GROIN PULL		(See GROIN PAIN on PAIN CHART)	

Myotherapy Exercise	Exercise #	Extra Exercise #
9, 13, 14, 15	35, 83	Chair 132 Weights 165 Rope 183 Pulley 191
7, 8, 12	All bilateral exercises	
7, 8, 10	1, 2, 27, 37, 39	Bed 100
(see ROUND BACK)		
See ROUND BACK	See SPREAD LEGS and also PAIN CHART for LOW BACK PAIN and GROIN PAIN	
20	All floor progressions All foot exercises	Walking Race Walk
9, 13, 14, 15	35, 83	Towel 172, 174 Pulley 191
(See GROIN PAIN on PAIN CHART)		

Condition	Test	Map Figure #	Myotherapy
HEAD TILT TURN	None	29, 36	31, 37, 38, 39
HEEL FLEXIBILITY	16	49	Do Myotherapy to the calf muscle according to the map
LIMP	None	51, 52, 21, 25	Do Myotherapy to *both* legs and calf. 22, 26, 27, 28, 50 18 and 19
MINCE	(See SPREAD LEGS and also PAIN CHART for LOW BACK PAIN and GROIN PAIN)		
PIGEON TOES	None	51, 21	Do Myotherapy to the entire leg according to the map and especially 22, 52, 53, 54, 55
SHOULDER FLEXIBILITY	14	31, 40, 44, 45	24, 32, 41, 44, 46
SPREAD LEGS	None	51, 52	Do Myotherapy to the entire leg on the outside from waist to ankle
TOE OUT	None	51, 52	Do Myotherapy to the entire leg on the outside from waist to ankle

Myotherapy Exercise	Exercise #	Extra Exercise #
11	32, 33, 35, 47	Chair exercise 125
18	25, 29, 57, 82, 83 All floor progressions	All foot exercises Stairs 175, 178, 179, 180
7, 10	All floor prgressions	119
	Walking	Walking
7	All floor progressions 65, 70, 71, 75	Chair exercise 124, 128 Bed exercise 98
13, 14, 15	21, 22, 23, 26, 35, 62	Chair exercise 132 Towel 172 and 174 Pulley 191
None	64, 70, 75	Stairs 178, 179, 180
None	64, 70, 75	Stairs 178, 179, 180

Condition	Test	Map Figure #	Myotherapy
TOE WALK	15	51	Do Myotherapy to the calf muscles according to map
UNEVEN "BUTTONS"	(see BACK PAIN on PAIN CHART)		

KNOW YOUR DYSFUNCTIONS

We all have parts of us that don't work as well as they once did, or that don't work as well as we would like. There is always the temptation to say, "Oh well, what can you expect at my age?" That's a cop-out. If you'd known what to do at the first sign of dysfunction—and done it—you wouldn't be faced with it now.

The following is a partial list of dysfunctions. There are many others that answer to Myotherapy, but these are the most prevalent. Not all dysfunction produces pain, but that potential is ever present should stress enter the picture. If your dysfunction is accompanied by pain, check with the Pain Chart on page xx for help in relieving that pain with Myotherapy and the exercises needed for retraining the muscles into healthier function.

BACK WEAKNESS WHEN LIFTING

The first thing to throw out is the word "arthritic." It goes without saying that the back will be a little stiff once you join the after fifty crowd, but the pain is almost always muscular. Check the Pain Chart and make the side-lying exercise a daily must.

TROUBLE GETTING OUT OF BED, THE CAR, OR A CHAIR

Do you have to use your hands and push? You are out of shape. You suffer from "jelling pain," and the name speaks for itself. The antidote is to raise your fitness level. As you get out of your car, bed, or chair check for the slightest pain and then look at the Pain Chart. Begin a program and keep it going even if you are stiff for a year. As a matter of fact, you'll be stiff all over again with each new thing you try. There's a happy side: you are very much alive and trying. You are also improving. One day, six months from now, when some old buddy huffs, puffs, whoofs, and groans getting out of a chair, you will realize it's been months since you did that. Be proud of yourself and then tell "Ol' Buddy" what to do.

Myotherapy Exercise	Exercise #	Extra Exercise #
18	29, 75, 82, 93	31
(See BACK PAIN on PAIN CHART)	(see BACK PAIN on PAIN CHART)	

CHEWING CRACKING NOISES, OR OCCASIONAL SUBLUXATION (TMJD)

TMJD means temporomandibular joint dysfunction, or jaw trouble. That problem usually has its roots in the groin, or seat, or both. Check the Pain Chart first and find the trigger points. Then check the Dysfunction Chart (page 104) for the exercises. One note: TMJD is stress connected. Reread the section on stress and understand what the warning pain means. It is a warning. Don't ignore it.

COMBING HAIR, SHAVING, OR RAISING ARMS (DIFFICULTY WITH)

You can't get that arm up where it belongs? That's not age; you have trigger points in your chest, upper back, shoulder, arm, neck, and probably in your hand. Look up shoulder on the Pain Chart and then use the Dysfunction Chart to design a daily program.

CURBSTONES—THEY WORRY YOU

There are usually two causes for this: weak legs and eyesight problems. Eyesight is often corrected with bifocals which cut vision at curbs and stairs into two sections, making you uncertain. If you can get along without eyeglasses when walking around, leave them off. If you need glasses get two pairs—one set for walking around and bi-focals. Check legs, low back, and groin in the Pain Chart, even if there is neither pain nor weakness (that you recognize—it's there). See the Dysfunction Chart for your exercises.

DOG WALKING

If it's a little dog, that's no big deal. If the dog is a big one you will need to understand that the dog is actually walking you. If the leash hurts, see hands in the Pain Chart. If you feel uncertain about balance, check legs. Do the cross-the-floor progressions. If a dog is important to your happiness—as mine are to me—you want to keep that asset safe. Your dog, like yourself, is yours as long as you can care for both of you. Incidentally, if your dog has "arthritis," use Myotherapy. It works.

DRIVING

The usual problem encountered by the after fifty crowd when driving is seeing what's behind. The inability to comfortably turn your head is not age, it's a stiff neck. See the Pain Chart for neck even if there's no pain. There is limitation, as you will see when you use the neck test. Get rid of the trigger points and do your neck exercises daily. There may be an old injury (or a present occupation) working against you. Combine your exercise with some activity you do often throughout the day. Also be aware of the stress in your life. Stiff necks are often a sign of intolerable stress.

GARDENER'S BACK

"Gardener's back" usually accompanies the coming of spring when the robins and balmy weather pull us out of our winter sloth and into unaccustomed activity. We rake and lift and carry, we dig and plant and weed. We do everything our hearts (or sometimes nagging spouses) tell us to do and then by eventide we can't get out of the chair. "Gardener's back" can apply to *any* unaccustomed work—putting the boat in the water, getting the trunks out of the cellar. The best way to avoid "gardener's back" or any other back problem is to stay in shape year round with at least a half hour of calisthenics daily. Walking will not do the whole job.

LIFTING WITH WEAK OR PAINFUL HANDS

Painful, weak, or stiff hands will usually be called "arthritic." Check the Pain Chart and get rid of the trigger points in the arms, armpits, chest, and upper

FIGURE 18. DYSFUNCTIONS—PROBLEMS AND CORRECTIONS

Condition	Test	Map Figure #	Myotherapy
BACK, WEAKNESS	K-W	21, 25	22, 23, 26, 27, 28
BED, CAR, or CHAIR: getting out of	K-W	21, 25	22, 23, 26, 27, 38, 31
CHEWING, CRACKING NOISES, (TMJD) or OCCASIONAL SUBLUXATION	None	21, 25, 30, 36	22, 26, 27, 28, 31, 34, 35, 38, 39, 41
COMBING HAIR, SHAVING, or RAISING ARMS	14, 16	29, 31, 44, 45	24, 31, 44, 46

back. Use the exercises daily and at intervals throughout the day.

KNEE BENDS
If you have injured the thigh and calf muscles your knees will hurt, snap-crackle-pop, feel weak, and occasionally lock. Check the Pain Chart and make knee bends a part of your life.

STANDING STRAIGHT
This is the bottom line of posture. Get after it now and stick with it! Discover the faults in your posture and retrain your muscles.

STAIRS—GOING UP AND DOWN
That's not age, that's trigger points in your legs. Check the Pain Chart first and then the stair exercises in the section on Extra Exercises (page 330).

TOENAILS—YOU CAN'T GET DOWN TO CUT THEM
There are several reasons for this and one is inflexibility. You will need the Pain Chart for low back, groin, and legs, even if there is no pain. Then you will have to consider the hips. That's less easy to fix if you have post-traumatic "arthritis" of one or both hips. If you begin early to keep the legs free of spasm, you may keep that condition under control, but you may eventually need a hip replacement. Try everything else first! But if you are for it, get my book *Pain Erasure* and do the preparation just as though it were an Olympic event and the money was all on you ... it is! See the Dysfunction Chart for the exercises, and do them every time you go to the bathroom. This "interval training" will serve as a regular reminder.

Myotherapy Exercise	Exercise #	Extra Exercise #
7, 8, 9, 10, 18	33, 34, 42, 43	Weight bags
7, 8, 9, 31	All floor progressions	
7, 8, 9, 10, 11, 13, 14, 15	None	None
15	14, 28, 30, 41, 45, 53	Pulley series 183, 187, 188, 190, 191, 192 Towel ex. 172, 174

Condition	Test	Map Figure #	Myotherapy
CURBSTONES	15	49, 51	Do Myotherapy to both legs—hip to heel. Add Gluts and Groin.
DOG WALKING	None	21, 25, 40, 49, 51	22, 23, 26, 27, 28, 41, 50
DRIVING	None	21, 25, 30, 36	22, 26, 27, 28, 31, 34, 35, 38, 39, 41
GARDENER'S BACK	K-W	21, 49	22, 23, 32, 50
LIFTING (WEAK HANDS)	None	21, 44, 45	13, 22, 23, 44, 46, 47
KNEE BENDS	52	49, 51	55
STANDING STRAIGHT	None	21, 25, 40, 49, 51	22, 23, 26, 27, 28, 31, 34, 35, 38, 39, 41
STAIRS	52	49, 51	55
TOENAILS	None	49, 51	Do Myotherapy to the entire leg, according to the map

Myotherapy Exercise	Exercise #	Extra Exercise #
All floor progressions 29, 49, 57, 58		Stairs 175
7, 8, 9, 10, 13, 14, 19, 20	Floor progressions 63–78	
6, 7, 8, 9, 10, 11, 13, 14, 15	14, 19, 22, 25, 28, 30, 41, 43, 53	Weights, Towel exercise, Pulleys, Elastics
7, 8, 9, 81	33, 34, 39, 42, 43 Limbering series	Weights
7, 8, 9, 16, 17, 19	81	Towel exercise 178 Stairs 175 Weights 160, 163
118, 120, 121, 123	24, 25, 27, 29, 52, 64, 65, 67	164, 182
7, 8, 9, 10, 13, 14, 19, 20	Floor progressions 63–78	
118, 120, 121, 123	24, 25, 27, 29, 52, 64, 65, 67	Stairs 175 All floor progressions
112 through 123	29, 49, 57, 58 All floor progressions	39, 81

STRESS, THE KICKER FOR CHRONIC PAIN

You are all of a piece. Your physical well-being depends on your mental and emotional well-being, and they in their turn depend on the physical. You have tested your physical self; now ask the emotional self some questions. Test yourself—for stress, for physical problems, for any of the physical discomforts which, you now know, can be fixed with Myotherapy. Start by taking this test.

I. Where do I live?
Is this my choice or someone else's?
Am I in agreement?
If I'm not in agreement, is it worth what it costs me?
If the choice were mine, where would I live?

II. What is my work at present?
Is this what I want to do?
What would I do instead if the choice were mine?
What activities would I like to add to my days?
What am I planning to do when I retire?

III. What do I look like?
Is this the way I want to look?
What would I change (within reason)?
What are my physical limitations, if any? Are they fixable? (Answer this one again after doing therapy procedures and the exercises for awhile!)

IV. Who are my immediate family?
Do I enjoy being with them?
Would I rather enjoy them from a distance?
If I don't like them, why am I here?
Where and with whom would I rather live?
Why don't I?

V. Who are my friends?
What do I share with them?
Do I take time to enjoy things?
What do I really enjoy?
When did I do that last?
What would I enjoy if things were different?
What do I get out of life?
What do I give to others?
As my life is right now, is it worth living?
How would I change *me* if I could?
Have I really tried to make things different?
Am I satisfied with things the way they are?
Given the ways things are going right now, what do I see five years from now? What do I see in ten? Longer?
If I could have a dream what would it be?

The questions in Part V are different from the ones in Parts I through IV; they take longer to think about and answer. Pick up your notebook; take some time.

MYOTHERAPY, A WAY TO ERASE PAIN

I n this chapter you will learn how to get rid of pain. If you have suffered a long time or if you have a problem that has been given a distressing name or have developed symptoms similar to those a relative suffered and possibly died from, you may be inclined to think we are not talking about *your* pain; yours is different. Well, over 90 percent of the time we *will* be talking about *your* pain—but with a new way to get rid of it.

Most names for pain are merely descriptive. I like to call them geographical because they state location rather than cause. A couple of good examples are "sacroiliac" and "sciatica." What does "sciatica' mean to you? It's a pain running down the leg. Legend has it that the sciatic nerve is being frayed as

it exits the spine. Maybe, once in a blue moon, that could be the case. Actually it's being squeezed (which is just as painful) as it passes through the gluteus muscle (located just under the back pocket of your blue jeans). The "sacroiliac" is that bony area of the pelvis made up of the sacrum in the center of the back and the two ilia on either side. The name doesn't tell you anything about your pain except where it is, which you already knew. The problem there is almost always a muscle in spasm and, again, it's the gluteus muscle—which in this case *is* where the pain is. "Tendinitis" means inflammation of the tendon or tendon-muscle attachments. Whenever you see *itis* know that it means inflammation. According to the dictionary *inflammation means localized heat, redness, swelling and pain as a result of irritation, injury, or infection.* Before we go any further we must examine that explanation as it applies to you. Inflammation need not mean infection, but it can mean injury, and the injury is frequently not new. Old injuries of *any* magnitude can cause pain at any time and later is more likely than earlier. You could have had a fall, or been injured in a sport, or sewn too many seams on an old fashion-treadle machine several decades ago. The same kind of strain can be sustained even 50 years after driving a car, bus, tractor, van, or plane.

"Cervical arthritis" sounds pretty impressive and is a mainstay of chiropractors; orthopedists like it too. If you are in the after fifty crowd and you have a stiff and painful neck, you will probably be X-rayed and, sure enough, there will be some "arthritis." However, it is rarely the cause of the pain or stiffness which is usually due to muscle spasm and its boss, something called a *trigger point.*.

Various diseases cause pain: *rheumatoid arthritis, lupus,* and *multiple sclerosis* are just three villains that can be counted on to do just that. However, no matter what rascal is at work, don't think *disease* . . . think *pain.* Don't say, "My *arthritis* is killing me today," or "Damn, my *bursitis* is bad!" Or "ouch,

the *tendinitis* in my wrist hurts." If you take that complaint to enough doctors one is sure to label it Carpal tunnel syndrome. That might put you in danger of an operation and you don't want that, certainly not if there's a simple, inexpensive way to take care of it. Remember, 30 percent of your medical costs come out of your own pocket, and the price is rising.

If you have back pain think, "My back hurts." Of course, if you've been in an accident and have *acute* pain and one doctor tells you your back is broken and the second doctor tells you your back is broken, it's probably broken. That's different. But when you've had back pain for a long period, do not think disc. There *are* problems requiring "heroic" (you are the hero!) measures, like almost *any* operation, but most pain signals muscle spasm. At the end of this chapter you will find a list of pain areas (page 172). Check your own against that list and use the suggested Myotherapy patterns and exercise designed for each area.

It is pain that ages people, not years. No matter who else says so, the years in front of you really are the best; or you can make them the best. The one thing that might stand in your way would be pain and its buddies, infirmity and dependency.

Here comes the way to beat all three.

PAIN AND CHANGE

Pain is the prime ager of mankind. It is also a thief. Pain steals looks, vitality, strength, joy, sensuality, love, youth, intelligence, and independence. Most of our armaments against pain are aimed at the symptoms and are merely palliative. Naturally, they fail, and on the

way they cause further damage which leads to more pain, more destruction, and more despair.

The after fifty crowd is about to be faced with yet another change—that of handling its own pain and getting rid of it. Not only that, we are going to be given the means of preventing pain in the first place.

Never in the history of the world has a single generation been forced to adapt to as much change as we have. I was born in the opening year of the first world war. It was called "the war to end all wars," but it certainly didn't. The guns of August did usher in new ways of killing, thinking, and acting. A popular song of the times aptly described what happened once the smoke cleared after that war:

How ya gonna keep 'em
   Down on the farm
   After they've seen Pareeeeee?

They couldn't, of course, and a tremendous unrest took over the country. The slow, comfortable pace of nature's cycle in an agricultural era disappeared. We took to wheels, the air, movie houses, speakeasys, cigarettes, and cities. Jazz, flappers, rolled stockings, hip flasks, and "Twenty-three skidoo" became what rock, pills, bikinis, sex, and "Right on, man" are for today's young people. We thought we were tremendously daring and so do they. We thought we had the world by the tail. The bomb has *them* by the throat.

After eleven years of wild gaity and madman economics the bubble burst and we entered the Great Depression. That changed many of us painfully, but we weathered it and faced World War II. We came out of that war, too, with the unwarranted feeling that we had won. And, like all wars, it changed us and our way of life.

There were more changes ahead for us. The movies left their houses and came into our homes and we sat down to watch, never noticing that it became harder and harder to get up. Korea and Vietnam took our children, and neither we nor they could understand why.

Dorothy Parker once said, "Candy is dandy but likker is quicker." Those last two wars encouraged our children to go us one better: they discovered drugs. We tore our hair when we saw what was happening to them, never realizing that we too were addicted. We didn't see that substances we called "medicines" had hooked *us* and that we were the role models for our children.

And now we have reached the Space Age, a momentous time for youth, but not the first pioneering time for many of us. We came from generations of adventurers who left everything behind and set out to discover what lay beyond the here and now. Today a few men and women will get the chance to soar into the firmament and, in time, will be followed by others. We might be inclined to think, "Too late for me." But wait, there is a new frontier beckoning and you won't have to be an astronaut to be a pioneer. There's something wildly new that has never been possible before and you, who have been the recipient of so much change, are just the ones to be pioneers—again.

When the Chinese marry they start a new life called "The Red Happiness." They must leave all old things behind and start afresh. Everything must be new—furniture, pots, clothing, underwear, even toothbrushes. Beginning that way does give a different perspective to life. It could happen to you if you read one page further.

If you were now as agile and painless and filled with energy as you were at fourteen, you too would be thinking of starting afresh. Fourteen-year-olds dream of adventures but with many years of study and experience ahead before those adventures can be undertaken. You have all that study and experience behind you and you are about to be given a chance to take off.

Step into an airlock in your mind. Close the door on your old ways of thinking about pain, stiffness, weakness, and fatigue. Take a magic shower to wash away all limiting ideas, put on a gleaming new space suit, and afix your helmet. Now turn the handle on the door into the unknown. Step through into a new dimension where *you* will control your pain, where *you* will control what you do with your life, where *you* will decide where you want to live, how you want to live, and, to a degree, even how long. What have you got to lose?

When you reenter, the world may be the same, but *you* will be very different. You will have more reasons for getting up in the morning than you have ever had. You will be in control!

To prepare for that, here are some lessons to learn.

LESSON 1: FAITH IN YOURSELF

Before you learn to erase pain, you require a course in cobweb clearing and the injection of self-faith. Recently, the *AMA Journal* came out with a very helpful statement which said that most problems people bring to their doctors are self-limiting. That means that the problems would probably go away by themselves. It went on to say that 10 percent of the problems were beyond the capabilities of the medical professionals. Those could range from the common cold through any number of unpleasantnesses. While that 10 percent will undoubtedly make you un-

easy, how about the other 90 percent? Those problems are the ones you and Myotherapy will be dealing with.

If they would go away by themselves, you may ask, why not let them? Why bother?

Why bother, indeed? We bother because of *pain*. Pain, which at first is only a symptom, can become a disease in its own right. Pain exhausts. A person suffering even low-grade pain never gets the kind of sleep that knits up the ravell'd sleeve of care. Then too, when you hurt, you stop reaching out and taking in, you stop giving, enjoying, even laughing. Pain alone can do you in.

What you do want to know from your doctor is something well within the capabilities of medical professionals. You want to know if your pain is caused by some form of anatomical pathology like a tumor, an aneurism, tuberculosis, or a fracture, or some other condition requiring medical help *before* you are free to do muscle work.

Twenty years ago, pain was pain. Its only gradations were both subjective and suspect. "It's a kind of an ache, Doctor." "It's a sharp pain right over here." "It's unbearable, Doctor, help me." The doctor might have added words like "intermittent" or "unremitting," but pain, if it didn't lead to a diagnosis, was basically uninteresting to any but the sufferer. Twenty or more years ago you took a couple of aspirin or rubbed on some Ben Gay, or went to bed with a hot water bottle. Then pain, as a business, was discovered. Now there are "pain clinics" all over the country. For several thousands of dollars you can spend weeks and even months at such clinics being observed, probed, and tested. You can have your choice of palliative modalities, but in all probability you will leave with your pain intact, having learned "to live with it."

Unfortunately, "living with pain" may be possible in a protected environment, but the "lessons" don't do much good when you get back into the rat race. In addition, you may have picked up a drug habit. If you are female, Valium addiction is not only a very real possibility, it is a probability. There are new drugs coming on the market now that Valium is outliving its patent. They are supposed to be less harmful, but then so, once upon a time, was Valium. If you are male, you may have absorbed the conviction that you can't work anymore. For many that is tantamount to an execution order. Or you may have picked up a drug that will put a lid on your sex life. This time it won't be pain that limits your pleasure in bed; it will be lack of interest. YOU CAN DO BETTER THAN A PAIN CLINIC; BELIEVE IT.

LESSON 2: REAL KNOWLEDGE ABOUT PAIN

In every one of my Pain Erasure seminars someone gets up and says, "But I thought pain was supposed to be a warning . . . if you get rid of it, what about the warning?"

The answer to that is simple: there are two kinds of pain—*acute* and *chronic*. If your hand is on the radiator, acute pain says, "Hey! Your hand is burning, DO something!" What you do is get your hand off the radiator and run cold water over it. Acute pain tells you that when you have been rear-ended and your knee has been rammed into the dashboard, you've probably been hurt. It says quite clearly, "Don't move a muscle. Don't even help them get you

onto the stretcher. You are busted." Acute pain is a great informer and a good commander. You *will* obey. Acute pain cannot be ignored.

Chronic pain is something else. It too has a message, but few people understand its language, or ever have. That is why so little is known about it or has been done to alleviate it. Chronic pain says quite simply, "Your life is too stressful, you must make some changes and until you do, I will be here to remind you." A little further on in the chapter you will learn about the three ingredients necessary to bring on chronic pain, but for now, please accept the fact that chronic pain carries a warning.

LESSON 3: WHAT MYOTHERAPY IS

Myotherapy℠ is a service provided by an outfit called Bonnie Prudden, Inc. At its best it is done by Certified Bonnie Prudden Myotherapists℃ᴹ, who are trained in Myotherapy and are also Certified Bonnie Prudden Exercise Therapists. That sounds like a lot of Bonnie Pruddens, but that name is a guarantee. In 1976 I developed Myotherapy, and within months there were untrained people using the name, giving lectures and workshops, and calling themselves "myotherapists." Some of these were massage people who didn't like the taint adhering to the word "massage" at the time of the sexual revolution. Most, however, were just the usual camp followers who attach themselves to anything new that looks like it "works." Be sure, if you have occasion to go to a Myotherapist, that he or she is Bonnie Prudden certified. We stand behind our graduates and if they don't measure up, they're out! A letter or call to Bonnie Prudden, Inc., Stockbridge, MA 01262 will get immediate clearance or denial. Also, if you need a C.B.P.M. our office will find you the nearest one.

Myo means "muscle" and *therapy,* in my book, means "fix it." Most pain is muscle-related, and if it is muscle-related, Myotherapy has a good chance of relieving it. It should be a joy to you to learn just how many conditions such as arthritis, calcium deposits, bursitis, carpal, tarsal, and cubital tunnel syndromes, tendinitis, backaches, headaches, and even diseases like multiple sclerosis are "muscle-related." One of Myotherapy's chief contributions to happiness, however, is in the cause of preventing pain. Most of the aches and ails of aging are due to mis-use, dis-use, and non-use. As such they can be prevented altogether.

I have been enjoined by Dr. Desmond Tivy, who has written the all important afterwords to each of my books on pain, (all-important since they explain to the medical world what Myotherapy is), not to put forth any theories. There have been numerous theories on pain and most have been proven at least partially wrong. I hasten to obey. I don't *know* why Myotherapy works, but if a wave casts a drowning man onto dry land, it doesn't make sense to question the wave. It does make sense to be grateful to it. I can wait until someone who makes a livelihood from research and has the funds to sustain that interest finds out the reason for Myotherapy's success. For the present, let it be enough that it came in time, along with the other four pluses, for our after fifty generation.

LESSON 4: ALL ABOUT TRIGGER POINTS

A trigger point is a highly irritable spot in a muscle that is left behind after that muscle has been injured (or, in medicalese, "insulted"). Its unpleasant and unhealthy function is to throw its host muscle into spasm. Some spasms are so mild as to go unnoticed; others are so horrendous that they literally cause the muscle to tear itself apart while under attack. Trigger points are thought to be electrical or chemical in nature or some of both. They can lie "doggo" in muscles for years—as in the case of many young athletes who sustain the usual shoulder, back, and knee injuries but get over them in a matter of days or weeks. The same goes for battered children: They get over the *acute pain* fairly quickly, but the potential for crippling *chronic pain* later, when stress levels rise, is great.

Acute pain has to do with the immediate injury. *Chronic pain* seems to require three things: 1) a *trigger point* picked up at some time along the way; 2) a rise in the stress level *or* a point of exhaustion from continued stress; and 3) "the precipitating incident."

A precipitating incident is anything that brings on weakness, stiffness, limitation of function, substitution, or pain. It could be as seemingly unimportant as some stiffness after a long drive or a headache that just "came on." It could be back pain after spring cleaning or a sore shoulder after a game of catch. Usually stiffness following unaccustomed activity will disappear in a day or two, but sometimes continues long after the precipitating incident and becomes chronic. When that happens you will have to become a detective. Try and connect the precipitating incident with something that bothered you. Did the backache appear after the long drive the day you moved in to your new office or out of the old house? There certainly could have been some emotional stress in those situations. Then start looking for the original source. You'd hardly be likely to connect today's backache with the day you ran into a stone wall during the Dartmouth-Cornell game, but that kind of old injury may be the cause.

The after fifty lady wading through menopause might connect her abdominal distress with adhesions from her long-ago appendectomy or blame it on menopause itself, but she would hardly recall the real cause: the lithotomy position plus the episiotomy when her babies were born.

Practically no one coping with chronic pain would say, "What is this stress you are telling me about? I don't have any more stress than the next guy. Sure, we have money troubles, and keeping the girls in college is worrisome, and sure, John is tense about retirement and yes, I'm tense about John ... but none of those things are unusual." No, they aren't unusual, but you left something out of the recitation ... you.

Some people go broke over and over and it doesn't seem to bother them at all. But it does worry *you.* Some people lose their businesses and go bankrupt; no big deal. But not *you.* Some people can say to their kids, "We've done all we can for you, now you are on your own." Or they can say, "So, you want to drop out of school ... go ahead, it's your

loss." Not *you;* you are a worrier and these things distress you. All that's needed to bring on the chronic pain are time, an old injury, and one little extra strain—which is what you will pin it on.

Any old injury will do. How do you get one?

• Birth

Birth is very hard on women, but it's hard on babies too. People with a poetic bent talk of the long struggle down the tunnel leading to life. The birth canal isn't long at all; the problem lies in getting the damn door open. We butt our heads against stone walls all our lives, but we learn how while trying to get born. Little heads pick up lots of trigger points during birth. They lie in the muscles under the scalp. Sometimes they go to work immediately, causing what looks like colic. Sometimes they wait a few months and make teething a disaster. Sometimes they wait much later and become "migraines."

• Accidents

Accidents are second in line when it comes to trigger points and any accident will do. There are all kinds. Little boys used to fall out of trees (when there were trees and little boys climbed them). Little girls did, and still do, fall off horses. All Americans sooner or later collect whiplash injuries one way or another, mostly in cars. If the huge muscles of the neck, the sternocleidomastoids, take on a crop of trigger points, anything can happen from headaches, eye, ear, and sinus pain, to toothache and "the dizzies." These muscles can even cause tinnitis (ringing in the ears).

If "the dizzies" cause you to fall down and break a hip or pelvis, you could be in for real trouble. So, rather than trust yourself to an antivertigo pill, which is a stop-gap measure at best, find the trigger points in the sternocleidomastoids. You will find all these problems *and* what to do to get rid of them listed at the end of the chapter.

Whiplash is a very influential accident. It snaps the neck, leaving it stiff and sore. In a few weeks the pain and limitation seem to go away, but if you put on a sweater and stand with your back to the mirror and turn your head hard to the right, you will find that the sweater creases in long lines running from your left shoulder to a spot over your right hip. The immediate pain will be in the left side of your neck, but twenty years later the anchor for that pull in the muscles of the right hip will bring on your low back pain. Injuries are lavish with trigger points and trigger points are equally lavish with muscle spasm. Jaw pain, for example, usually starts in the seat and groin. Carpal tunnel syndrome and hand and finger pain begin in the upper arm and armpit, shoulder, and chest. Unless the injury just happened, don't think that the place that hurts is housing the cause of the pain. It is probably somewhere else, and just *where* else is what you need to know.

Jaw pain is interesting for a lot of reasons; not the least is the increase in reported incidences of battering. About four million cases of jaw pain, called TMJD (temporomandibular joint dysfunction) are reported each year and 3,800,000 are reported by women. A lot of dysfunction is caused by the gritting and grinding, not to mention gnashing, of teeth in frustration, but some of it is unquestionably due to a "right to the jaw." Just what part of the head will sound off in later years seems to be anybody's guess. If it's eye pain, the sufferer heads for the opthalmalogist. If it's an earache then an eye, ear, nose, and throat doctor will be consulted. If headaches take over there are specialists for that too. I know one headache doctor who boasts thousands of returning patients. To me that would mean he hadn't been all that successful.

Eventually most TMJD sufferers end up with the dentist, who calls it "the mystery disease." Dentists have tried everything from splints, retainers, tooth grinding, extraction, to root canal work. Since the major sufferers are women, psychiatry has also been offered, and Valium, lots of Valium. Certainly, this pain is *really* in their heads! But those measures won't get it, because the treatment is being given where the pain is. The *source* of the pain is somewhere else. When you look up TMJD at the end of this chapter remember that the head is attached in many ways to the groin, lower back, even the legs. The problem might be far from the pain.

• Sports

The third major way to amass trigger points is through sports. Nobody in the after fifty crowd can really say, "I never did anything in sports" the way today's young people can. Once upon a time the whole world of children was a sports arena. We climbed trees, hung from our knees, jumped rope to school and then skipped double dutch in the schoolyard. We rode bikes, pushed scooters, roller skated, ice skated, skied, tobogganed, turned cartwheels and somersaults. We went fishing, clamming, scalloping, crabbing, hunting beechnuts, horse chestnuts, and mushrooms. We went camping, hiking, rowing, canoeing, sailing, stilting, pogoing, riding, and climbing. We played tag when we didn't have a ball and if we had a ball and a board we played baseball. For most American children those things have disappeared. Now play has to be "organized" and it's very different. No kid ever got "pitcher's elbow" until "Little League" took over baseball and little kids had to do the same thing over and over at some adult's direction. The very lack of concentration that belongs to children used to send them off every few minutes in a different direction and a different game. Today it's no use playing basketball unless you can make the team, and for that you have to be very tall, and very young. That doesn't happen except to a very small minority. The guys who make the football team are another minority. Most of the baseball team are Little League graduates, and girls don't count at all, although that *may* change.

Today's sports are expensive too. In the "olden days" they didn't cost must of anything. If you had a boat, fine; if you didn't you made a raft. If you had a scooter, fine; if you didn't you made one from a skate, three boards, and a milk bottle box. Everybody played in the street or backyard and there were very few fat kids. Most of us had skinned knees until we were fourteen. Most of us had dogs, cats, frogs, white rats, raccoons, fish and snakes. Some had ponies, calves, pigs, donkeys, ducks, geese and we were free. We had

the run of our neighborhood with its rocks and wood lots. We could visit other neighborhoods and be welcome. We were free to be children.

We played what are called lifetime sports, but the new sports are not lifetime sports; they are limiting and often dangerous. First, there is running. If you run cross-country, that's one thing. The changing terrain is like the diversified activities we enjoyed. You don't hit pavement to begin with and then you don't keep hitting the same way mile after mile. But jogging is something else. Six years ago we had 30 million registered runners. Today, half of them can no longer run due to foot, leg, and back injuries. The same problems have been decimating aerobic dancers.

Each sport chooses its own area for trigger point collection. Soccer players get the points in the "quads" or thigh muscles which in later life can cause knee pain. The knees are treated and don't get better because the trouble isn't *in* the knee, but in the muscles pulling *on* the knee. Skaters get trigger points in the adductors in the thigh. They too pull on the knee and the floor of the pelvis. Since skaters often fall flat on their seats, they have probably sustained trigger points in the muscles surrounding the coccyx or tailbone. Then they may develop what could pass for hemorrhoidal pain.

Many ex-athletes suffer from low back pain. Racquet sports enthusiasts, basketball players, and any others who indulge in spike sports which demand quick starts and stops, have knee and groin pain. Impotence and spastic vaginas are very real possibilities as the floor of the pelvis sustains recurrent damage. Football and ice hockey aren't really games; they are legalized mayhem. While knees and shoulders take the all-the-time beatings, the rest of the body may load up on trigger points contributing to terrible posture, pain, and exhaustion.

The good news is that those trigger points respond and you can be in control. But be careful what you call for. Don't have an operation unless it is absolutely the last resort. The disc operation, once so popular among ex-athletes as well as ordinary people, is not done these days by reputable surgeons because it didn't get rid of pain. The six-inch-long incision made on the side of the knee, done for a "meniscus injury," didn't work either and has gone by the board. Arthroscopic surgery which has taken its place, sounds innocuous and the tiny scars it produces look innocuous, but nobody really knows what the long-term effects will be. One doctor I know said of such surgery, "We just go in and do a little vacuum cleaning." But the instrument that travels around in there isn't so harmless, and while it "looks around" it creates a catacomb of wounds. Those wounds heal and produce scar tissue. Scars attract trigger points.

If you have such pain, try clearing the muscles of your leg, starting in the groin and ending with your second toe, which is probably long. Get rid of every complaining trigger point, and then see what your knee says. (See the end of this chapter). Better than that, use Myotherapy to *prevent* knee pain, which is called "growing pains" in children, Osgood-Schlatter's disease in teenagers, chondromalacia patellae a little later, and "arthritis" in the after fifty crowd.

• Occupations

The fourth part of life that contrib-

utes trigger points is your occupation . . . *all* your occupations. If your job entails driving *anything* many hours a week, you'll have trigger points in your arms and hands, shoulders, chest, lower back, and legs. In all probability, the muscles of your groin will be foreshortened and your hamstrings tight.

Doing the same motion over and over again, day after day, and often under stress, injures muscles. So does repeating actions like tightening pipes, shoving logs, and using a pneumatic drill. Violinists and dentists have similar patterns and similar pain. Dental hygienists have the same—plus "tennis elbow." Machine operators have pain patterns to match the pattern of their job. Overhead reachers will match the pain patterns of house painters. People who rotate their hands, turning or tightening objects, will have carpal tunnel syndrome (wrist pain) or tennis elbow (elbow pain) or both, and hand pain as a bonus. It could go the other way as easily and cause shoulder, chest, neck, jaw pain, and headaches. When any of these workers are older they will be said to have "arthritis." What they really have is muscle pain from overuse and trigger point collection.

• Disease

Last comes disease. Diseases affect trigger points in two ways: they lay down new ones and heat up old ones. Every time you ache with flu, your illness is "turning on" old trigger points. The good news is that a great deal can be done about disease now that wasn't possible before Myotherapy. Myotherapy plays a very important role in treating the pain accompanying diseases that are cyclic (recurring or moving in cycles). When diseases are active they are often said to be "in flare." When they are quiet they are said to be "in remission." People with these diseases often take powerful medications that can be very dangerous, yet many patients can thrive on exercise and take only aspirin. When a disease is in remission, medication should be discontinued to allow the body to rebuild itself. The trouble with continuing the medication is that with trigger points jumping all over the place in response to the disease (and to the medication which often acts to cause more pain and therefore more medication) the pain doesn't stop; remission is wasted. If, however, the trigger points are erased, "flare" will be easier to bear and remission time can be used to regain health. We have some MS patients whose remission states have gone on and on. When pain creeps in, Myotherapy seems to discourage it at once.

It is very unpleasant to be told that a medication that isn't helping must be continued anyway "because the pain will be worse if you don't." Probably not true, but it's the rare person in great pain who's going to risk "worse."

The drug designed for the disease is only the beginning. People in pain sleep so badly they are given sleeping pills. But sleeping pills can actually interfere with sleep. They are much like alcohol in that respect. You can pass out or into a kind of not-really-awake state and then, a couple of hours later, you are wide-eyed, sleepless, and in pain again. Somehow that's worse at 2 A.M. than at 11 P.M., so you take another pill.

If your sleeping pill is a barbituate, your chances of falling down the stairs and fracturing yourself on the way to the bathroom at midnight are quite good. Add your sleeping pills to the muscle relaxants and the tranquilizers you were given to relieve the anxiety attached to the disease and the pain, and you are a good candidate for depression. For your depression you may be given antidepressants, a very dangerous group which, taken with other medications, seem to cause *more* depression. If you are on them now, get off before you start Myotherapy; they even interfere with that.

When you read about "new" drugs or see them advertised on TV, know that millions of dollars are being spent so that you will read and see. Almost nobody reads the list of side effects that go with the drug. Most of us just figure that if the druggist sells these products, they must be all right. Not so. If a pharmaceutical house mounts an ad campaign, the product will be on the shelves—usually from coast to coast.

When I was a frequent guest on television in the sixties, promoting fitness and exercise, people wrote thousands of letters to me. Suddenly I began getting letters about "that great diet pill you are advertising." I began watching the shows on which I appeared. Sure enough, there was the spot—right after mine, exactly as though we were connected. I went to the producers and explained my position, and asked them to move the ad. But the terms of their contract said "connected with Bonnie Prudden," and I was given a choice: allow the implication, or leave. I left. I left the biggest and best-paid job I'd ever had, and the best way to reach people. Six months later, the two models using the pill died. The station dropped the ad, and the diet pill company went on to other things—not a whole lot less lethal, but a bit harder to trace.

You can't count on anyone to be responsible for you, other than yourself.

What we really have to do is get out of The Valley of the Dolls. Lord knows, we have enough object lessons available to us, if we'd just look for them. *Our* drug addiction began in our parents' medicine chest. Our children's drug addiction and that of our beloved grandchildren began in *our* medicine chests, and with *our* habits.

LESSON 5: FINDING AND FIXING THE TRIGGER POINTS

Remember, a trigger point is an irritable spot in a muscle. What you will be looking for is just that—a spot that feels uncomfortable, irritable, maybe even sore.

The body isn't as big a mystery as you may think. You are put together much like Ma Bell. You have trunk lines running from your trunk out to the hinterlands—your hands, feet, and head. You can call out from headquarters, or back in. There can be a disturbance anywhere along the line and going either way. While you have pain in your foot, the real trouble may be back at the main office, the seat or groin. Or, you could have a damaged foot which refers pain to your knee or possibly up into the hip. Your fingers begin in your shoulder and a dislocation of that important joint could eventually lead to hand or wrist pain.

What you will learn here is how to do a "quick fix." It can relieve the pain or lessen the pain for a while and maybe permanently. If Myotherapy causes any change at all, including making you stiff the next day, it will probably work.

In Myotherapy we look for trigger points by pressing on the complaining muscles with a thumb, a finger, a knuckle, or for large muscles, an elbow. First

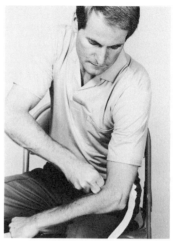

Figure 19.

you need to know how a trigger point feels. Place your left arm on the table in front of you and bring the middle knuckle of the right hand down on a point on your left forearm about ¼ inch below the crease made by your elbow bend. Press straight down as if to go through the arm to the table. You will probably find a very irritable spot on your first try. If not, simply keep the pressure on and move your knuckle north, south, east, and west on your arm (compass technique) until you find it. It's there; it's almost always there.

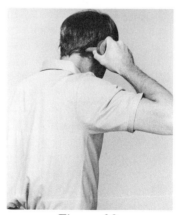

Figure 20.

Hold the pressure for five seconds. If you had arm or hand pain you would hold it a little longer, seven seconds. If for any reason your knuckle can't do the job (sometimes the after eighty bunch have arthritic knuckles), use a bodo, a wooden dowel with a handle, designed to provide maximum leverage. I take one with me when I travel alone in case I wake up with a stiff neck or one of my overused hands develops an ache.

The pain you feel when you press on a muscle tells you where at least one villain is hiding. Don't go for broke. Take only as much pain as you can stand easily. Repeated attention to trigger points over a period of time gets much better results than trying to get it over with in a few agonizing minutes. Besides, too much pain is always counter-productive. It can throw other muscles into spasm—the jaw muscles, for example. If you are working with a friend, set up a code using the numbers 1 to 10. When you find a trigger point and your partner says, "One, two, or three," she's just feeling pressure. When he says, "Wow! That's a good six or seven," you are getting up there. If the "Wow" sounds more like "Ow!" and is followed by "TEN!" or perhaps "TWENTY-TWO!" or "OH, LORD!" *don't press any harder.* Just hold the pressure steady for the count. Agree that if the person getting "fixed" says, "Hold it, no harder," or words to that effect, the "fixer" will *never* go any harder. That removes the stress of uncertainty. Expectation always makes pain worse. That's the problem dentists live with. Their patients' tension gives them the highest rate of backaches in any profession except perhaps that of truck drivers.

#6 Arm Rotations

The next and all-important step is to stretch the kinked muscle and reeducate it. Follow these steps.

- Stretch the arm straight out to the side and rotate your hand counterclockwise so that the thumb points straight up toward the ceiling.
- With the arm in this position, stretch it as long as possible and hold the stretch. This will bring in the whole shoulder, which also needs to stretch.
- Next, rotate the hand clockwise so that the palm faces up and the thumb straight back. Stretch the arm as far as possible to bring in the chest muscles. Stand tall.
- Repeat the arm rotations three times, and then let your arm hang down. It will feel both looser and

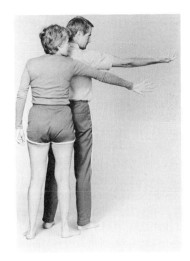

warmer than the other arm. That means that even the minor spasm (which you didn't even feel) has "released" and the circulation has improved.

And that was just one trigger point to a limb that wasn't complaining. In a painful arm or hand you might find *thirty* trigger points! To know more, read one of the books written specifically on pain. (See Sources.)

People who are newly introduced to Myotherapy often ask, "How many pounds of pressure do I apply?" Don't think in terms of pounds; think pain. If your friend says "TEN!" that's the limit. Go no further. If you are pressing on yourself, understand that pressing too hard will not help. You have time. Do a little every day. If the sensitive area is terribly painful, start quite a distance away and hunt down every trigger point you can find. Do the stretch exercises and next day, begin again . . . but a little closer to the painful area. Little by little you will cut the supply and feedback lines until you can do that area as easily as you did its outskirts.

THE FINAL LESSON: A WAY TO ERASE PAIN

Backache is the most common pain we have in America. Most of it is due to sedentary living, stress, and old injuries. It costs individuals, employers, and insurance companies billions of dollars and ruins millions of lives. If the bottom line in business is production, and between 60 and 80 percent of the work force is rendered less competent by back pain, there's a major drain on the economy. Fortunately, back pain is the easiest pain to erase.

Different kinds of back pain have different names, such as the already mentioned sacroiliac, or lower back pain. Then there is the cover-all name, "arthritis of the spine." There are more erudite names like *spondylalgia*, which is a combination of spondylos meaning

"back" and algia meaning "pain." *Ankylosed* usually means fused, but all too often it merely means stiff until the patient looks it up and starts to accept and *act* "fused." We often try to live up to names, even of diseases. Don't.

Spondylitis means inflammation of the vertebrae and so does *spondolodynia*, and both mean back pain. Even arthritis sounds more exciting (and dangerous) when called *spondylarthritis*. *Spondylolisthesis* means that one vertebra has slid forward on top of another and looks magnificent on an X-ray. It responds just as magnificently to Myotherapy. *Spondylosis* is a general term for degenerative changes in the spine said to be due to arthritis. Then come the real scary words, usually connected with discs—"degenerating," "disintegrating," and "slipped." The latter doesn't even exist, but it's used all the time because the patient can see it so well with the mind's eye.

Disc surgery used to be the big moneymaker until open-heart surgery came along, but today it is used less, because along with the fee came the sad fact that the operation, while a howling success, did not get rid of the pain. One of the reasons it didn't was explained by Bellevue Hospital in New York. There they do thousands of autopsies every year and they discovered that literally millions of us have faulty discs, but far fewer have back pain. The faulty discs are not discovered unless there's pain, which leads to an X-ray or myelogram.

If an operation is undertaken for excruciating pain (and it's easy to go that route if you are in it, I've been there) and the pain has gone *forever*, then the operation really was necessary. If, however, the pain remains, a second and perhaps a third operation may be done.

Those, too, are usually unsuccessful, but now you have three wounds, all gathering trigger points. If the problem was muscular and nothing is done about those muscles, then the pain will go on and on until you run out of vertebrae. If you try Myotherapy and the pain goes away, you have saved time and money, not to mention discomfort and calcium-leaching, muscle-atrophying bed rest. Once the doctor has said, "No, you don't have tuberculosis of the spine, a tumor, or a fracture," ask if it's all right to have your friend plant an elbow into the back pocket of your pants, a long way from the spine, and push. It's one of medicine's new tools. A medical director at one of the country's largest auto manufacturers has been using the procedure on injured workers for three years. NONE of the workers required further medication or physical therapy. They needed only one Myotherapy session and almost none needed to be switched to lighter work or time off. That doctor had had one day of training with me. If he can do it, you can.

BEFORE YOU BEGIN . . .

Before you start to apply Myotherapy for lower back pain, look at Figure 21, the Back. That is an accurate diagram of *your* back and the backs of all those around you. Wherever you see a circle, there could be a trigger point lurking. If you have back pain, it *is* lurking. Wherever you see a grid, there are

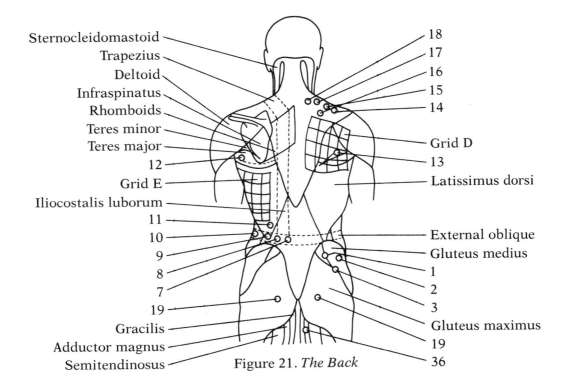

Figure 21. *The Back*

bunches of trigger points, and they can cause all sorts of miseries. For example, #13 is right on your shoulder blade, the *scapula*. It is the major trigger point for shoulder pain and often for headaches and stiff necks. If you are in a hurry to get rid of a pain so you can attend to the day's business, pressing on #13 may be enough. However, if you have the time and want to get rid of the pain permanently it will take more time and effort. Every square in the grid needs to be addressed for a trigger point as well as other muscles which might be influencing the ones indicated with circles.

> When you learned your first Myotherapy technique (on the arm) you did the stretch exercise for that area immediately afterward. That must always be the rule: Myo-Stretch. That's not all. Do the exercises often for the first days after you've begun Myotherapy, then include them in your daily series. It isn't a big price to pay for being pain free.

LOWER BACK

The person with the backache lies prone on a table or desk.

- Reach across the person's back and place your elbow on trigger points #1, #2, or #3 (see Figure 21).
- Press down into the muscle and then draw your elbow toward you.
- To generate more power, clasp your hands together and use both arms to direct your elbow.
- When you find a tender spot, hold for a slow count of seven and then ease up very slowly.
- Hunt for two or three more trigger points in the same area.

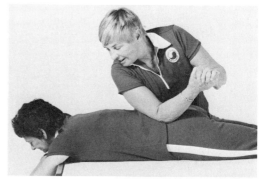

Figure 22.

- Do the other side. *Always* do the other side of everything—arms, legs, shoulders, chest.

#7 Side-Lying Stretch

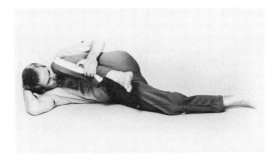
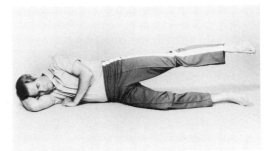
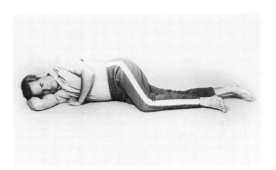

Lie on your side with both legs straight.

- Draw one leg up as close to the chest as possible. Use your arm or hand to help with the stretch.
- Extend the leg straight, about eight inches above the resting leg.
- Rest the working leg on the resting leg and relax for a slow count of three.

> If there is pain anywhere, back, groin, or thigh, check with the Pain List at the end of this chapter and do the suggested Myotherapy before going on. Pain means "glitch." There's a spasm interfering with smooth function. Find the trigger point and get rid of it.

MID-BACK

Have your partner lie face down in the prone position. The next trigger point in line for Myotherapy when doing a Quick Fix on any part of the back is #11 on Figure 21. It is about four inches out from the spine between the crest of the pelvis and the rib cage.

- Reach across the body to the other side.
- Place your elbow on #11.
- Press down and then pull in. People who have played golf, tennis, basketball, in fact any demanding sport, or whose job demanded rotation of the upper body, will have a nasty trigger point in that area.
- Hold for seven seconds and release *slowly.* Do both sides.

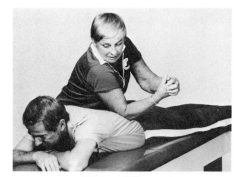

Figure 23.

#8 Angry-Cat-and-Old-Horse Stretch

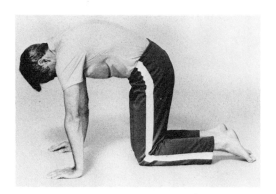
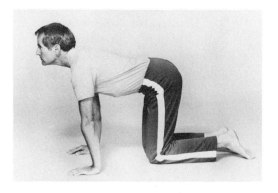

- Get on hands and knees and press his or her back upward like the back of a furious cat.
- Drop the head and hold the press for a few seconds, feeling for tight places that might need Myotherapy later.

- Keeping the arms stiff and straight, bring the head up and let the back fall in like the sagging back of a very tired horse.
- Do this exercise four times.

You can pick up the next one, #13 on the shoulder blade, by having the subject lie prone again and reaching *across* the back to place your elbow on the seam where sleeve meets shirt midway between the shoulder and armpit. Press down and then pull toward you.

- Drop again to the prone position

for the third trigger point needed when doing a Quick Fix on the back—#13. *Everybody* hurts at that spot, so go easy.
- Reach across to place your elbow right on the seam where sleeve meets shirt and midway between shoulder and armpit.
- Do both sides.

More often you will be called upon to relieve a headache or shoulder pain on the job. Then the search will have to be conducted in a chair. The subject sits, leaning forward, and the searcher stands to one side.

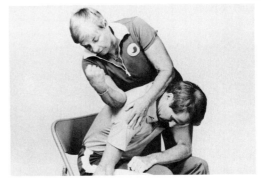

Figure 24.

- Lean over and find the spot with the working elbow while anchoring the subject with the other arm.
- Press down and pull in.
- Hold for seven seconds.
- If at first you don't succeed then try a little compass work, moving your elbow *slowly* north, south, east, and west. *Expect* to hit pay dirt so be ready to halt in mid-press when the yelp comes.

- Don't release your pressure, but don't go any harder, either.
- See if you can locate two or three trigger points in the area.
- Remember to do both sides.

SHEPHERD'S CROOK

A half-inch wide aluminum conduit, bent to curve over the shoulder or around the waist or pelvis, can be used to reach trigger points in the back, shoulders, hips, and thighs. It allows you to administer Myotherapy to yourself whenever you need it. This is especially helpful for those who live alone or whose work is a constant threat to muscles already housing trigger points. At risk are computer operators, dentists and dental hygienists, desk workers, hairdressers, salespeople who drive long distances, teachers, psychiatrists, nurses, and performing artists, among others. If used at once, when the first sliver of pain sends a warning, this action can interrupt the Pain-Spasm-Pain cycle and prevent the ache that turns the evening to misery.

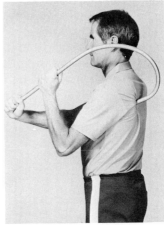

Figure 24A.

#9 Thread Needle Stretch

Start on your hands and knees

- Reach the right hand through between knee and left hand as far as possible and then draw the arm back and up.
- Follow the hand with the eyes
- Do four on each side.

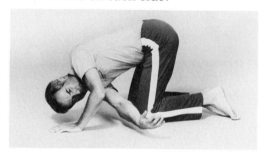

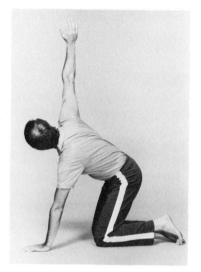

After you have worked on your friend's back, or your friend has worked on yours, there should be "Show and Tell Time." If the former is the case ask your friend to sit up with legs hanging over the edge. Ask this question, "Where has the pain moved to?" DO NOT ASK IF IT HAS GONE. You could get lots of answers such as, "It's better," or, "It's moved to the other side." Best of all is, "It's gone." Those answers might also come from you if you were the one on the table. If it's better, *some* of the trigger points have been found. If the pain has moved, then further work will surely get rid of it. However, if you find or your friend finds that there has been no change, read on.

THE GROIN

The groin is on the opposite side of the back but connected by many muscles. If any one of them is in spasm it can pull either way or both. If a woman has menstrual cramps, her major pain will be felt in the front of the body, as would be the case in "spastic colons" or the pain often attributed to "adhesions." The major trigger points however, may be in the back, in the gluteus muscles. The reverse is also true: The pain may be in the back, but the trigger points lodged in the abdominal and groin muscles. Always remember that you are intricately connected and from time to time your wires may get crossed, eliciting pain in places remote from the cause. For permanent pain erasure you must find all, or at least most, of your trigger points.

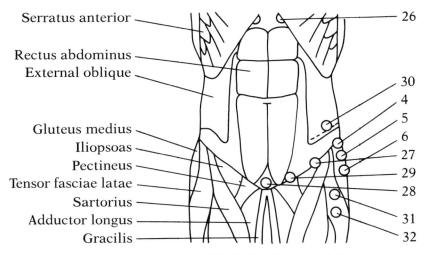

Serratus anterior ——
Rectus abdominus ——
External oblique ——
Gluteus medius ——
Iliopsoas ——
Pectineus ——
Tensor fasciae latae ——
Sartorius ——
Adductor longus ——
Gracilis ——

26
30
4
5
6
27
29
28
31
32

Figure 25. *Abdominals and Groin*

Groin trigger points are almost universal for the After Fifty Crowd and are responsible for the bent posture of Hansel's witch. If you are going to work on your friend have him/her lie supine.

- Place your fingers on the rim of the pelvis nearest you.
- Pressing the skin into the abdominal cavity, pull back to catch the trigger points between your fingers and the bone.
- Hold each sensitive spot for the re-

quired 7 seconds. If there is no sensitivity, there is no trigger point. Move on.
- Reaching across, make the same search on the other side of the pelvis, using the thumbs. (The points you are covering are #30 on each side, see Figure 25.)

If you are the one with the problem, you can lie in bed and hunt for the groin trigger points, using a Bodo. (See page 120.)

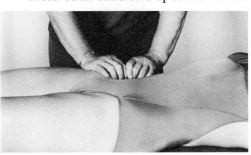
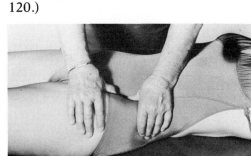

Figure 26.

The abdominal muscles have several functions. They support the organs and, should you wish to lean forward, it is they that contract to accomplish that move. They attach at the bottom to the pubic arch.

- Place your fingers *on* the arch.
- Press the skin back into the abdominal cavity and then pull *down* to catch trigger points #28 and #29 between your fingers and the bone.
- This is a very sensitive area, so go easy. Remember, every athlete has insulted this area over and over; so has any woman who has given birth to a child. Sitting postures limit the muscle's potential to

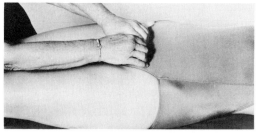

Figure 27.

stretch normally, and driving a car both limits and overworks them.

If you are working on yourself, use the Bodo to press along that lower rim of the pelvis. Go slowly and don't press too hard. You have lots of time and it doesn't all have to be done at once.

- Find the ribs, even if they are well padded. The abdominal muscles anchor at the top to the ribs.
- Reach in under them to find the trigger points and squeeze them between your thumb and the bone. (There are usually nasty points on the right sides of people who run. If you get "stitches" in your side, here's the answer. Get them detriggered before you run.)

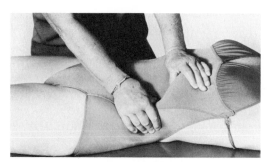

Figure 28.

#10 Groin Stretch

- Hang first one leg and then the other over the side of a table.
- Press down on the knee in short easy bounces.

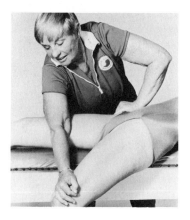

At night, if I watch TV from my bed I hang my right leg over for the first commercial and the left for the next, alternating till I turn it off. Commercials are great reminders to *do* something!

HEADACHES

The next pain suffered by many, many people, including the after fifty crowd, is a headache, and it has even more and fancier names than backache. If it shows up on one side of the head it's called a *migraine* and occurs more often in women. *Cluster headaches* are particularly nasty: if your headache comes in bunches and is the worst pain you can imagine, it's a cluster. More men have that one. If it's the all-over kind it's usually called *tension*. If it shows up on Mondays it's called *a Monday headache*, and is tied to hating your work. *Friday headaches* are said to come when tension is released. If your head aches when you have menstrual cramps, it's a *menstrual headache* and if you are simultaneously depressed, a *depression headache*. When you feel it in front, it's a *sinus headache*. There are a couple that are sometimes overlooked: the *hangover headache* and the "*Not tonight, George headache*." There is, of course, the *drug headache, skip-lunch headache, I-can't-stand-this-another-minute headache*, and the *changed-schedule headache*. What all those designations boil down to is . . . a pain in the head.

A lot of headaches are said to be vascular, which means related to blood vessels. The pain is to blood vessels what sciatica is to the sciatic nerve. In the case of sciatica the sciatic nerve, descending through the huge gluteus muscles, gets its tail in a crack. Spasmed glutes squeeze the poor nerve, which yells bloody murder loud enough to be heard (felt) as far down as the toes.

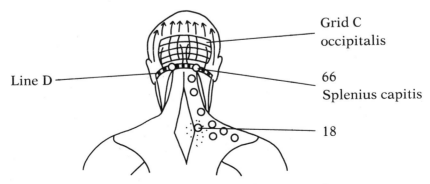

Figure 29. *Back of Head, Neck, and Upper Back*

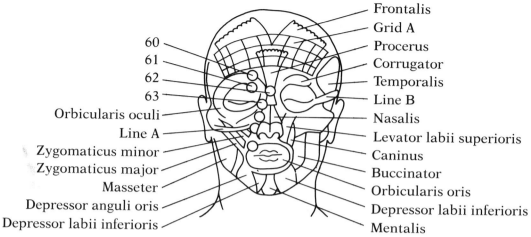

60 — Frontalis
61 — Grid A
62 — Procerus
63 — Corrugator
— Temporalis
Orbicularis oculi — Line B
Line A — Nasalis
Zygomaticus minor — Levator labii superioris
Zygomaticus major — Caninus
Masseter — Buccinator
Depressor anguli oris — Orbicularis oris
Depressor labii inferioris — Depressor labii inferioris
— Mentalis

Figure 30. *Front of Head and Face*

There are many muscles, and nerves in the head, face, and neck. When one or more of those muscles shouts "Uproar," they have a family gathering. They squeeze everything in sight. Any old trigger point is welcome to crash the party, and usually does. Most headaches follow the lead of the muscles in the shoulders, back of the neck, and head. Even when the pain is behind the eyes, a powerful old *pater familias* called *splenius* (#66 in Figure 29) can start the ball rolling and rolls right over the top of the head to settle in an aggra-

vated *orbicularis oculi*, (#60 and #61 in Figure 30).

Modern medicine depends mostly on medication to relieve headaches, which usually means that the source of a headache is overlooked. That, in turn, means that when the body gets used to it the medication must be replaced by another one, equally expensive and equally foreign to the body. Wouldn't it be better to get rid of the cause, the medication, and the need to waste time lying in a darkened room? Follow these steps.

- Place two fingers on your spine at the back of your neck, right in the hairline.
- Slide fingers outward on a horizontal line to a point halfway between your spine and your ear. You will find a little hollow just under the curve of the skull (#66, in Figure 36, the *splenius*).
- Press up against the skull to trap the trigger point between your fin-

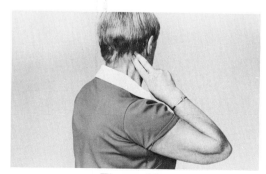

Figure 31.

gers and the bone. You need not be so gentle this time.

- Hold the trigger point for five seconds.
- Slide your fingers halfway down your neck on the same vertical line
- Press in and hold.

For the next trigger point, your leverage will be better if you use a bodo.

- Slide your fingers down your neck to the point where it joins your shoulders.
- Press in again.

Here's the last stop on the *splenius*— and for this one you may need a friend.

- Sit sideways in a chair and have your friend stand behind you.
- Lean over and drop your head to put the muscle on the stretch. (The base of the *splenius* is #18 on Figure 29.)
- Have your friend support your chest as he or she puts an elbow into #18 and captures the trigger point.
- Hold for the required seven seconds.

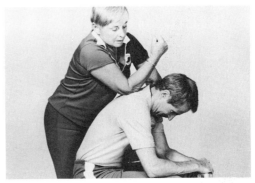
Figure 32.

- Do the other side.

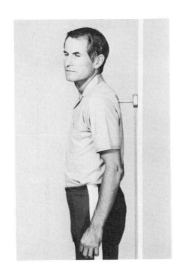
Figure 33.

If you don't happen to have a friend handy, but you do have a headache, fasten a bodo to the wall (at #18 level) and back into it. If you do not yet have a bodo, hold a wooden spoon against the wall and back into that.

You have now covered the back of the head and neck for a Quick Fix. Move to the front of the head, the face, and the forehead.

Check with Figure 30, the front of the head and face, and note that the *orbicularis oculi* is a muscle encircling the eye. A great way to fill it with trigger points is to squint, overuse your eyes, and laugh a lot. Since you *will* squint and overuse and laugh, you'd better know how to clear up those trigger points and soften your face.

- Place the middle finger on the top edge of your eyebrow near your nose.
- Put pressure on and then push your eyebrow down over the edge of your eye socket.
- Pull back up to trap the trigger point between your finger and the bony socket. (Do it gently; it's a sensitive area.)
- Hold for a count of five.
- Move your finger outward one finger-breadth toward the outside of the eye.
- Repeat four times, until your finger is at the edge of the eye.
- Do the other eye.

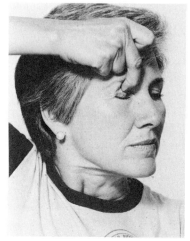

Figure 34.

There is one more bit of work for the head.

- Put your finger on your temple and push in.
- Keeping the pressure steady, push the skin north, south, east, and west. Every time you find a sensitive spot keep the pressure for five seconds.

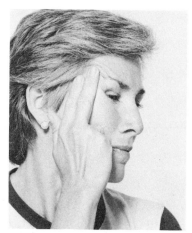

Figure 35.

EYE EXERCISE

Close your eyes and keep them closed. Raise your eyebrows as high as possible. Scrunch your whole face, like a kid eating a lemon. Repeat three times. Keeping your eyes closed, roll your eyeballs first right, then left, then up and down. Do that three times.

THE NECK

Figure 36 shows the neck and the SCM (sternocleidomastoid). Trigger points hidden anywhere in the neck can send pain in any direction. The neck is endangered because of the diagnosis "pinched nerve," which can lead to an operation. It would be wise to be sure first that any neck pain you have is not caused by trigger points left behind after a fall or an accident.

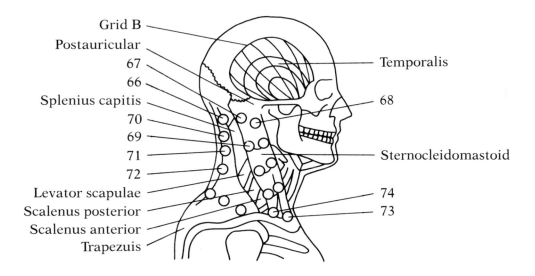

Figure 36. *The Neck*

- Start with trigger point #67 and #68.
- Grasp your earlobe in your thumb and forefinger.
- Twist the lobe counterclockwise and press your fingers down against your neck.
- Let go of the lobe and your forefinger will be on point #68 while your thumb will be on the other side of the huge muscle.
- With your first two fingers, press back *into* the muscle.
- Hold for a count of five.
- Use your thumb or fingers to press *forward* into the back of the muscle. (This will probably hurt.)
- Hold for five counts.

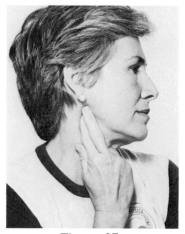

Figure 37.

- Drop your fingers down a half inch and repeat.

The following procedure, the Squeeze, looks mean, and is, but it is a sure way to find, trap, and eliminate trigger points.

- Tip your head toward your hand, which makes the neck muscle easier to grab.

- Squeeze the muscle at half-inch intervals all the way down your neck.
- Wherever you find a sensitive spot, hold for five counts.
- Do both sides of the neck.

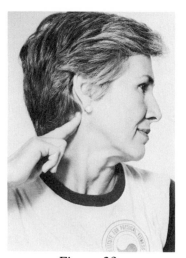

Figure 38.

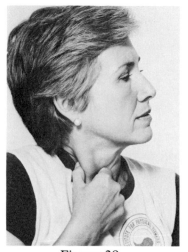

Figure 39.

#11 Neck Resistance and Stretch

- Place your right hand on your right cheek. Giving yourself a *little* resistance, "fight" your hand as you turn your head to the right.
- At the furthest reach of the turn, keep the pressure on and bring your left hand to your left cheek.
- This next step is crucial: Don't release the pressure of face to right hand until the left is in place and can push the turn a *little* further without any resistance.
- From the furthest point of the turn, put pressure on with the left hand and turn the head to the left against resistance.

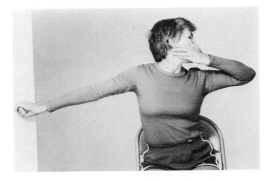

- Repeat the crucial shift at the other side.
- Do four.
- To get more resistance, do the exercise holding onto a door handle.

The neck can be a good or bad neighbor to the head, and vice versa. If your headache is not gone after doing both the back and the front of the head, do the neck. If your stiff neck is still cranky, do the back of the head. Then consider that the problem may lie in the chest.

THE CHEST

Chest muscle spasm often causes mock angina. It can make your asthma worse, give you heartburn, and make you think you have a hiatus hernia. Spasm in the chest muscles can refer to the upper back and give you the feeling that your old gall bladder is back in operation. It will ruin your posture and drop your bust into your lap. Better clear out the trigger points.

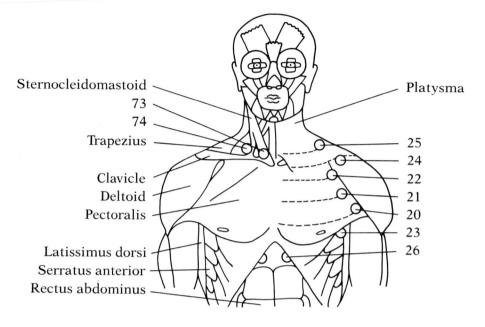

Sternocleidomastoid
73
74
Trapezius
Clavicle
Deltoid
Pectoralis
Latissimus dorsi
Serratus anterior
Rectus abdominus

Platysma
25
24
22
21
20
23
26

Figure 40. *Torso, Front View*

This is another procedure you can do for yourself although it's easier if someone else does it for you.

- Start at points #20 through #25 (Figure 40).
- Work your way to the center of the chest, a half inch at a time.
- Hold each sensitive spot for seven seconds—and take your time. If you have had a mastectomy and have sensitivity around the scars, use gentle fingers and go softly around each scar. The trigger

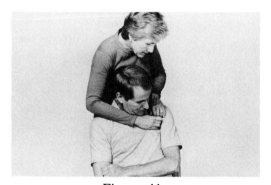

Figure 41.

points are there and they can cause pain and swelling.

Emphysema is a particularly mean disease, and you can help.

- Have your friend lie on his or her side.

- Using very gentle fingers, search between the ribs in the *intercostals* for the trigger points. There are lots of them, but if you can get rid of them, you may get your friend some more lung space.
- If you are the sufferer, you can do the *intercostals* on the front and sides, but you will need help with the back.

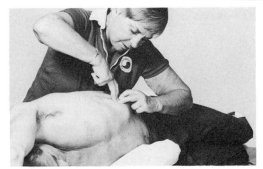

Figure 42.

#12 Chest Stretch

- Lie on your side with a folded pillow under your waist.
- Hold a weight bag in your free hand.
- As you raise the arm overhead, inhale.
- As you bring the weight to your thigh, exhale.
- Start easy and increase as you feel stronger.
- Do both sides.

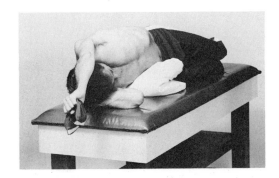

#13 Snap and Stretch

- Stand with feet apart and elbows bent.
- Snap the elbows back on the count of "one."
- On the word "and" bring the arms back across the chest to stretch your upper back.
- On "two" swing straight arms wide.
- On "and" cross in front once more.
- Do eight as a set.
- Try to do four sets.

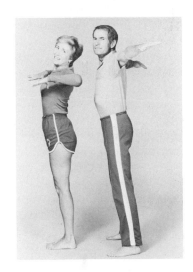

#14 Back Stroke

- Stand with feet apart.
- Place the back of your right hand against your right cheek and press your elbow back as far as possible.
- Keep the elbow back, and at its furthest reach, carry the hand and arm around in a wide circle.
- Alternate arms for a count of eight.
- Do *both* arms at the same time for a count of eight.

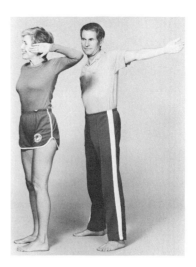

THE ARMS

Fifty percent of the people who have arthritis don't know they do. "Arthritis" is often self-diagnosed, and even when the doctor diagnoses it, he or she may mean myofascial pain, or muscle pain. There are many kinds of arthritis and the one that affects the after fifty crowd most is osteoarthritis. Most of us have it and most of us can keep it under control. If I'd known about Myotherapy twenty years ago I think I could have kept my hip joints. The main effort should be toward keeping all muscles free of spasm, and in particular any muscles that have once been injured. They will go into spasm if they get a chance—and that chance comes with stress.

Our hands, fingers, feet, knees, and neck seem to be most vulnerable to arthritis. Fingers have their roots in shoulders. Soaking fingers, rubbing them with liniment, or wearing splints to prevent painful movement won't get at the cause—trigger points. See Figure 44 and use every small circle as a starting point for a search. Move up or down the arm doing trigger points every inch. The dotted lines give you a path to follow. The empty circles come first and are for a "Quick Fix." The black circles are secondary.

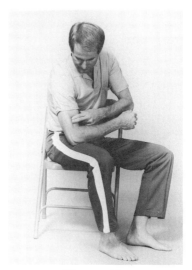

Figure 43.

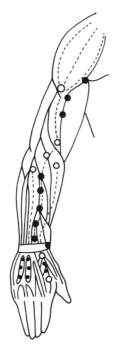

Figure 44. *Arm and Hand, Posterior View*

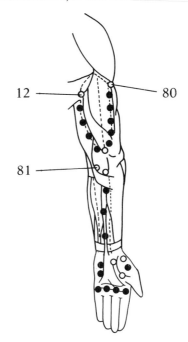

Figure 45. *Arm and Hand, Anterior View*

The anterior view (Figure 45) doesn't show how very important this side of the arm is, but believe me, it is. Points #12, #80, and #81 cover the kinds of trigger points that cause carpal tunnel pain, hand and finger pain, "trigger fingers," hand weakness, and the inability to close or open the hand.

To find these arm trigger points, you can use either your fingers or a bodo. I prefer the bodo. I have "skier's thumbs" as well as a "baseball finger" and several broken fingers left over from when I was supposed to be breaking horses (once in a while they broke part of me). My grip on the bodo is good, but without it my angle is wrong.

The armpit is a nest of trigger points, and since there's no telling where these trigger points will be, you won't need a diagram. Just lie down and put one

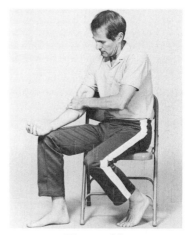

Figure 46.

hand behind your head and, with bodo in hand, go at it. Armpits are very sensitive, so treat yourself like your very best friend. Go easy. Then do the other side.

#15 Shoulder Rotation

- Stand with feet apart for balance.
- Reach straight forward and rotate the arm and hand counterclockwise until your thumb points to the ceiling, then clockwise until the thumb turns back toward the wall.
- Do eight for a set (three sets should be in your program).
- Later in the day, do the same exercise with arms reaching to the side.

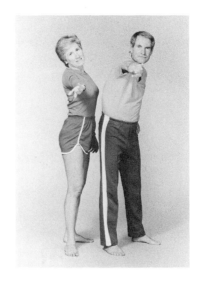

THE HANDS

After you have done your arms you can take care of your hands. If the hands are very painful or weak, the arm work should ease the pain and allow you to start strengthening them and making them more flexible. Use the bodo front and back. Remember, if the hand hurts, hunt first around the elbow and then the hand. If there is still pain, move higher up the arm (the inner surface yields the most trigger points). The armpit is a gold mine, and the chest and upper back are also sources of hand pain.

THE FINGERS

The best way to hunt trigger points in each finger is to squeeze top and bottom together, then the sides, like pincers. Do *not* squeeze the joints.

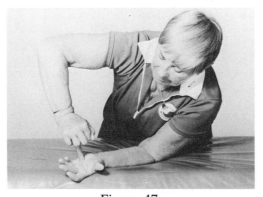

Figure 47.

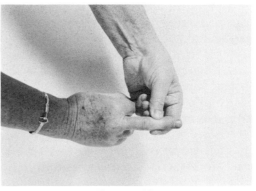

Figure 48.

#16 Hand and Finger Exercise—The Ball

Squeeze a small sponge or rubber ball to strengthen hands and fingers. Keep one next to the telephone and another next to the TV. Once you are free of pain . . . squeeze.

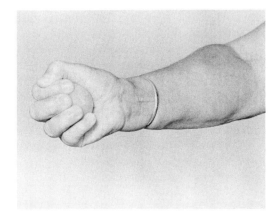

#17 Hand and Finger Exercise—Rubber Band

- Slide your fingers into a rubber band and open them as far as you can.
- If this is too easy, add another band.
- If movement is too hard, get a thinner band. When you work against resistance, you improve range as well as strength.

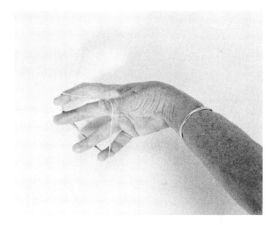

Finger numbness may come all the way down from your neck, but first think trigger points. When your hands are cold, don't plan on a warm heart, although you probably have one. Think trigger points causing spasm and therefore lack of circulation. When your nails keep breaking, also wonder about that circulation.

THE LEGS

Legs are the auxiliary pump for the heart. Healthy legs squeeze the blood back up into the body when their system of pipes and valves is in good order. If, however, legs are loaded with trigger points, toenails look awful, feet are cold, ankles are swollen, achy, and tired making walking difficult, disaster is ready to strike.

To help a friend with these problems, you can use a bodo for the backs of the legs, but it's not as good as an elbow

- Have your friend lie down on a table and put a rolled-up towel under the ankles.
- Start with the calf at point #47 (Figure 49), the edge of the soleus, one of the trigger points noted for calf cramps in the middle of the night. The back of the leg is impor-

tant, since the hamstrings run down that surface and always house a myriad of trigger points.
- Place your elbow on that point in the leg nearest you.
- Press down, draw in, and hold for seven. There *will* be a trigger point there.
- Follow the dotted line in the diagram down to the heel, at inch intervals.
- Next, do the middle line in the diagram.
- Do the outside line standing at the other side. This allows you to pull toward the mid line as in the back. Anyone prone to night leg cramps, or whose legs feel weak, or who is troubled with swollen ankles, will find this procedure helpful.

#18 Calf Stretch

To stretch the calf muscle you have just worked over, bend the knee and press down on the ball of the foot. If your friend says this hurts, go back and hunt for more trigger points. Keep in mind that the leg has probably been damaged, without any relief, for many years. Don't hurry. The trigger points are always their most painful the first time you find them. It will get easier with time.

The standing calf stretch exercises (half knee bends with heels tight to the floor) will help enormously. Use the door-held knee bends as well (see Exercise #31).

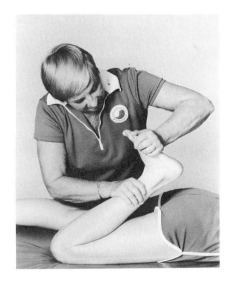

The line starting at point #36 (Figure 49) in the upper leg will be very sensitive on ex-atheletes, people who stand on cement (or tile over cement) for long hours, and runners.

- You can help stimulate and relieve the backs of the thighs by pressing with an elbow or bodo along the lines shown in the diagram. Start from the top and work toward the knee at one-inch intervals. Always start from the outsides of the leg and work in.

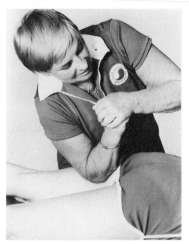

Figure 50.

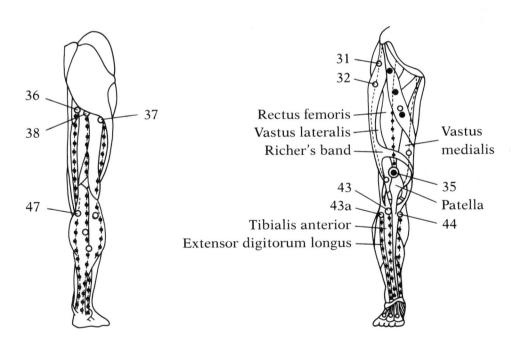

Figure 49. *The Leg, Posterior View*

Figure 51. *The Leg, Anterior View*

#19 Hamstring Stretch

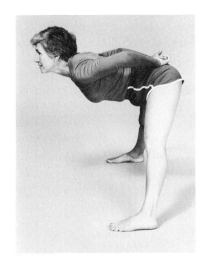

- Spread legs wide and clasp hands behind back.
- Keeping head up and back as flat as possible, bounce the upper body downward in eight *easy* bounces.
- Turn the upper body to the right and repeat the bounces.
- Turn left and do the same. (To this exercise add the Hip Shift on page 257 to stretch the inner thighs.)

Do this exercise often throughout the day. Sitting and stress shorten hamstrings; combating both must be a daily effort.

The anterior view of the leg shows the magnificent pillar of muscle arrangements and proves how important the legs are to you. Learn as much as you can about the legs (in my books on pain) and keep this pair of good soldiers in working order.

People seem to be able to endure leg pain even when it is excruciating (which is no longer necessary most of the time). However, the knee is something else. If it doesn't work, walking becomes very difficult and walking safely, an impossibility. Most people think that knee pain comes from a condition *inside* the knee. Most of the time it comes from muscles pulling *outside* of the joint. First, look at Figure 51 and note how many of those muscles attach at the knee. Then check with Figure 49, the back of the leg, and know that they too attach at the knee *and trigger points in any one of them could cause knee pain*, never mind the diagnosis "arthritis."

To note just two of the muscles that cause knee pain, recall when you were a little kid and someone grabbed your thigh just above the knee joint and squeezed really hard. You went straight up in the air and were laughingly told—"that was a horse bite." What that person did was press on the trigger points closest to the knee in each of those two muscles. You can use those

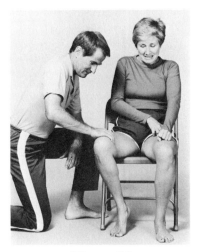

Figure 52.

two points as direction finders whenever you want to get rid of your own pain or someone else's. They are at the base of the *vastus medialis* on the inside of the thigh and the *vastus lateralis,* on the outside. You will also have to work on the calf and even perhaps the seat and upper thigh. Everything going and coming in the leg has something to do with the knee.

Knees are often sinned against by sports, long periods of sitting, extra weight, and inappropriate footwear, not to mention the unavoidable structural anomaly "long second toe."

- To work on yourself, sit on the edge of a bed or table and bend the knee needing care, outward.
- Start at the spot of the "horsebite" on the inside of the thigh, just above the knee.
- Keep to that line, which is just under the inside seam of your slacks, and move at one inch intervals, pressing with either bodo or elbow from knee to groin.

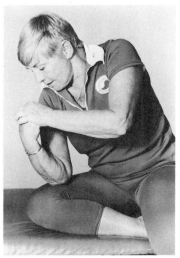

Figure 53.

Using the bed, table, or a chair, go after the trigger points on the outside of the leg, starting at that "horsebite" spot and working up the outside of the leg to your waist at one inch intervals. That line is right under the outside seam of your slacks. For this work you will need a bodo.

Follow that with work to the calf either with the help of a bodo or a friend.

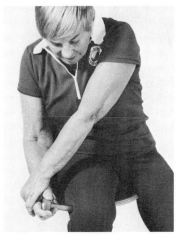

Figure 54.

When you have removed the trigger points from the three areas, then start with a series of *half* knee bends while keeping the heels on the floor and feet together. As soon as you can (which will be almost immediately) start walking stairs, starting with a few at a time. See the section on stair exercises (page 330) and also the floor progressions (page 260).

If you have a friend who needs help, sit side by side in chairs. Have your friend drop her leg over your nearer knee while you, using the nearer elbow, start to press on the inside of the leg right at the "horsebite" spot and press at one-inch intervals up to the groin. To get at the outside of the leg change places and have your friend cross the leg over your lap, exposing the outside surface to your nearer elbow.

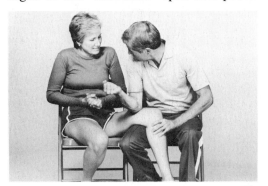 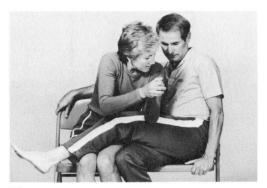

Figure 55.

Don't neglect knees due to the misunderstanding that the knee is either "arthritic" or just plain old. Cared-for knees do very well, as do cared-for legs.

Feeble walking is due to neglect and not knowing the answers. You now know the answers; it's up to you to apply them.

THE FEET

Anyone who has tired, burning, aching, throbbing, swelling, miserable feet is miserable all over. Most of you already know that corn and bunion plasters, arches, orthotics, specially molded shoes, "sensible" shoes, supported shoes, and hot soaks really are not the final answer. You may even have "arthritis," fallen arches, flat feet, the works, but that isn't the end of the world by any means. You can still have strong, painless feet.

Use your bodo to get at all the trigger points shown in Figure 56. That's just for starters. Next, check for a long second toe. You can start by looking at your feet, but if they are like mine you will not see that the second toe is any longer than the first. However, if you bend all your toes down and then, with a felt-tipped pen, circle the first joints of the first two toes, you'll see that joint of the second toe is farther forward in your foot than that of the big toe. This means that all your life you have been landing on your heel like everybody else but, while others were stepping forward onto a three-point landing, with weight evenly distributed on both sides of the front of the foot, you were landing on the *middle* of the front of the foot, right in the middle of the metatarsal arch. That's why women who wear high heels or tight shoes get a callus on the middle of that arch right under the second toe joint. Athletes with this problem usually get a callus on the outside of the big toe. The Greek models for statues all had this problem (which is sometimes called "the classic Greek foot"), but wore sandals that allowed the muscles free play. Thus, though they had the structural problem, they didn't develop the side effects. (Another reason why wearing sneakers for dance is counter-productive.)

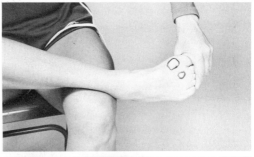
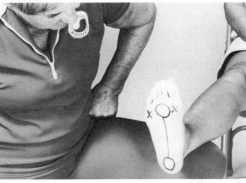

Figures 57 and 58.

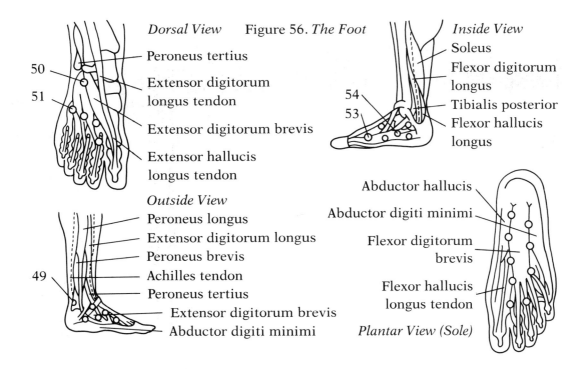

Dorsal View   Figure 56. *The Foot*   *Inside View*

50
51

Peroneus tertius

Extensor digitorum longus tendon

Extensor digitorum brevis

Extensor hallucis longus tendon

Outside View

Peroneus longus
Extensor digitorum longus
Peroneus brevis
Achilles tendon
Peroneus tertius
Extensor digitorum brevis
Abductor digiti minimi

49

Soleus
Flexor digitorum longus
Tibialis posterior
Flexor hallucis longus

54
53

Abductor hallucis
Abductor digiti minimi
Flexor digitorum brevis
Flexor hallucis longus tendon

Plantar View (Sole)

OK, so you've got a long second toe. What has it caused besides corns, calluses, hammertoes, and bunions? Instability in your ankles for one, as you may have noticed with frequent sprains. It has also caused knee instability which refers upward to cause hip pain. Every muscle in your legs has been working overtime to keep you going and every one, especially the tibialis anterior on the outside of the front of the lower leg, is loaded with trigger points. You need to repair the structure of the foot by lifting the weight off the second toe joint that has kept you walking an unstable knife edge for too many years.

Get an innersole for your shoe and a sheet of adhesive foam (available at any drugstore). Cut a circle the size of a quarter and one the size of a nickel from the foam. Stick the larger circle to the underside of the innersole just

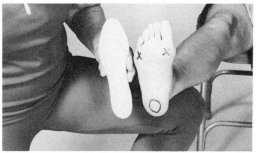

Figure 59.

under the ball of the foot. Then stick the second circle on top of that one. If you are heavy, add another pad. If you want to wear sandals but still want to straighten out your bunion and hammer toe and take the pressure off your leg muscles, stick the pads directly to your foot. Do the exercises on page 296 and blame the whole problem on your grandparents: long second toe is hereditary.

#20 Foot Exercises

For these exercises, you should have a partner who can provide resistance. If a partner isn't available, you can probably manage to do these yourself.

- Plantar Flexion: Sit in a chair and, placing the instep on the floor, slide your foot back until the weight is on the toes and instep. Press down *gently* three times and relax. If you get a cramp while doing this, there is still a trigger point lurking. Go after it in the sole. Repeat with other foot.
- Supination: Sitting on one folding chair, place the ball of your foot on

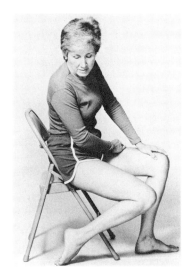

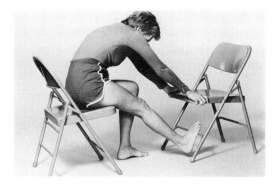

the rung of a chair opposite you. Holding onto the seat for leverage, press the heel down three times and relax. Repeat with other foot.

- Inward Rotation: Lay the side of the foot on the floor just in front of your chair. Press down on your knee to stretch the outside edge of the foot. Press three times and relax. Repeat with other foot.
- Outward Rotation: Push the foot backward but turned on its inside edge. Press down on the knee three times; relax and do the other foot.

Do three sets of these exercises every day as long as feet are painful or weak. Replace with walking as soon as you can. Then use the series twice a week to maintain flexibility.

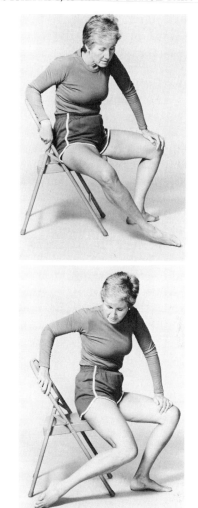

DELILAH'S STORY

There are still two things you need to know about pain. One of them is the story of Delilah. Delilah is a 200-pound English mastiff. She is brindle in color, angelic of disposition, and when I met her, her condition was "crippled."

I had lost my closest friend, a brindle mastiff named Elizabeth, the summer before and just wanted to see mastiffs again, so I stopped off in Virginia to visit Eve Olsen Fisher, who raises them. We had been friends for years and we spent some time catching up. Then I told her about Myotherapy and said,

"Too bad you don't have a dog that hurts." "But I do," Eve said. She sent the kennel master down to get Delilah. I couldn't believe what I saw. The dog was swaybacked, bent-legged, and spastic. "She's much better since we put her out in the kennel rather than in the house," Eve said. "There she just dragged herself across the floor."

Eve held the dog's head and I did five minutes' worth of work on Delilah's back legs, and, by golly, she walked better. "I'm sending a Myotherapist down as soon as I get home," I said. They were going to "sacrifice" the dog to see why she couldn't walk. The Myotherapist arrived and Eve gave her Delilah to bring north to me. After a month of treatment the dog was leaping, strong and pain free across the fields.

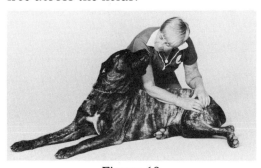

Figure 60.

Delilah will never be a deer, but a happy, healthy, wonderful dog she is. And we learned, working with her, that dog muscles, horse muscles, and cat muscles respond to Myotherapy in exactly the same way as human muscles do: they get well. Now many of my Myotherapy students have become interested in helping animals; I send them down to the Bilmar Kennels in Great Barrington and they work on the dogs there. If your dog hurts, use the same trigger points as you would for yourself. You may see a difference in minutes.

THE NO PAIN CLUB

I recently lectured to a large group of health professionals at the Springfield (Massachusetts) Technical College. The group was made up of nurses, dentists, doctors, and dental hygienists. As I talked I wondered why, with their backgrounds, they couldn't help each other. "You ought to get together and form a No Pain Club, I suggested. I promised to send them a Myotherapy instructor once a week for eight weeks if anyone would be interested. They were, and we began. Myotherapy then became a part of their college curriculum.

All very well, I thought, for health professionals, but why couldn't regular people have a No Pain Club, too? I applied for a chance to talk to a group of older people in Lenox, Massachusetts, near my home.

"I know how to get rid of the muscle spasms that cause pain," I told this group. "Is anyone interested in giving us a chance to teach you how to do that for yourselves?" It took me half an hour to explain the basics and show them, on themselves, how Myotherapy worked. They were interested; they formed a No Pain Club.

My associates and I started teaching Myotherapy for headaches, backaches, knee pain, arms that wouldn't go up, necks that wouldn't turn, tinnitis, jaw pain, fingers that wouldn't bend, and even double vision and hearing loss. All of these "students" got better and better—and they were helping each other! In addition, we were teaching exercises, including everything in the floor progressions and chair exercises you'll read about in the next chapter. We didn't get down on the floor because they weren't dressed for it and there wasn't time. At the end of eight weeks it was the Osborne Home all over again, except that this time we also knew how to get rid of pain, and these people were not sequestered—they were right out there, living in the real world.

Of all the people to join the group, only two were housewives. That should be some kind of warning. People who are used to working outside the home continue to stay active and take on new activities; it's habit. If you are housebound, make a break for it . . . now! Then later, when you *need* friends, you'll have access to them. Another mention of networking should come in here: a No Pain Club will give you a Myotherapy partner who knows the techniques.

PROBLEMS OF A (MOSTLY) EVERYDAY NATURE

> Look up your pain in the Pain Chart at the end of this chapter (page 170) for the Myotherapy patterns, exercises, and extra-exercises (278) you'll need to help you erase the pain, control the pain, and in some instances, *prevent* the pain.

For many ills no "cure" has as yet been discovered, but there is always tomorrow. Be cheered by what has been discovered in our lifetime and prepare for future discoveries by being as healthy as possible. Put aside the name of the problem, and look up the "pain." It is what hurts that counts with Myotherapy, not the name of the pain.

AMPUTATION

A limb that has been amputated is like a lost love; it never really goes away, but leaves a phantom of itself which often aches, burns, itches, or growls with pain. Treat the remaining stump with Myotherapy *as though the limb were still there*. Do every muscle, on all four sides. Then, pretend to lay a cloth on which a crossword puzzle has been printed, over the stump, and using a small bodo, press on every single square of the "puzzle," holding for seven seconds at each sensitive spot. Do stretch exercises that might apply if the limb were still there; and if the prosthesis irritates, give the stump a rest for three days while you work. Do the stretch exercises every couple of hours.

ANGINA

Real angina signals an insufficiency of blood to the heart; *mock* angina signals trigger points in the chest muscles. Since many things can put those trigger points there, one should not be conned into thinking that the pain is in one's head just because all heart checks are negative. The problem is probably where you feel it—in your chest.

A muscle in spasm is grateful for release from its agonizing clasp, no matter what the cause. Check the Pain Chart for *chest pain* and you will find that the work needed must be done to the upper back, groin, arms, and neck, as well as the chest muscles.

ANKLE PAIN

To rid the ankle of pain and/or swelling and weakness, start in the groin and seat muscles with Myotherapy and proceed in a methodical fashion down all sides of the leg; include the foot (see page 148). The muscles in the lower leg on the outside, the tibialis anterior, will be the worst. See the Pain Chart for *ankle pain.*

ARM PAIN

Arm pain takes in everything from shoulder to armpit (where most arm pain has either its start or its support), and includes the constantly worked biceps and triceps of the upper arm and the pectoralis in the chest. The elbow must not be considered a cause of most arm pain of the chronic variety; it is merely the anchor for muscles in spasm. The lower arm, due to constant rotation, is also a nest of trigger points, as is the hand. Repetitious movements, *over and over* such as knitting, can cause pain at any point along the arm, and even chest pain that passes for angina.

ARTHRITIS

There are many kinds of arthritis, but *Osteoarthritis* is most prevalent in the after fifty crowd. Put the diagnosis to bed, forget about it, and go after whatever hurts. You must keep your circu-

lation in good repair and you must keep the muscles out of shortening spasm that can jam the joints together until they are destroyed. In the end it will be up to you. Blessings on Doctor Charnley, who developed the first total hip replacement, but like your teeth, there is no replacement quite as good as your own real thing. Help yourself keep yourself together.

ASTHMA

Asthma has as many causes as there are people. For better health, you need relaxed chest muscles, but the asthmatic's chest and upper back are loaded with the trigger points that cause spasm and make breathing harder to accomplish simply because of the terrifying strain they have worked under for years. The stress is ever present in the form of apprehension. "When will an attack come again?" "Will this breath be my last?" "Is there enough air in the whole world?" Myotherapy, used at the onset of an attack, has been known to abort it. Used between attacks it can make the next one less arduous. Used during an attack it helps ease the muscles and keep them from turning more muscles into bands of steel. See *chest* in the Pain Chart; in addition, as you lie in bed or watch TV, do the Myotherapy pattern for the chest and pay particular attention to the trigger points along the breast bone and the collar bones.

BACK PAIN

The best way to look at back pain is to view it as merely back pain and not as something mysterious or esoteric. There are numerous muscles in the back, and the back is used enough to provide plenty of simple reasons for pain in the form of trigger points. True, the spine is somewhere in there, but we have been brainwashed to believe that most back pain comes from the spine. Chiropractors are taught that just about everything unpleasant comes from the spine. This is simply not so. A way of life has caused the American backache which afflicts between 65 and 85 percent of the population. The active Austrian population had a 10 percent rate of back pain when I tested there; it may be higher now, as they've achieved a higher level of affluence, but it could never approach ours, because the Austrian is trained from early childhood to *walk*. If you don't walk from necessity, walk for pleasure and health. It is the cheapest and safest medicine in the world. Get rid of the pain, and then stick with the exercises.

BELL'S PALSY
Myotherapy works for Bell's palsy. Check the Pain Chart for *facial pain* even if there isn't any pain there. The trigger points that cause pain for some people can cause numbness, tingling, weakness, and lack of control for others. The cause is the same even when the effects are different.

BONE SPURS
See Spurs, Bone.

BUNIONS
Bunions are caused by a long second toe. Long before thinking "operation," try the "cure" suggested on page 150. In addition, rid your overtaxed feet and legs of trigger points and kick off your shoes as often as possible.

BURSITIS
"Bursitis" is the name usually given to shoulder pain. The treatment is often injections of cortisone. The pain is in the shoulder, but the cause is very rarely the bursa, a little sac containing lubrication for the joint. The real cause is usually spasmed muscles in the arm, chest, upper back, and axilla (armpit), which tell you where to look for trouble.

CARPAL TUNNEL SYNDROME
This is a comparatively new name for wrist and hand pain. The operation usually performed for this condition consists of reaming out the osseofibrous passage for the median nerve and the flexor tendons. It rarely works because the real trouble is usually somewhere else—in the muscles of the shoulder and upper arm. Before you try an operation try Myotherapy to the arm.

CELLULITE
Cellulite is an expensive word for *fibrositis* which came first, but is a controversial word. What both stand for is the thickened flesh that appears on the thighs, hips, shoulders, and upper backs, mostly of women. It is stress-related and, of course, diet-related: if you eat a lot, those are the places that are waiting for it. Different from abdominal fat pads, which are more like what you clean out of your chicken (!), fibrositic (cellulitic) fat is hard. It requires pinching massage and exercise (see *Pain Erasure*, in Sources).

CEREBRAL PALSY
Cerebral palsy is a motor disorder which appears before the age of three. Muscles cannot be made to do what they should. The earlier Myotherapy is applied, the better the results. Remember that Myotherapy helps ease mus-

cles that cannot ease themselves at any age.

CERVICAL ARTHRITIS

Most of us have arthritis in our spines by the time we get into the after fifty crowd, but as it says under Arthritis, treat it as a pain in the neck, think of it as a pain in the neck, and get rid of your pain in the neck. (That was said that way advisedly. Do you have a "pain in the neck" around the house?)

CHEST PAIN

Chest pain is just that, yet every man feeling a pain in the chest, even on the wrong side, will think, "My heart!" Most women think, "Cancer . . . there's got to be a lump!" A pain in the chest means check it out and when heart, lungs, and breast have been okayed (but you *still* have chest pain) think, "I have a pain in my chest *muscles*." Check *chest* in the Pain Chart.

CIRCULATION

See the Pain Chart for *arm* and *leg pain*. The same spasm-causing pain also limits circulation. See also Dizziness.

CLUSTER HEADACHES

Quite the worst kind of headache. See the Pain Chart for *headaches*.

COLON, SPASTIC

A spastic colon means a bellyache—not a stomach ache. Lower down. That same pain is sometimes blamed on adhesions.

CONSTIPATION

A nursing home was amazed to discover that it had a surplus of ten thousand dollars in its drug budget at the end of the year. Since there had been no change in the clientele, it investigated the cause of the good fortune. A new dietician had added fiber to the diets, and that was it. The patients had not required laxatives—which to my mind are one of the chief curses of America. Fiber and exercise, especially pelvic exercises, should put more money back in your pocket and a bloom on your cheek.

CUBITAL TUNNEL SYNDROME

See Elbow, and leave the high-priced operation alone until you have tried everything else.

DIABETES

Diabetes is a nasty disease that puts about two million people in the hospital each year. The people I know who have handled it best *exercise* every day. Exercise is like a prayer in reverse; mostly we say, "Dear God, help me; if you do I will. . . ." That's unsmart. It would be better to say, "Lord, I'm doing my part, do you have time to look over the results?"

About 20,000 diabetes patients are said to suffer from leg and foot cramps. Cramps slow circulation, and if there is one thing a diabetic can't afford, it's poor circulation. See the Pain Chart for *leg* and *foot pain;* see also Dizziness. Eyesight is another problem for diabetics and you don't need impaired circulation to the head. See Eye exercises.

DISCS OR DISKS

These are the cushions between the vertebrae. We have already discussed them in relationship to back pain. When you are told you have discogenic disease (slipped disc, degenerated discs, etc.), it's quite possible; most people do.

However, it is rarely the cause of your backache. Check the Pain Chart for back pain.

DIZZINESS

First of all, don't think "brain tumor" when you suddenly get dizzy for no reason. Think about the fall from the horse, the wrestling team in college, the whiplash last year that "only" gave you a stiff neck. See the Pain Chart for *neck pain* even if yours doesn't hurt.

DUPUYTREN'S SYNDROME

See Hand Pain.

ELBOW PAIN

There are many ways to get elbow pain but the most common is overwork. The carpenter or electrician with his screwdriver or the dental hygienist with her scaler are good examples. If you understand that the elbow, like the knee and shoulder, are at the crossroads of busy intersections of muscles, and that any one of those muscles, like roads, can be closed off to cause trouble at the intersection, you will be safer. Stop thinking "joint" (unless you just dislocated it) and think "muscles pulling on it."

EMPHYSEMA

Emphysema means your lungs have been affected to the point where they don't draw in enough oxygen. If you take the trigger points out of the intercostal muscles between the ribs, your chest will relax somewhat and make more room for the lungs to expand. (See the Pain Chart for *chest pain.*)

EYE STRAIN

Sometimes eyes play tricks: they blur, burn, itch, and ache and you can't separate the lines of print when you try to read. When the doctor says you have no pathology and you should rest your eyes, think exercise. There are several eye exercise systems available, and the Bates System is one of the better ones. While you are investigating exercise systems use Myotherapy for the neck, head, face, chest, upper back, and arms. (See the Pain Chart for *eye strain* even if your eyes don't hurt.)

FACIAL PAIN

Facial pain is sometimes called *neuritis*, sometimes *tic douloureux* or *trigeminal neuralgia* (which is the same thing). All are awful and all respond to Myotherapy, although you may need a Myotherapist to help you. Those trigger points hide in the most unlikely places. For more information read *Myotherapy* (see Sources). Check your memory for a slap or blow to the face or even a box on the ear. Perhaps some recent dentistry turned it on.

FIBROSITIS

See Cellulite.

FINGER PAIN

Finger pain, unless you just whapped one with a hammer or closed the car trunk on it, probably comes from high in the arm, shoulder, or armpit. "Arthritis" may well be present, but it is rarely the reason for constant pain. Palliative measures will ease the discomfort, but until you find the trigger points causing the muscle spasm, pain will continue. There is a condition found in fingers and toes called *tingling* or *numbness* or a combination which we call *"numbling."* This usually has the same cause as pain: muscle spasm.

Treat the condition like pain and don't think "pinched nerve in the spine." See also Trigger Finger.

FLAT BACK

This is a posture fault covered in the Taking Stock section (page 67). See the Problem Chart for exercises (page 172).

FLAT FEET

These are covered in the Taking Stock section. See the Problem Chart for exercises.

FOOT PAIN

There are a lot of names given to foot pain such as *plantar faciitis* which is foot sole pain, or *heel spurs*. Keep in mind that whatever the name for a pain, it is still a pain, and look up the area. Feet and toes begin in hips and groin, so don't be surprised when the Pain Chart starts your search for cause in those areas—you have every reason to hunt there if you want to get rid of the pain, weakness, imbalance, and "aged walk."

FRACTURE

Any fracture leaves trigger points in residence. Spend a little time doing Myotherapy around yours even if your trigger points are quiet and giving you no trouble.

GALL BLADDER DISEASE

It's bad enough when you really have it. Sometimes you don't. The same kind of pain can be caused by extreme stress. The pain is usually in the stomach area and upper back. If Myotherapy gets rid of the problem permanently, you may avoid the X-rays you don't need. See if you can erase the pain; at the same time look around and say, "*Who's* the matter with me?" (See the Pain Chart for stomach *chest* and *back pain*.

GOUT

This is a form of arthritis and can spoil your day. Before you settle for that diagnosis, however, do Myotherapy to the entire foot while avoiding the painful big toe joint. Do the entire leg with special attention to the calf. Give the leg a day of rest, and repeat.

GROIN PAIN

This pain is usually a sign that abdominal, back, and leg muscles are in spasm. It is another muscular crossroads being tugged at by several muscles, some coming from opposite directions. Groin pain ruins lots of athletic careers because trainers don't know what to do about it.

For the after fifty crowd, groin pain comes on sneakily. See the Posture section on bent-over people (page 98). Check with the Pain Chart and do lots of groin stretches.

HAMMERTOE

This often accompanies a long second toe, which has been covered extensively since it is responsible for extensive damage. See *foot pain* in the Pain Chart.

HAND PAIN

Chronic pain in the hand, or finger pain, usually stems from trigger points in the arm. If the injury is recent, use the same system to clear the arm of spasm and to increase circulation, which speeds healing. There is a condition called Dupuytren's syndrome which is a contracted state of the fingers and palm due to injury of the palmar fascia. You probably developed the condition by pounding can openers into cans; you can hardly miss it. The tendons foreshorten and you cannot lay your hands flat on a surface either to get up or down, or to do push-ups. Do the work suggested on the Pain Chart, and stretch the hands back by pulling on the fingers whenever you think of it.

For "Arthitis of the hands" consider the diagnosis to be "Hand pain." See the Pain Chart.

HANGOVER
A hangover is a headache from drugs or alcohol. In the alcohol crowd it is often referred to as being "hung over." Among druggies who know they are druggies, it's called "crashing." Among druggies who don't know they are druggies, it's called by whatever problem for which they are taking medicine. By whatever name, it is a form of poisoning with very unpleasant side effects.

HEADACHE
The only pain problem that comes close to backaches in number is headaches. They are dangerous because, aside from opening up the head and taking a peek, there is little help available but drugs. There are warnings connected with head pain, but very few headaches signal tumor, aneurism, fracture, or hematoma. If you've had a concussion, you will be watched very carefully until any danger is past. Once pathology has been ruled out, treat a headache for what it is—a pain in the muscles strapped over and around your head. See Pain Chart.

HEARING
When was your last hearing checkup? If your hearing is suffering—which will be much worse in the next generation's time due to noise pollution—beat the mythmakers (and sundry friends and relatives who will whisper to others, "Speak a little louder, she's hard of hearing, you know") and get a "deaf button," politely known as a hearing aid. Myotherapy often improves hearing when some lack is due to poor circulation and spasm. (See also *headache* in the Pain Chart.)

HEART
This is the star actor of our particular show right now. When our parents were the after fifty crowd there wasn't nearly as much heart disease around, partly due to diet and exercise, but also due to the fact that the diseases that have been vanquished in our lifetime carried so many of them off. Our parents ate "real" bread, ingested few additives, breathed less pollution, and exercised. With a little more protection, a lot of them would still be with us, lasting until we got the sense to see them as they really were . . . and to thank them for the things we were too young to realize were gifts.

There've been a lot of bad "heart" years lately, but it's getting a little better, except for the women who (and I will *never* understand this) have taken up smoking. We can make it still better for the after fifty crowd with more attention to diet and exercise. Just don't put all your exercise eggs in one basket. Running may be "in," but it's not "it." Vary your program every day and listen to your body. That's something runners do *not* do and the first sign of a heart attack that they might have listened to, has been sudden death. See the Pain Chart for *chest, arm, back, groin, leg, arm,* and *neck pain.* (Did I miss something? If I did, find the spot and apply

Myotherapy to that area—your heart labors to serve all of you.) There need be no pain; just check for trigger points. As you already know, trigger points can be quiet as mice until your stress level reaches the boiling point.

HEARTBURN

This is an uncomfortable burning sensation in the chest which can rise right up to your ears and make it impossible to lie flat. It is often referred to as "indigestion" and sometimes confused with hiatus hernia. Your pharmacist will offer you half a dozen antacids which aren't all that harmless. A better way to handle and prevent heartburn is to apply Myotherapy to the areas in question and their neighbors.

HEART PAIN

See Chest Pain.

HEART SURGERY

This is another specialty of our time and one which grows in controversy. Once you've had it, the controversy ends, but the chest, neck, upper back, and even head pains may linger on. If the job was a bypass, the sites of the removed veins are also prone to pain. See the Pain Chart for the areas still causing discomfort.

HEMORRHOIDS

Myotherapy can't "cure" hemorrhoids, since they are varicosed veins. However, it has been known to ease the pain.

HERNIATED DISCS

This is another way of saying "slipped" or "degenerated" and probably means muscle spasm. Unless there is some *very* unusual reason, your doctor will prescribe rest and exercise before sug-

gesting surgery. If that is not the case, get a second opinion. If exercise *is* suggested, ask if you may try Myotherapy.

HERPES ZOSTER

Terribly painful when in action—and Myotherapy doesn't help then. Later, however, it does. Check the Pain Chart for the area that hurts.

HIATUS HERNIA

If the diagnosis is right, that is one thing. If it isn't, then there's a good chance Myotherapy will get rid of the pain (see Heartburn).

HIGH BLOOD PRESSURE

This is one of the stinkers for the after fifty crowd. The disease is bad enough, but some of the medications are worse. Exercise does bring down high blood pressure, and weight loss combined with a salt-free diet helps. Myotherapy may also help. We found that patients having Myotherapy done on legs for low back and leg pain brought their blood pressure down dramatically by the third session. It stands to reason that when the spasm in the huge gluteus muscles and quadriceps in the legs is relaxed, the heart has a much easier time pushing blood along. Do prescribed seat, groin, and leg exercises. See the Pain Chart for these areas.

HIP PAIN

Hip pain is gruesome. At first, it is just ache and limitation, but if it is going to progress to the hip-replacement stage, we usually put it off long enough to become drug-sick and exhausted. The famous phrase "Pain will dictate" is right, but don't wait too long. Myotherapy can keep the pain within bounds and prevent drug sickness and addiction, but your best bet is "Aqua-ex" (see page 345). If you have Myotherapy done before and after a hip operation (avoiding the suture line) recovery is faster. For more information, read the section on hips in *Pain Erasure* (see Sources).

HYSTERECTOMY
Even done vaginally, this operation leaves a scar somewhere. If there is abdominal pain administer Myotherapy to the groin and gluteus muscles as for low back pain and menstrual cramps.

JAW PAIN (TMJD)
Jaw pain is mostly called TMJD.

The main point to remember about jaw pain or TMJD is that even if it comes as a result of a pop on the jaw, dentistry, or controlled fury, it is attached to the groin and the seat—that's where you start hunting trigger points!

"JELLING PAIN"
That's the kind of stiffness you encounter after sitting for a long time. It is also ornately described as "post inertial dyskinesia," which means the same thing, but looks far more impressive. What it amounts to is sedentary living, not age. Get cracking with your program ... daily.

KIDNEY PAIN
A kidney problem can contribute to muscle spasm. If you can ease the muscles of the back with Myotherapy, so much the better. Who needs multiple pain? Sometimes the pain in the lower back is not due to kidney spasm, but to aerobic dancing and other strenuous exercise. Always question tests and procedures, and know that group physicians order *twice as many* tests as do physicians working alone. Results,

however, are the same. See Pain Chart for *back pain*.

KNEE PAIN
The knee is another crossroads where many muscles pull on a joint and cause pain in the joint. Ask yourself: what could pull on my knee? Then detrigger those muscles.

KYPHOSIS
That's a *really* round back. The pain will be in the upper back, but the cause can be found in the chest and arms. Check the Pain Chart for those areas.

LEG PAIN
The pain may be *felt* anywhere along the leg and the trigger points can be anywhere, too. Remember for your trigger point hunt that the muscles tie into the pelvis and start high in the groin and seat.

LONG SECOND TOE
See page 148 and Figures 56 through 59 for suggested treatment.

LUPUS ERYTHEMATOSUS
Our patients who do best with this autoimmune disease do so with exercise and small amounts of aspirin. Systemic lupus erythematosus causes dysfunction of many organs, including the heart and kidneys. Myotherapy works well with any pain connected with the disease that we have seen. It is especially useful in correcting the leg spasms that are drug-induced and that cause ulcers, leg and foot pain, and swelling. See the Pain Chart for the area needing attention.

MASTECTOMY
There are now several choices when it

comes to mastectomy operations, but for most of the after fifty crowd there was only one—radical surgery, which left painful swelling and scarring. Check with the Pain Chart and do the exercises.

MENIER'S DISEASE
See Dizziness.

MENISCUS
Check Knee Pain and don't think cartilage—think muscle spasm. For more information, see the book *Myotherapy* (listed in Sources).

MIGRAINE
Migraine is a headache ... period. While more men have cluster headaches, more women have migraines. When we work to get rid of clusters, they often progress to the migraine stage before they give up and go away. Medication is the conventional way of handling migraines, but Myotherapy has been successful with most of the ones we have seen and we see them by the hundreds. See the Pain Chart for *head,* and don't make your self-image turn you into a "Migraine invalid." There is also the "WHO's the matter with you?" question to be asked.

MULTIPLE SCLEROSIS
There is no "cure" yet for MS, but we have had great success with Myotherapy and exercise. Once the muscles are clear of spasm, they begin to obey again. The exercises are essential and those patients who do best, exercise as though their lives depend on it ... because they do. Use the Pain Chart and look for spots that hurt. The sooner you start exercising (after diagnosis), the better.

NECK PAIN
Neck pain is usually due to an old injury which may have occurred as long ago as birth. Such an injury can cause all sorts of problems—pain, stiffness, dizziness, jaw, eye, ear, and tooth pain, difficulty in swallowing, hoarseness, laryngitis, facial pain, wryneck, torticollis—you name it, your neck can be at the bottom (or the top) of it. Check with the Pain Chart and after you have taken care of your neck, see which symptoms are left and then follow up on them.

OBESITY
That's a pretty general problem in America, and, yes, it is a disease. And, yes, it can shorten your life, and, yes, it can make life difficult, and, no, it's not all that hard to lose weight. Crash diets don't work, but you already know that. What you may not know, however, is that every time you quickly take off weight and just as quickly put it back on, you make it harder to lose the next time. Follow the directions of a reputable diet plan, plus the right exercise, and the extra weight will come off.

OSTEOPOROSIS
This is one for the after fifty crowd.

Osteoporosis is a thinning of the bones, which become brittle and breakable. Much of it is preventable. The prevention lies in calcium and exercise. Also, check any tight muscles that might be pulling anywhere. You can become knock-kneed, bow-legged, bent over, pulled sideways, or short. It will be up to you, so check with the exercises and get started.

PARKINSON'S DISEASE
Myotherapy will help with pain and

loss of balance which accompany this degenerative brain disorder. Exercise helps, plus it helps overcome the despair. Keep in mind that any day now there could be a "cure," and you want to be as high on the ladder as possible when that day comes.

PIGEON TOES
Feet turn in when the muscles in the hips and insides of the legs are in spasm. Do the Myotherapy and then the exercises, even if your legs don't hurt.

POLIO
The danger of polio is past for most people, but those who contracted the disease when younger still have the trigger points set into the muscles. These trigger points cause pain, decrease in height, poor coordination, and deteriorating balance. They can set the individual up for a fracturing fall which could cause loss of calcium and muscle atrophy. Handle each pain using the Pain Chart as reference.

RAYNAUD'S DISEASE
That's described as intermittent attacks of ischemia of fingers or toes and sometimes ears or nose. Ischemia means "deficiency of blood to a part due to functional constriction or actual obstruction of a blood vessel." Muscles in spasm do exactly that. They constrict everything from blood vessels to nerves to lymph glands. If your fingers turn pale and are constantly cold, you have a constriction. Mine used to do that when I was in the water too long, but since we have used Myotherapy on my arms it no longer happens. Ask yourself, "When did I injure that arm or that leg?" Another question: "What

drugs am I on?" Drugs, too, cause constriction. Do Myotherapy on and exercise those body parts that seem to be constricted.

ROTATOR CUFF
This is usually in pain due to an old football or hockey injury, but it can also be hurt in an auto accident or fall. See the Pain Chart for *shoulder pain.*

SACROILIAC PAIN
See the Pain Chart for *back pain.*

SCIATICA
This pain usually begins in the lower back and radiates down the leg. It is rarely due to a "pinched nerve" anywhere near the spine, but rather a squeezed sciatic nerve in the seat muscles. See the Pain Chart for *back* and *leg pain.* This can be quickly treated.

SCOLIOSIS
This is a lateral curve or curves in the spine. Very fixable for your beloved grandchildren, and certainly a condition that can be rendered painless for you. See the Pain Chart for *back* and *groin pain.*

SHIN SPLINTS
Pain in the front of the lower legs often signals the presence of shin splints, usually caused by abuse or exercise without preparation. They are thought to be caused when muscle tears away from bone, but actually it's your old friends, trigger points. See the Pain Chart for *leg pain* and then look at what you are doing for yourself. If you are "aerobic hopping," change your program before you get so discouraged you give up on fitness.

SHOULDER PAIN

Shoulders, like knees and elbows, are crossroads where many muscles meet. Check the Pain Chart to get rid of the trigger points and then do the exercises *often* to prevent the return of *trigger points,* should your sport or occupation bring them on.

SKIER'S THUMB

This thumb is something many skiers have as souvenirs of their wilder trips down snowy slopes. They come to us because our thumbs were either dislocated or subluxated (not quite dislocated) by the ski pole straps when we fell at high speeds. The trigger points are in the arms as well as in the areas around the thumb joints.

SPURS

Spurs here and there are scare words. If you are told you have bone spurs on your spine or heels, the pain you are having for whatever reason begins to feel even worse. One patient who came to me had been told that her neck spurs were so bad they could cut her spine, and she had to wear one of those awful collars for the rest of her life and was afraid to move. It took fifteen minutes to get rid of the spasm that was causing the pain. The "spurs" are usually rounded and couldn't cut cheese. The ones on the heels usually shut up once the trigger points in the calves have been neutralized. Treat spur pain as "pain" and see the Pain Chart.

STROKE

Here's another biggie that has been on the decline of late, but even so, general conditioning should always be on our minds. If you walk across the street and are hit by a car, your chances of sur- vival depend on the help you get, the speed with which you get it, the extent of your injuries, *and your general condition at the moment of impact.* You can't decide you need a better muscu- lature as you bounce off the fender. Strokes, too, demand that you be in combat-ready shape, because illness, like injury, is a form of combat.

If you have been "hit" with a stroke, the road back should start *in your head.* Even before you can lift a finger, *see* yourself lifting that finger. Give whole speeches in your head and *feel* the words in your mouth. As soon as you can, get at the Bed Ballet and Gym in a Chair and Round the Clock Exercises on pages 278–330. When the doctor says, "Full range of motion," ask for My- otherapy. Naggers who know what they are talking about, get their way far more often than do "veggies" who don't want to bother anybody. When you, your parent, or your friend gets to the leg dangle stage, you'll need three chairs to change sitting posture. Don't just lie there in bed all day waiting for meals or a bed pan; get cracking and start exercising, if only with one hand, one foot—or an idea.

TARSAL TUNNEL SYNDROME

This is similar to carpal tunnel syn- drome, only it occurs in the foot. See the Pain Chart.

TEETH

There are a couple of ways to help pre- serve teeth: one is to have the plaque removed often (I go to the dentist every three months). The second is to keep the circulation to the jaws flowing by administering Myotherapy to your neck, head, and face. A general exercise program is far more important than those funny face exercises, so often suggested by today's exercise teachers. About 45 percent of all Americans have lost all or most of their teeth from gum disease by the age of sixty. Prevent that.

TENDINITIS
Tendinitis is a compound word, *tendon* plus *itis* which means inflammation. It means that there is something wrong with *something* in an arm or leg as a rule and that something hurts. You are covered with muscles and tendon-muscle attachments, and chronic pain usually means there is pain due to spasms caused by trigger points. See the Pain Chart for the part or area that hurts.

TENNIS ELBOW
See Elbow. "Tennis elbow" is merely a name for a place that hurts.

THORACIC OUTLET SYNDROME
That's another "new" name for shoulder pain and calls for a truly dramatic operation. *Thoracic* pertains to the chest; in this case, nerve trunks are compressed, leading to pain in the arms, paresthesia (numbness or tingling), and *Raynaud's* disease, which you know as cold hands and/or feet. Check the Pain Chart for *shoulder pain* and you'll know just what to do. Add *chest pain* for good measure, and always remember that "heroic measures" means *you* are the hero!

TINNITUS
Tinnitus is the sound of ringing, hissing, clanging, even roaring that seems to come from inside the ear. Actually, most of it is caused by trigger points in muscles adjacent to the ear, or others at some distance. Anything that might cause jaw pain might also cause tinnitus. An operation, especially one connected with large muscles like the SCM (sternocleidomastoid) in the neck, or muscles connected with the neck in any way, could contribute to tinnitus. Violinists or cellists who contort their bodies to support their instruments are susceptible. So are the players of reed instruments who must do the same thing to facial muscles.

Although tinnitus doesn't cause pain, it is intensely annoying, especially at night when day noises are still. Use the Pain Chart; you will be referred to the Myotherapy pattern for the neck. To those trigger points, add a ring of them completely surrounding the ear, about ¼ inch apart.

TMJD (TEMPOROMANDIBULAR DYSFUNCTION)
See Jaw Pain.

TORTICOLLIS
Torticollis is neck spasm. Babies are often born with the potential for it, and even a mild whiplash accident can get it started. Treat it as *neck pain* on the Pain Chart.

TRIGGER FINGER
One finger or another cocks inward and cannot be stretched. Looking for the cause in the finger is a waste of time. Cutting the tendon for release is a waste of finger. Check the Pain Chart for *arm, armpit, shoulder,* and *upper back*. The most likely place for a trigger point will be on the inside of the upper arm.

VARICOSE VEINS
You can thank one or both parents for these since they are hereditary; you were born with faulty valves in the

veins. When these valves are efficient they allow blood to flow back toward the heart with ease. When the valves break down, the blood pools and the veins become stretched like old rubber bands. Leg muscles in spasm make it even harder to get the blood back up into the body, the veins then swell, break down further, and become limp cords. For health reasons as well as for cosmetic ones, keep the legs free of spasm so the veins can lie flatter. See the Pain Chart for *leg*, *groin*, and *lower back pain*.

WHIPLASH

This is an injury to the neck, but since the neck is a part of the head, face, chest, shoulders, and arms, a whiplash can cause pain in any of these areas. If I say it often enough you will remember that the neck is also in communication with the seat and groin muscles. See the Pain Chart for all of the above mentioned parts and areas.

WRIST

See Carpal Tunnel Syndrome.

EMERGENCY MEASURES FOR WRIST AND ANKLE

The preceding section listed physical problems of an everyday nature. For the after fifty crowd, some of the most common problems incurred are sprains to the wrist and ankle. Here are some steps to follow when treating sprains.

IMMEDIATE MOBILIZATION SERIES

Immediate mobilization is what you use when the doctor has said the wrist or ankle is not really busted, merely strained or sprained. It is also what you use if the wrist or ankle were ever strained or sprained and is still swollen, weak, or painful. A sprain is a temporary dislocation after which the damaged joint goes back to its normal position, but the sinews holding and operating it have been damaged. There is usually leakage of blood from torn vessels and it is this leakage which gives the injured joint its carnival col-

oring. The swelling comes from the activity of many trigger points all up and down the limb. These are activated whenever there is injury anywhere along the limb. The trigger points set up a clamor from shoulder to fingertips, if there has been an injury to fingers, hand, wrist, or elbow, work should begin in the shoulder. Forget the end of the road and remember that fingers and everything else in that arm begin in the shoulder and armpit. Remember, too, that the toes, foot, ankle,, and knee begin in the groin and the hip. Begin your work there. The object is to erase the trigger points causing spasm which is preventing fresh blood from reaching the injury in sufficient quantities for fast healing. The trigger points are also preventing the flow of body fluids from the injured area. In addition, the leaking blood and other fluids are compressed into the injured area causing swelling and pain.

FOR THE ANKLE

If you have ever sprained an ankle and had to walk on it, you know you could manage somehow. Everything was if not OK, at least functioning until you sat down. Then the ankle swelled quickly and became so painful you couldn't use it. While you were walking your muscles were squeezing the blood back up the leg in a fair semblance of normalcy. Once they stopped squeezing, fluids pooled. As pressure increased, movement decreased. What should be done?

Old-fashioned, conventional sports medicine would have you rest the ankle. What's wrong with that? You were doing fine *until* you rested. Then sports medicine practitioners would have you put ice on the ankle. Ice is nice, but it's only a palliative, and doesn't get at the cause of the present pain—trigger points in action. The third thing they will suggest is taping. That will further inhibit free flow of fluids and increase swelling and pressure . . . and pain. The last thing usually suggested is elevation which is what you have to do if you did those other three things. What *should* you do?

Let's say you've turned your ankle. Your first move would be to take the trigger points out of the hips and groin and all four sides of both the upper and lower leg. For this you really do need the help of a friend, although it can be done with a bodo. Be sure to get all the trigger points adjacent to the ankle. Do the foot and then you will have to approximate what the leg did while walking. The muscles must be helped to squeeze the fluids out of the injured area. Pain and swelling will begin to decrease before you even reach the ankle. Then point the toe downward, upward, inward and outward. If there is pain, find the trigger point causing it. Then exercise with a friend.

Resistance Exercises for the Ankle

- Pronation. Your friend supports the ankle at the heel and places his or her fist against the ball of your foot. You then press the foot down against resistance. Resistance must not be so hard that you can't push, nor so light as to prevent a real squeeze of the muscles. Do this four times.

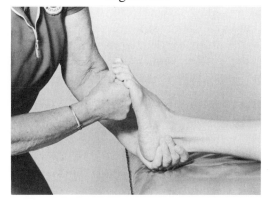

Figure 61.

• Supination. Still supporting your heel, your friend places his or her hand across your instep as you pull your toes upward toward your nose. Alternate with Pronation four times.

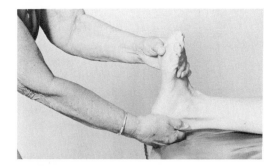

• Inward Rotation. Still supporting your heel your friend offers resistance to the inside of the front of your foot as you try to rotate it inward.

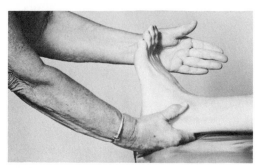

• Outward Rotation. Have your friend apply pressure to the outside of the foot as you try to rotate outward. Alternate four times.

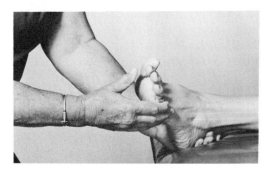

You may have to go through this series twice to get rid of enough fluid for comfort. If a friend is not there when you damage your ankle, use the self-administered resistance exercises on page 150.

Another reason to do Myotherapy after an ankle is sprained is to get going again. You never want to be in a dependent position if you can help it.

• Stand with both hands resting on a table and feet together.
• Do *gentle* half knee bends, eight for a start. If there is still pain, look again for the trigger point causing it. It will probably be in the calf.
• Then do some *gentle* toe rises.
• Now sit down and elevate your legs.
• Every five minutes do the foot exercises you started with.
• In an hour, repeat the resistance exercises.
• You may have to do this series every hour on the hour. It's a small price. You should be walking pain-

lessly (though colorfully) the next day. Even if the insurance company is paying your doctor bills, how much is your time worth? Wouldn't you rather be busy about your life than waiting in a doctor's office?

FOR THE WRIST
Suppose you've sprained your wrist. First, get the trigger points out of the armpit, the shoulder, and down the entire arm. Then do these resistance exercises.

Resistance Exercises for the Wrist

- Pronation: Lay the damaged arm on a table for stabilization. Press the fingers down against the resistance afforded by the other hand.

Figure 62.

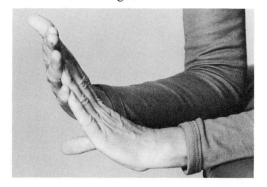

- Supination: Place the fingers of the good hand on the backs of the fingers of the sprained one and lift them against resistance. If a spasm announces its presence with a pain anywhere in the arm, stop and erase it with Myotherapy. (See hand pattern on page 142.)

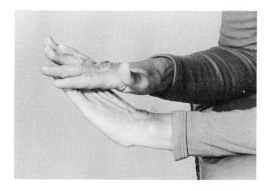

- Inward Rotation: Place the uninjured hand against the inner side of the injured hand and provide resistance as the hand is pressed inward toward the median line. Then do the next exercise

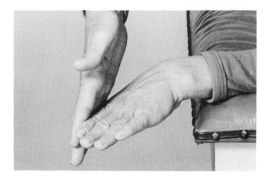

• Outward Rotation: Place the uninjured hand along the outside edge
of the injured one and provide
gentle resistance as the hand is
turned outward. Alternate with the
above (inward rotation) four times.
Do these exercises every hour
throughout the day.

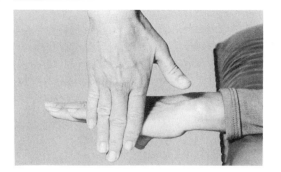

IT'S TIME FOR ACTION

The chart that follows will tell you
which Myotherapy patterns to use for
each problem and which exercises you
should put into a daily program. After
you've filled out your pain chart and
planned your course of action, you'll
want to go and discover what your occupation and your sport are doing to
you (as well as for you!).

If you have only a few pains and minor limitations, your program will not
be a difficult one. If, however, you were
forced to let yourself go for a long time,
as I was, through immobilization or injury or illness, you may feel despair,
particularly if you look back at your
Take Stock section and see that the road
ahead is a long one.

Don't despair. Select something—

one area—that you want to improve,
and work on just that. I began with sit-
ups (for abdominal strength) and side-
lying flexibility (following Myotherapy
to the seat). At first, my knee was eight
inches from my nose. Both of them now
touch, but it took months. I really
wanted to be able to walk—the way I
used to, mile after mile. I can do that
now, but that, too, took months. I rev-
eled in each small improvement—and
so will you.

Take three steps:

1. Basic to your program is *painless-
ness*. That is where you begin. Start
with the Pain Chart and do the recommended Myotherapy patterns and the
easiest of the exercises—and take it
from there.

Figure 63. PAIN CHART

Pain	Map Figure #	Myotherapy
AMPUTATION, LEG	21, 25	22, 23, 26, 27, 28 Do Myotherapy to the entire stump
AMPUTATION, ARM or HAND	40, 44, 45	21, 22, 23, 28 Do Myotherapy to the entire stump

2. Next in importance is repairing the current damage that's been done, probably by your occupation or your sport. Check the Occupation Chart (page 198) and see what it is doing to you and what exercises you will need to do on a daily basis. Then, check the Sports Chart (page 214). You need to be protected at play, too. Do not give your sport up; that's not what life is all about. Just protect and prevent.

3. Finally, work to prevent future damage. Assemble your whole picture by mastering your pain, occupation, and sports. Go back to Take Stock and check your posture, weight, measurement, and diet statistics.

One last reminder: Myotherapy doesn't "cure" anything. What it does is get rid of pain, improve circulation, and make it possible for your body to get at its very important task—that of making and keeping itself well. Your body *can* do this—with a little help from you!

Your first concern is to relieve your pain wherever you feel it. Do not be discouraged by the name of your pain, the prognosis, or what happened to Cousin Mae or Uncle Roger. This is a new time and you have a new tool in your hands. Remember what they said about the horseless carriage—it would never catch on? Myotherapy *has* caught on and you might as well be one of the first to "own one"—an educated elbow, thumb, and knuckle.

Once you have rid your muscles of the trigger points and done the exercises that have been given with each Myotherapy pattern, add the suggested exercises. You will also find additional exercises that apply to each problem. You can't do everything in one week and probably not in several months, but with time and trying, you will find what works for you and what you enjoy the most. Then you will have a program tailored just for you.

If you will watch TV or listen to music while you do Myotherapy (on yourself, on someone else, or while someone else is doing it to you) the pain will be less irritating. Remember, take it easy—you have time. Trigger points hurt the most the first time you disturb them. It gets easier with every succeeding session. I do Myotherapy when something hurts, but I exercise every day to prevent pain. As you try for ever higher levels of fitness, you may be a little stiff. Use Myotherapy on those stiff spots every day and follow with warm-ups.

Myotherapy Exercise	Exercise #	Extra Exercise #
7, 8, 10	25, 27, 31, 33, 37, 38, 44, 45, 49, 51, 52, 54	Chair exercises Walker series Weight training series
9, 13, 14	21, 22, 23, 24, 28, 30, 62	None

Pain	Map Figure #	Myotherapy
ANGINA	See CHEST	
ANKLE	21, 25, 49, 51	22, 26, 27, 28, 50
ARM	29, 36, 40, 44, 45	Do trigger point work as shown on Map 44, 45 also 24, 32, 37, 38, 39, 41, 43, 46
ARTHRITIS	Go by the pain, not the name, and do the trigger point work according to the maps for pain. Follow with corrective exercise.	
ASTHMA	21, 40	24, 31, 32, 41
BACK	21, 25	22, 23, 26, 27, 28, 32
BELL'S PALSY	29, 30, 36, 40	24, 31, 34, 35, 37, 38, 39, 41
BUNIONS	See LONG SECOND TOE	
BURSITIS	See SHOULDER	

Myotherapy Exercise	Exercise #	Extra Exercise #
See CHEST		
7, 10, 18, 31	20, 117, 118, 119, 120, 121, 122, 123	Foot massage (p. 292) Foot exercise (p. 296)
11, 13, 14, 15	21, 22, 23, 28, 30, 35, 83	Pulley exercise Towel exercise Weight training exercise
Exercise according to tolerance		
9, 13, 14	Any, according to tolerance	Chair exercises Floor progressions
7, 8, 10	1, 2, 5, 33, 35, 36, 37, 40, 42, 43, 106, 107, 108, 109	Floor progressions
9, 11, 13, 14, 15	Do all arm and hand exercises	Chair exercise
See LONG SECOND TOE		
See SHOULDER		

Pain	Map Figure #	Myotherapy
CARPAL TUNNEL		See WRIST
CEREBRAL PALSY	Do Myotherapy work and exercise according to spasticity and pain	
CERVICAL ARTHRITIS		See NECK
CHEST	21, 40, 44, 45	12, 22, 23, 24, 32, 41, 42 Do all the trigger points in the arms and in the arm pit
CIRCULATION		See ARM and LEG
COLON, SPASTIC	21, 25	26, 27, 28
CONSTIPATION		See COLON
CUBITAL TUNNEL		See ELBOW
DIABETES	21, 25, 30, 36	22, 26, 27, 28, 31, 37, 38, 39, 49, 51 Do Myotherapy to the entire leg and foot on both sides

Myotherapy Exercise	Exercise #	Extra Exercise #
See WRIST		
Exercise according to tolerance		
See NECK		
7, 8, 9, 11, 12, 13, 14, 15	21, 22, 23, 26, 30, 35, 62	Chair exercises Floor progressions Pulley exercise
See ARM and LEG		
10	1, 2, 3, 4, 5, 8, 27, 37, 47, 56, 106, 107, 108, 109, 140	Chair exercises
See COLON	32, 33, 35, 36, 40, 44	Chair exercises
See ELBOW		
7, 10, 11, 15	27, 31, 39	Floor progressions

Pain	Map Figure #	Myotherapy
DISCS or DISKS	See BACK	
DIZZINESS	See NECK	
DUPUYTREN'S SYNDROME	See ARM	
ELBOW	44, 45	Do all trigger points in the arms 43, 46, 47
EMPHYSEMA	See BACK and CHEST 40, 41, 42	
EYE STRAIN	30	31, 34, 35, 37, 38
FACIAL	29, 30, 36	24, 32, 34, 35, 37, 38, 39, 41
FINGER	Remember that the fingers begin in the shoulders and arms See ARM and SHOULDERS	
FLAT BACK	See FLAT BACK in Posture Chart	

Myotherapy Exercise	Exercise #	Extra Exercise #
See BACK		
See NECK		
See ARM		
15	13, 14, 21, 22, 23, 35	183, 187, 188, 189, 190, 191, Weight training, Elastics
12, 13	See BACK and CHEST	
11	All upper body exercise to improve circulation	
11, 13, 14	Do all arm and hand erercise to tolerance	
See ARM and SHOULDERS		
See FLAT BACK in Posture Chart		

Pain	Map Figure #	Myotherapy
FLAT FEET	See FLAT FEET in Posture Chart	
FOOT	21, 25, 49, 51, 56	22, 23, 26, 27, 28 Do all trigger points in the legs and feet
FRACTURE	See location of the pain and then do the trigger point work above and below the injury	
GALL BLADDER	21, 25	22, 23, 24, 26, 27, 28
GOUT	See LEG	
GROIN	21, 25	22, 23, 26, 27, 28
HAMMERTOE	See LONG SECOND TOE	
HAND	See FINGER	
HANGOVER	See HEADACHE	

Myotherapy Exercise	Exercise #	Extra Exercise #
See FLAT FEET in Posture Chart		
7, 8, 10, 20	Foot Massage (p. 292) and Foot Exercise (p. 296)	All floor progressions
See location of the pain and then do the trigger point work above and below the injury		
8, 9, 10	1, 2, 3, 4, 5, 21, 22, 23, 25, 26, 27, 28, 32, 33, 106, 107, 108, 109	All chair exercises
See LEG		
7, 8, 10	19, 25, 27, 31, 33, 37, 39, 42, 83, 84, 90, 91	All floor progressions
See LONG SECOND TOE		
See FINGER		
See HEADACHE		

Pain	Map Figure #	Myotherapy
HEADACHE	21, 29, 30, 36	24, 31, 32, 34, 35, 37, 38, 39 See also CHEST, BACK, and ARMS
HEARING	See HEADACHE	
HEART	See CHEST	
HEARTBURN	21, 25, 36, 40, 44, 45	22, 23, 24, 26, 27, 28, 31, 32, 37, 38, 39, 41, 42, 43, 46, 47
HEART SURGERY	See CHEST. Treat trigger points along site of operation.	
HEMORRHOIDS	21, 25, 49, 51	22, 26, 27, 28, 50, 53, 54 Pay special attention to #19 and to the floor of the pelvis
HERNIATED DISCS	See BACK	
HERPES ZOSTER	See affected area	
HIATUS HERNIA	See HEARTBURN	

Myotherapy Exercise	Exercise #	Extra Exercise #
11	None	None
See HEADACHE	None	None
See CHEST		
7, 8, 9, 10, 11, 12, 13, 14, 15	All chest and back exercises to tolerance	Pulleys Chair exercises Floor progressions
See CHEST		All chair exercises and floor progressions as tolerated
7, 10, 25, 35	1, 2, 4, 5, 18, 34	All chair exercises, often
See BACK		
See affected area		
See HEARTBURN		

Pain	Map Figure #	Myotherapy
HIGH BLOOD PRESSURE	See LEGS, BACK, and GROIN	
HIP	21, 25, 49, 51, 56	22, 23, 26, 27, 28, 53, 54 Do any other area of pain in addition to the above
HYSTERECTOMY	See BACK and GROIN	
JAW (TMJD)	21, 25, 29, 30, 36, 40, 44, 45, 49, 51, 56	22, 23, 24, 26, 27, 28, 31, 32, 34, 35, 37, 38, 39, 53, 54
KIDNEY	See BACK	
KNEE	21, 25, 49, 51	22, 26, 27, 28, 50, 53, 54
KYPHOSIS	See ROUND BACK in Posture Chart, Figure #12	
LEG	25, 49, 51	Do all the trigger points on all three maps
LONG SECOND TOE	56	57 Erase all trigger points from Maps 51 and 49

Myotherapy Exercise	Exercise #	Extra Exercise #
See LEGS, BACK, and GROIN		
7, 8, 10	1, 3, 5, 18, 21, 22, 23, 24, 25, 26, 27, 31	All chair exercises All floor progressions as tolerated
See BACK and GROIN		
7, 8, 9, 10, 11, 13, 14, 15, 19	All warm-ups 21–30	Pulley Floor progressions
See BACK		
5, 7, 18	82, 86, 118, 120, 121, 123	31, often Stairs
See ROUND BACK in Posture Chart		
10, 18, 19, 31	20, 25, 33, 34, 36, 38, 42, 46, 58	All chair exercises All floor progressions as tolerated Stairs
20, 57, 58, 59	29, 57 All foot massage All foot exercise	All floor progressions

Pain	Map Figure #	Myotherapy
LUPUS	Do Myotherapy according to the pain. Follow with the appropriate exercise.	
MASTECTOMY	21, 25, 36, 40, 44, 45	22, 23, 24, 26, 27, 28, 31, 32, 37, 38, 39, 41, 42, 43, 46 and all around the edges of the scar.
MENIER'S DISEASE	See NECK	
MENISCUS	SEE KNEE	
MIGRAINE	See HEADACHE	
MULTIPLE SCLEROSIS	See areas of pain, weakness, and dysfunction	
NECK	21, 29, 30, 36, 40, 44, 45	22, 23, 24, 31, 32, 34, 35, 37, 38, 39, 41, 42, 46
OSTEOPOROSIS	Use gentle exercise to all areas, increase to toleration	

Myotherapy Exercise	Exercise #	Extra Exercise #
According to the site of the pain		
7, 8, 9, 10, 11, 13, 14, 15	21, 22, 23, 26, 28, 30, 31, 83	Pulley exercises Weight training
See NECK		
See KNEE		
See HEADACHES		
	See areas of pain, weakness, and dysfunction, and follow with the exercise that goes along with the Myotherapy patterns	
7, 8, 9, 11, 13, 14, 15	Same as Myotherapy exercises	Chair exercise 125, 126, 129, 130, 131, 132
	Use gentle exercise to all areas and increase to toleration	

Pain	Map Figure #	Myotherapy
PARKINSON'S DISEASE	See areas of pain, weakness, and dysfunction	
PIGEON TOES	21, 25, 49, 51	22, 26, 27, 28 Do every trigger point on the inside and middle lines All points in 49 and 51
POLIO	Do Myotherapy according to the areas of pain, weakness, and dysfunction. Follow with the exercise that goes along with the Myotherapy patterns.	
REYNAUD'S DISEASE	See ARM	
ROTATOR CUFF	See SHOULDER	
SACROILIAC	See BACK	
SCIATICA	See BACK; also work the trigger points on the outside of the leg	
SHIN SPLINTS	21, 25, 49, 51	26, 27, 28, 50 Do Myotherapy to all sides of the leg

Myotherapy Exercise	Exercise #	Extra Exercise #
See areas of pain, weakness, and dysfunction, and follow with the exercises that go along with the Myotherapy patterns		
5, 7, 10	49, 51, 65, 70, 71, 75	Chair exercise Bed exercise 98 All floor progressions
See area of pain, weakness, and dysfunction, and follow with the exercises that go along with the Myotherapy patterns		
See ARM		
See SHOULDER		
See BACK		
See BACK		
18, 19, 20	Same as Myotherapy exercises	All floor progressions except skips or jumps

Pain	Map Figure #	Myotherapy
SHOULDER	Use Tests 14, 15 and Maps 21, 29, 30, 36, 40, 44, 45	22, 23, 24, 31, 32, 34, 37, 38, 39, 41, 42 Plus all trigger points to be found in the armpits
SKIER'S THUMB	See ARM and HAND	
SPURS, BONE	See Myotherapy according to the area of pain. Follow maps and exercise directions.	
STROKE	See Myotherapy according to the pain, spasticity, weakness, and dysfunction. Follow with the Myotherapy patterns.	
TARSAL TUNNEL	See LEG	
TEETH	See JAW (JMJD)	
TENDINITIS	Do Myotherapy according to the pain and dysfunction. Follow with the exercises that accompany the myotherapy patterns.	
TENNIS ELBOW	See ELBOW	

Myotherapy Exercise	Exercise #	Extra Exercise #
7, 8, 9, 11, 12, 13, 14, 15	21, 22, 23, 26, 28 Straps 183	165, 166, 167, 168, 170 Towels 172 and 174 Straps 183 All pulley exercises Weight training
See ARM and HAND		
Do exercises according to pain area and tolerance		
Do exercises according to pain, spasticity, weakness, and dysfunction. Follow recommended exercises often throughout the day.		
See LEG		
See JAW (TMJD)		
Do recommended exercises according to area of pain		
See ELBOW		

Pain	Map Figure #	Myotherapy
THORACIC OUTLET	21, 29, 30, 36, 40, 44, 45	24, 31, 32, 41, 42
TINNITUS	See HEADACHE and NECK	
TMJD	See JAW PAIN	
TORTICOLLIS	See NECK	
TRIGGER FINGER	See HAND	
VARICOSE VEINS	See LEG, GROIN, and LOW BACK	
WHIPLASH	See NECK	
WRIST	21, 40, 44, 45	Do trigger points in the entire arm 22, 41, 43, 46, 47, 48

Myotherapy Exercise	Exercise #	Extra Exercise #
7, 8, 9, 10, 11, 12, 13, 14, 15	15, 21, 22, 23, 26, 28, 32, 35	All pulley exercises Weight series to tolerance
See HEADACHE and NECK		
See JAW PAIN		
See NECK		
See HAND		
See LEG, GROIN, and LOW BACK		
See NECK		
13, 14, 15, 16, 17, 20	43	Weight training

OCCUPATIONS

There is no such thing as retirement from history, and your occupations are part of your personal history. Every one of them has laid down *trigger points*. Every one of those points has the potential to cause you chronic pain. Next to each occupation in the following chart are the Myotherapy patterns most likely to be needed, the exercises that should become part of your daily program, plus Extra Exercises you might enjoy. Be sure to check the chart on page 198 for *each* occupation you've had throughout your lifetime, and then check the Pain Chart for the location of the pain.

ACCOUNTANT

Accountants sit at desks, lean over, drop their heads, strain their eyes, round their shoulders, foreshorten their hamstrings, and often grind teeth or tighten jaw muscles. In April many of them get pains in their stomachs.

ACTOR

These people are always under stress, whether they are on the ladder to success and working overtime to get higher, at the top and working hard to stay there, or trying to make up their minds where they want to be, should be, or ought not to be. It's exciting, fun, wonderful . . . and devastating. Any sport or accident will come back to haunt actors as their stress levels rise. One of their chief dangers is the drugs that will get them through a performance. Myotherapy may save some of our future greats from needing the Betty Ford Center by making the drug/alcohol support unnecessary.

ARTIST/ARTISAN

People who use their hands for demanding or repetitive work will usually develop chronic pain. See the Pain Chart for *hand, arm, and finger pain* and be kind to your body, the one that allows you your skill.

ASSEMBLY LINE OPERATOR

What did you do when you worked on the assembly line? Did you stand a lot? That means leg, groin, and low back pain now. Did you sort things or pull levers? That may be the reason for your "arthritis." Whatever the action, it could be the reason for your distress right now. Think about it and consult the Pain Chart.

BABY TENDER

Half of us were baby tenders. That means back strain. We lifted babies off the floor, we lowered them onto potties and into cribs, we grabbed them away from danger, and we lugged them everywhere. Check for both *back* and *shoulder pain* in the Pain Chart.

BARTENDER

Bartenders, whether male or female, will have the same trigger points suffered by those in any profession that requires standing for long hours. In addition, people who have worked in bars have listened a lot to people in pain. There is also the stress of rush hour and the need to be quick and pleasant to the customer. What you did as a summer job to get you through college can come back as chronic pain fifty years later. Check the Pain Chart for what hurts.

BOOKKEEPER

See Accountant.

BUS BOYS AND GIRLS

My daughter Suzy was a bus girl at the Log Cabin in Lenox, Massachusetts. The trays gave her back pain but she refused to quit. She was seventeen. She still has occasional back pain from those trays and only Myotherapy gets rid of it. Many of you could trace your pain that far back and come up with the same answer . . . heavy trays. See the Pain Chart for *back* and *shoulder pain* that now is called "arthritis" and for which you may be taking dangerous and unnecessary drugs. See also Cook.

CARPENTER

It doesn't matter whether carpentry was an occupation or a hobby; if you did enough of it, there are trigger points somewhere in your body. The usual places for the after fifty crowd, who used a saw and a screwdriver before there were many electrical tools, will be in the working arm. Of course, if something heavy got away from you and you rescued it with brute strength, the trigger points will be in the back, usually the mid-back (see #11.) Stop thinking "age" and start thinking "bacon and how you got it in order to bring it home."

CLEANER

It doesn't matter whether we cleaned house for ourselves or for someone else, the after fifty crowd did a lot of furniture moving, floor scrubbing, and waxing. When I got married I had a vacuum cleaner, an iron, and my mother-in-law's second-hand washing machine. The dryer was the clothesline. Will you ever forget six-foot-long sheets frozen solid? But they *smelled* better than anything we have today. The trigger points you picked up were put there by whatever you did most and whatever strained you most.

COMPUTER PROGRAMMER

See Secretary/Office Worker. Such workers have the same problems and often the same jobs. The only difference is the video screen, which makes the pull on the neck a little different from the one caused by copying from shorthand.

COOK

Cooks, like other restaurant workers, have back, leg, and foot pain. Check also for long second toe.

DANCER

See section on Sports.

DELIVERY BOYS

Our generation did a lot of odd jobs and delivery boys were very important when there were no family cars, shopping malls, or supermarkets. You went to the market with a list, or you phoned, and sure enough, a boy would arrive with your groceries. Those boys now have back and shoulder pain, all of which can be neutralized. Check the Pain Chart for the location of the pain, not its name.

DENTAL HYGIENIST

See Dentist, but also Electrician. The action of scaling teeth is the same as that needed for a screwdriver; both cause "tennis elbow."

DENTIST

Of all the people in the health field, dentists suffer most. They stand or sit at an awkward angle, their arms are held at an awkward angle, their patients do not love them, but are afraid of them. Dentistry is doing the same thing that medicine is doing: doctors are going in for group practice, and dentists for assembly line dentistry. Both interfere with the doctor-patient relationship which means *stress*. Dentists have low back pain almost to a man or woman. They also suffer (or will) from arm and shoulder pain.

DRIVER

Sitting in a car, bus, cab, truck, tractor, van, even an airplane requires a limiting position for the entire body and repetitive motion. The bus has a motion secondary to driving; that of opening the door. The truck needs a lot of clutch as the driver shifts both up and down. The tractor requires strength, and anything pushed through city traffic or the Los Angeles Freeways spells stress. Don't think age; think pain. Trigger points are usually found in the shoulders, arms, lower back, and quite often in the hamstrings.

ELECTRICIAN

Electricians often have "tennis elbow" (which tennis players rarely have, although they have "Little League shoulder" from serving). The rotation of the wrist, while using tools, causes the damage. See *elbow* and *wrist pain* in the Pain Chart.

ENGINEER

This is a desk worker, drawing board worker, and executive all rolled into one. Go for the pain in the back and shoulders and do everything possible to stretch hamstrings and chest muscles and strengthen abdominals.

FARMER AND RANCHER

Nature never really cuts out for the day; there's always more to do and none of it can be laid aside. These sturdy, hard-working people usually cannot touch the floor with their fingertips and many cannot turn their heads around to back up the car or truck. The Pain Chart will tell you how to get rid of sundry pain; the stretch exercises should be done daily.

FIREMEN

Whether they are active and collecting trigger points or retired and collecting pensions, firemen have a real potential for back pain—and very localized at that. They have tugged those huge hoses up ladders and stairs and around corners. They have rousted and wrastled them into improbable places and carried people down, out, and away. Never are they free from the stress of fear unless they are foolish, and firemen are not foolish. Fighting fires seems to attract a special breed of men. When was the last time you heard of a fireman in a scandal? Probably never. But they do get hurt. Many of our trained Myotherapists work with them on special exercises designed to make them not only strong, but agile. Firemen must be in shape *now*. If the fireman is over fifty he must get back into shape. He could be needed any time, for anything and he wouldn't have a moment's hesitation about getting into it. That means *be prepared*.

GARDENER

Gardening is three things in one: a hobby, a sport, and a good way to feed your family pure food. There are more people gardening today than engaging in any other "sport." Spring is backache time and more people "discover" they have "arthritis" between April and June than at any other time. Both backache and "arthritis" can be prevented. Real arthritis can't be prevented (yet), but pain that is said to be "arthritic" can be.

Gardening, like skiing and any other demanding sport, should be prepared for. You set up an exercise program that prepares the muscles that will be used and then, when you start the real gardening, you start easy. In addition, you garden "smorgasbordly" . . . with a watch: Rake the yard for ten minutes and not a minute longer. Carry the debris away; ten minutes. Spread fertilizer; ten minutes. Dig up the garden; ten minutes. Break up the clods and rake it smooth; ten minutes. Now sit in the sun for ten minutes admiring your work. That's an hour. Go in the house and do the side-lying exercise #7 on page 125. A few hours later you can repeat that performance if you are up to it. Every hour for the rest of the day do the side-lying exercise. You'll be stiff the next day, but not crippled. Check with the exercises and pain patterns at the end of this chapter. Keep to the "smorgasbord" pattern all summer and even carry it to freezing and canning. When your vegetables come up, pick enough for dinner plus three other dinners. Cook and freeze, or can, a little every day rather than slave over a hot stove for a week. By the time you must, you can.

HAIRDRESSER
Hairdressers have one of the most stressful jobs there is. They have awful schedules and must produce a work of art every hour. They eat badly and off schedule, they breathe hair lacquer, pick up hair dye by osmosis, *and they stand* with blood pooling in their legs.

They also hold their arms forward and their backs slightly bent, their shoulders rounded, and their heads bent. Not many things are worse. Since the job is the killer and the job is all day, it must be combated all day with exercises designed for the purpose. Don't forget, you can suffer from your job twenty, even thirty years *after* you have closed the shop door for the last time and moved to a warm climate where the only tourist you have to contend with is you!

HORSE TRAINER/RIDER
There are all kinds. Some horse people are as rich as Croesus and some work for them, but oddly enough, both do similar work. My neighbor is a horsewoman who owns a spread that would make a Kentucky bluegrass colonel turn green with envy, but this morning I met her on my trail. She had spent 3 months showing horses, getting up at 4 A.M., and getting to bed after midnight. Horses, like farms and ranches, belong to Mother Nature who doesn't keep shop hours. Also, *all* horse people have been thrown, one time or fifty. Check the Pain Chart. (A reminder: Myotherapy works on horses, too.)

HOUSEWIFE
Housewives are women of many trades, all of them hard. When *we* were housewives, and half of us were, we did the whole thing: washed, waxed, swept, vacuumed, dusted, polished, cooked, had the children, and cared for them. We were den mothers, Little League rooters, shoppers, gardeners, chauffeurs, carpenters, and painters. To discover what category your any-kind-of-pain-at-all comes under, look at the Pain Chart.

MANICURIST

Manicurists are usually bent over in later years. They have all the disadvantages that go with desk work, with the addition of having listened to other people's troubles. A really good manicurist is an artist of sorts and appropriately overworked. Check the Pain Chart for *back, shoulder, arm,* and *neck pain.*

MASON

Masons overlift and generally end up with low back pain. They, like sculptors, clobber their hands and fingers which could cause everything from carpal tunnel syndrome to cluster headaches. See the Pain Chart and clear suspicious areas.

MASSAGE THERAPIST

Massage has taken on new life in America—and high time. Masseuses and masseurs are now called massage therapists; they deal with people who are often in pain. They use their arms, hands, and shoulders, and most have shoulder and arm pain. In time, low back pain will be added. For people with such jobs, ongoing exercise is essential, as is a once-a-week session with Myotherapy.

MEDICAL PROFESSIONAL

Medical professionals are more at risk than their patients. Nurses lift heavy, often helpless patients and stand or walk all day on cement-under-tile hospital corridors. Surgeons stand on the same surface and lean forward. Lab workers perch on stools and peer into microscopes. Psychologists and psychiatrists sit all day and absorb others' pain. Medical professionals are beginning to understand the relationship between physical fitness and improved emotional health, but rarely apply this understanding to their own health. The aches will vary according to the demands made by the profession.

MUSICIAN

Musicians are at risk from the day they first lay hands on their instruments. Guitarists suffer from arm and shoulder pain which can take in wrist and fingers. While we were doing a study using biofeedback, Arlo Guthrie allowed us to apply the biofeedback machine to his shoulder and arm muscles after he had done his best to relax the muscles for a half hour. The machine registered over 20 microvolts at each part of his arm and shoulder. Half an hour of Myotherapy brought the tension in those muscles down to 4 microvolts. Harpists suffer the same syndrome, with the addition of low back and some leg pain. Organists and pianists, like secretaries, have upper back and shoulder pain that often refers to their hands. In addition, they have leg pain due to pedal work. Pianists are also like dentists, their pain invariably attacks their low back and neck areas and the spasms may even force their fingers to curl. Players of woodwind instruments will not be surprised to find that their jaw muscles are involved, but may be surprised to learn that groin and seat muscles are vulnerable. They also suffer from shoulder, arm, and hand pain. String instruments pose a variety of problems. Low back pain is quite usual, as is arm, shoulder, and neck pain, and mock angina. One of the worst things I ever saw was at a talk I gave for one of the world's greatest orchestras. Two violin players appeared with leather slings supporting their arms. What was their problem? They had arm and shoulder pain. What did the slings do? They limited *all* motion to the very motion that was causing the pain—playing. What would the outcome be? The loss of a career. Myotherapy done at the first twinge would have prevented the pain and in addition, often improves the skill.

NEWSBOY
Chronic pain is not dependent on what you did last week, but rather what you did last year, ten years ago, forty years ago, or even at the time of birth. The paperboy who wore a canvas bag that pulled on his shoulder, and threw folded papers up onto porches every day for years, may now find his arm stiff and aching. Check the Pain Chart and remember the actions that might have caused your pain. Muscles never forget an insult.

PAINTER
House painting calls for overhead brushing, standing on ladders, moving ladders, balancing, and repetition year after year. There is usually shoulder and leg pain, especially in the lower legs. The pain feels like shin splints because it *is* caused by shin splints.

PHOTOGRAPHER
Photographers carry heavy equipment and add insult to injury by standing *in* cement-floored darkrooms many hours of every day. They are also under the same stress as accountants and artists—the need for perfection.

PLUMBER
Plumbers do heavy work, but threading pipe is what usually gets them into trouble. They often have chest pain which feels like a heart attack. Take the trigger points out of the chest muscles, shoulders, and arms.

POLICE
We have already mentioned the firefighter who faces an emergency with every muscle cold and tense. Police officers must also maintain a high rate of fitness while active and should be aware that the job hurts many muscles over the years. Rather than think "arthritis" or at least a dozen other names for pain, think "police work" and check the Pain Chart.

SALESPERSON
Selling is part birthright, part acquired skill, and part compulsion. In any event, stress is attached to it. If on top of the stress, you insult muscles with long hours of standing, long hours of driving, and long hours of paperwork, there will ultimately be pain. Keep in mind that your selling days might have been when you were twenty. Low back and leg pain, foot pain, and even headaches can be tied to that long-ago job.

SECRETARY/OFFICE WORKER
Any job that limits daily action is as dangerous as digging up the street with a power drill. The only difference is that when you do small, repetitious work you damage small muscles which have direct connections to larger muscles. Together these muscles can cause very large pain.

SHIPPER AND HANDLER
This heading involves anyone who does or has done heavy work. They are the longshore men, the truckers, the people who work on loading docks, who fill the shelves of supermarkets, load the ma-

chines, and dig up the city streets. In other words, those who lift, shift, and carry, or who once did. There's no way of saying which job will cause which pain, but backaches are a pretty sure bet. Don't listen to those who say, "Never lift with your knees straight," or "Never sleep on your back or your front," or any one of a dozen old-time tales. Go to the Pain Chart and get rid of your trigger points, and your body will do whatever you ask it to, in whatever position you like best.

SINGER

Singers are musicians, except *they* are the instruments. Chest, upper back, shoulders, arms, hands, head, and neck will probably yield trigger points. Voices are very dependent on freedom from stress, so if yours sounds as if it is deteriorating, check your stress and then check the areas in the Pain Chart, even if there is no pain.

SOLDIER

Boot camp or basic training was hell. You survived, but many of you have left-over trigger points here and there.

Again, don't think "old soldier or sailor," think trigger points. As for the once wounded, old wounds often begin to talk about the weather. They are trigger point-loaded areas.

STEWARD/STEWARDESS

These workers are under constant stress. Handling the public is always stressful. Doing physical chores while unbalanced, such as handling trays from the aisle, picking them up, pushing the drink cart uphill from New York to Detroit, or any of a dozen chores done on a moving platform . . . will cause back pain to begin with. Menstrual cramps may get worse, and often lead to jaw pain and headaches. Problems with a long second toe will be aggravated. See the Pain Chart and have yourself "cleared" by Myotherapy once a month or once a week if necessary. *Remember . . . if you ever were in this line of work, take the same route.* Your muscles are still flying even if you aren't getting paid anymore.

TEACHER

This is certainly a stressful job, and one

Figure 63A. OCCUPATION CHART

Occupation	Map Figure #	Myotherapy
ACCOUNTANT	21, 25, 29, 30, 36, 40, 44	22, 23, 24, 26, 27, 28, 31, 32, 37, 38, 39, 41, 43, 46
ACTOR	Do Myotherapy according to pain. Follow with exercises that accompany the myotherapy patterns.	

that stays with you like everything else. The pain associated with the job is usually found in the upper and lower back, neck, and shoulders. You taught in the days when there was some sense to education and when reading and writing were important. If you still have a yen to teach, you are desperately needed. If you are wondering what to do "when you grow up," you may want to do some remedial work. It is needed even at the college level.

TELEPHONE OPERATOR OR USER

If the telephone is your job or ever was, there will be trigger points in your neck, face, lower and upper back, chest, shoulders, and armpits. Your legs will also have suffered from inaction. See the Pain Chart. Be sure to cover the work for *headache* even if you've never had one.

TELEVISION CREW

Whenever I do a TV spot, I almost never get away from the studio without "fixing" a cameraman's back or shoulder. Remember, the television crew almost always works on cement floors. That means painful knees, especially if you also jog or play a racquet sport. See the Pain Chart and get into condition to enjoy your job and your sport.

WAITRESSES AND WAITER

Doing such work was a great way to make money while you were in school or looking for your lifework; it was a good way to make a living. It was also murder on your back, shoulders, and legs.

WRITER

Writers are a special breed. They work at typewriters and word processors, but not always wisely. When the muse is on they roll, and that can be for ten, twelve, or more hours. Shoulders, neck, upper and lower back, arms and hands—all ache. See the Pain Chart and pay particular attention to the Extra Exercises. You *must* tie in your work habits with your preferred exercises. Tennis on the weekends simply will not be enough.

Myotherapy Exercise	Exercise #	Extra Exercise #
7, 8, 9, 10, 11, 13, 14, 15	1–6, 12, 17, 18, 12–31	Floor progressions Rope exercises Towel exercises Chair exercises
Do recommended exercises often and warm-ups before performance		

Occupation	Map Figure #	Myotherapy
ARTIST/ARTISAN	Same as for Accountant	
BARTENDERS	21, 25, 49, 51	22, 23, 24, 26, 27, 28, 32, 50
ASSEMBLY LINE OPERATOR	Same as for BARTENDER	
BABY TENDER	Do Myotherapy according to pain. Follow with exercises that accompany the myotherapy patterns.	
BOOKKEEPER	Same as for ACCOUNTANT	
BUS BOY and GIRL	21, 25, 29, 36, 40, 44, 45, 49, 51, 56	22, 23, 24, 26, 27, 28, 31, 32, 37, 38, 39, 44, 46
CARPENTER	Do Myotherapy according to pain. Follow with exercises that accompany the Myotherapy patterns.	
CLEANER	Do Myotherapy according to pain. Follow with exercises that accompany Myotherapy patterns.	

Myotherapy Exercise	Exercise #	Extra Exercise #
Same as for ACCOUNTANT		
5, 7, 8, 9, 10, 13, 14, 15	31 Plus all warm-ups	Floor progressions
Same as for BARTENDER		
Exercises recommended for painful areas		
Same as for ACCOUNTANT		
7, 8, 9, 10, 11	21, 22, 23, 24, 25, 26, 27, 28, 29, 30, 31	Floor progressions
Do exercises recommended after Myotherapy according to pain		
Do exercises recommended after Myotherapy according to pain		

Occupation	Map Figure #	Myotherapy
COMPUTER PROGRAMMER	Same as for ACCOUNTANT	
COOK	Do Myotherapy according to pain. Follow with exercises that accompany the Myotherapy patterns.	
DELIVERY BOYS	Same as for BARTENDER	
DENTIST	21, 25, 29, 36, 44, 45, 49, 51, 56	22, 23, 24, 26, 27, 28, 31, 32, 37, 38, 39, 44, 46, 47, 50, 53, 54
DENTAL HYGIENIST	Same as for DENTIST	
DRIVER	21, 25, 29, 36, 44, 45, 49, 51	22, 23, 24, 26, 27, 28, 31, 32, 37, 38, 39, 41, 42, 43, 46, 47, 50, 53, 54
ELECTRICIAN	21, 40, 44, 45	22, 23, 24, 31, 32, 41, 44, 46
ENGINEER	Same as ACCOUNTANT	

Myotherapy Exercise	Exercise #	Extra Exercise #
Same as for ACCOUNTANT		
Do exercises after Myotherapy according to pain		Chair exercises Floor progressions
Same as for BARTENDER		
7, 8, 9, 10, 11, 13, 14, 15, 17, 27	After each patient 13, 14, 15, 31 21–30 at end of day	Pulleys Floor progressions Chair exercises
Same as for DENTIST		
7, 8, 9, 10, 11, 12, 13, 14, 15, 17, 18, 19, 20	21–30 daily 31 often	Pulleys Towel exercise Chair exercises Weight training
7, 8, 9, 10, 13, 14, 15	Warm-ups 21–30 daily	Pulley exercise Rope series
Same as ACCOUNTANT		

Occupation	Map Figure #	Myotherapy
FARMER and RANCHER	Do Myotherapy according to pain. Follow the exercises that accompany the Myotherapy patterns.	
FIREMEN	21, 25, 29, 40, 44, 45, 49, 51	22, 23, 24, 26, 27, 28, 32, 41, 43, 46 Do Myotherapy according to pain and to prevent spasm during emergency
GARDENER	Same as for FIREMAN	
HAIRDRESSER	See BACK, ARM, GROIN, SHOULDER, and LEG in Pain Chart. Follow with exercises that accompany the Myotherapy patterns.	
HORSE TRAINER/ KEEPER	See SHOULDER and do Myotherapy according to any other pain. Follow with exercises that accompany the myotherapy patterns.	
HOUSEWIFE	Do Myotherapy according to pain. Follow with exercises that accompany the Myotherapy patterns.	
MANICURIST	Same as for ACCOUNTANT	
MASON	Same as for ELECTRICIANS	

Myotherapy Exercise	Exercise #	Extra Exercise #
Recommended exercises following Myotherapy		
7, 8, 9, 10, 11, 13, 14, 15, 18, 19	31 often 21–31 at least once daily	Pulleys Weight series Floor progressions
Same as for FIREMAN		
See BACK, ARM, GROIN, SHOULDER in Pain Chart		
See SHOULDER		
Do warm-ups 21–31 and floor progressions often throughout day		
Same as for ACCOUNTANT		
Same as for ELECTRICIAN		

Occupation	Map Figure #	Myotherapy
MASSAGE THERAPIST	Same as for ELECTRICIAN	
MEDICO	Do Myotherapy according to pain. Follow with exercises that accompany the Myotherapy patterns.	
MUSICIAN	Do Myotherapy according to pain, BUT to prevent lessening of skill, do the chair exercises during rehearsals and do WARM-UPS daily.	
NEWSBOY	See SHOULDER in Pain Chart. Do Myotherapy according to pain. Follow with exercises that accompany the Myotherapy patterns.	
PAINTER	Same as for ELECTRICIAN	See SHOULDER and BACK in Pain Chart.
PHOTOGRAPHER	See BACK and SHOULDER in Pain Chart.	
PLUMBER	Same as ELECTRICIAN	
POLICE	Same as for FIREMAN	

Myotherapy Exercise	Exercise #	Extra Exercise #
Same as for ELECTRICIAN		
Try to get warm-up exercises 21–31 into daily schedule twice		
Try to use warm-ups 21–31 before and after performance		
See SHOULDER		
Same as ELECTRICIAN		
See BACK and SHOULDER		
See CHEST in Pain Chart.	Same as ELECTRICIAN	
Same as for FIREMAN		

Occupation	Map Figure #	Myotherapy
SALESPERSON	Do Myotherapy according to pain. Do warm-ups twice daily and #31 throughout the day. Follow the Myotherapy with exercises that accompany the Myotherapy patterns.	
SECRETARY/ OFFICE WORKER	Same as ACCOUNTANT	
SHIPPER AND HANDLER	Same as for FIREMAN	
WAITRESSES and WAITERS	Same as BUS BOY AND GIRL	
SOLDIER	Same as for FIREMAN	
WRITER	Same as for ACCOUNTANT	

SPORTS

Sports *must* be a part of your way of life. Sports can include—or rather start with—walking to the corner or doing the Ten Penny series, Gym in a Chair, even Round the Clock (see the next chapter). There is no one sport. Every sport does something for you and some sports do several things. *Every sport can cause injury*, too, and precautions should be taken to see that your old sports aren't the reason you hurt today. Then, when you are painless, you will

Myotherapy Exercise	Exercise #	Extra Exercise #
Do exercises according to Myotherapy applied. Do floor progressions at home.		
Same as ACCOUNTANT Chair series regularly		
Same as for FIREMAN		
Same as BUS BOY AND GIRL		
Same as for FIREMAN		
Same as for ACCOUNTANT		

be able to engage in the sport or sports of your choice without letting small injuries add up to a big one that puts you out of business. Read about all the sports, find yours, and then consult the Sports Chart on page 214, which gives you preparation exercises, exercises to improve your performance during the season, and exercises to make up for what the sport is *not* providing. Together these exercises keep your program balanced.

AEROBIC DANCING

Dangers: You need more of a warm-up than is usually provided. The floor should be checked. If there is cement under the rug or tile, don't sign up for the class. Dancing on this type of surface will be as bad as running on a road.

Usual Injuries: Calf cramps; shin splints; knee, ankle, and foot pain; low back and groin pain.

BADMINTON

Dangers: Be sure you are well warmed up. Most badminton players think a rally is a warm-up. Check the floor. Don't play on cement or, if you do, take the same precautions offered runners.

Usual Injuries: Wrist and arm pain; knee pain due to spasm in thigh muscles.

BASEBALL

You probably don't play a lot of that today, but if you do, *warm up*. If you are sitting on the bench waiting your turn, don't. Warm up, gently but constantly.

Usual Injuries: Shoulder and elbow. Watch for Dupuytren's syndrome in which the tendons of the palm start to contract.

BASKETBALL

If you are still playing in the backyard, watch out for ankle turns and sprained knees. Keep the leg muscles clear . . . *before* you go out. If you are still competing, warm up before the game. The others will think a little lay-up practice will do it. It won't.

Usual Injuries: Knees and ankles. If you have a long second toe, try the "cure" on page 149.

BIKING

More and more of us are taking up the sport. My editor bikes to and from work through New York's busy streets every day. Be sure to start slowly and if weather or something else keeps you out of the saddle for any length of time, start easy.

Usual Injuries: Calf muscle spasm, shin splints, low back and shoulder pain.

BOATING

Canoeing: Get in shape before the trip. For starters, you can take your paddle to the pool and paddle under water against resistance. Warm up before you push away from land or dock. Keep shoulders in good shape all year.

Usual Injuries: Shoulders and elbows, lower back.

Rowing: A rowing machine for year-round use is ideal preparation for the season. Failing that, use weight bags. Remember, chest muscles foreshorten. A good exercise is "Falling" into designated corners of the house, placing hands on the two walls to stretch the chest muscles.

Usual Injuries: Upper back, shoulders, and chest.

Sailing: In this sport you have sudden actions to contend with. Wind is an inconstant companion. Pulling on ropes can strain back, shoulder, and arm muscles even when the stance is firm. When the sea is up, it's something else again. Keep the muscles free of spasm against the day when strength is needed.

Usual Injuries: Neck, shoulder, and arm strain.

BOWLING

Bowling is one-sided so it requires exercises that will work both sides. When you look for exercises other than calisthenics to offset bowling, use a bilateral program such as swimming or rowing.

Usual Injuries: Hand, wrist, elbow, and shoulder strain; low back pain; right knee injury.

BOXING

Most boxers have shoulder and arm pain, but whenever you take a blow anywhere, just as whenever you stick a needle anywhere, you cause some damage. Damage heals and leaves behind the scar tissue that attracts trigger points. The boxer's "cervical arthritis" usually comes from whiplash at the end of a power-packed glove.

Usual Injuries: Jaw, neck, face, and head. When there is pain over the kidney area, try Myotherapy before undergoing cystoscopy.

CROSS-COUNTRY SKIING

See Skiing.

DANCE

Dance is the most demanding of any sport or performing art except gymnastics, which is half dance. Today there are many forms of dance available and many activities called dance which are not. Most of the after fifty crowd danced in some way. We had ballet, tap, jazz, "aesthetic" or "interpretive" (which would now be called "modern"), folk, acrobatics, and square. We were raised on rhythm and now it is going to pay off. We probably won't take ballet again, and acrobatics is for bones like green sticks, but there's a lot of good stuff out there. Modern, *if* the teacher is good, is probably the best form of dance for women. Tap is fun but doesn't do much to make the body supple. Jazz *dance* is different from "Jazzercise," so you had better look at both before signing up for either. Again, the quality of the workout depends on the teacher. Most dancers and dance teachers stretch before class. That is the best way to cause muscle pain, and should *never* be done. You know about warm-ups; do them instead. "Aerobic dance" isn't dance at all, and you really don't need to hop around for an hour. Walking will do as much for you and is far safer.

Usual Injuries: Calf muscle spasm, shin splints, knee pain, low back pain, and later, upper back pain.

DOWNHILL SKIING

See Skiing.

FENCING

Fencing is a lovely sport, but teachers often overlook warm-up exercises. It is a unilateral sport and needs bilateral sport or exercise to offset it.

Usual Injuries: Right knee pain due to overwork of the thigh muscles. Since the spasm is in the muscles, think Myotherapy rather than trouble in the knee.

FISHING

Fishing is a varied sport ranging from dropping a line off the bridge and hauling in snappers in September to fighting a huge swordfish off the Florida coast. Check the Pain Chart for what bothers you when you do your kind of fishing. The main thing is, the pain can be erased so you can enjoy whatever you want to do. Trigger points, not age, may get in the way. Don't let them.

GARDENING

This is covered in the section on Occupations. It is the fastest growing "sport" in America and probably one of the best. Its problem is that it, like swimming, is seasonal. Start thinking now of something to take its place when winter comes.

GOLFING

The better your physical condition, the better your golf game. With the exercise programs in this book you can drop many strokes from your game. Do your warm-ups *before* you put your ball on the tee.

Usual Injuries: Back (at the waist line), shoulders, and elbows. Occasionally a wrist.

HIKING

Hiking is like walking—excellent for you and one of the few sports that are unlikely to injure you in any way—*unless* you have trigger points which can be activated on a trail that is too ambitious for your condition. Again, be warned: start below what you consider your limit—way below. If you have had any pain such as a backache, a "trick knee," or an ankle that "bothers sometimes," get rid of the trouble-causing trigger points *before* you hit the trail.

HOCKEY

There are two places for this game and while ice hockey seems to go on into middle-age, most people give up field hockey after they get out of school. Hockey doesn't give up on its players, however, and many old injuries come back to haunt them. Get rid of your trigger points, and if you intend to play, remember your warm-ups.

HORSEBACK RIDING

There are many ways to use horses in sports. Trail riding, ring riding, western riding, hunting, polo, and dressage. The main problem is the occasional failure of the mount to negotiate something or a disagreement leading to a parting of the ways. Falls from horses are expected and can cause a variety of injuries. Check your old injuries against the Pain Chart. As far as fitness goes, the horse is the one who gets the workout but it's great fun to get from here to there astride. There doesn't seem to be an age limit, except for the horse.

ICE SKATING

Figure skating improves with practice and is something you can learn to do better and better. Ice skating, especially to music, is as good for the soul as it is for the body. The better you are, the easier it is, so don't use it as your only fitness program.

Usual Injuries: Falls leading to back pain. Trigger points in the adductors, the muscles on the inner side of the thighs.

MARTIAL ARTS

This is a new twist for the after fifty crowd. Kung fu, karate, and half a dozen other forms require much practice and self-discipline but yield great dividends, since they require very real effort and cannot be faked. You can proceed at your own speed and need not compete to feel good about your progress. Check the Pain Chart for old injuries before you start.

MOTORCYCLING

This is a great sport so long as you stay on the cycle. Racing is not recommended.

Usual Injuries: Low back. If you fall off, anything goes and it's usually your head.

MOUNTAIN CLIMBING
One of the nice things about being a member of the after fifty crowd is that endurance improves with years. Mountaineering is an ageless sport and once the desire to climb is born, it never seems to wane. Only one warning, and it is the same as for everything else: prepare. Climbing, backpacking, and cross-country skiing have one thing in common—you have to get back to where you started. Always be in better shape than the proposed trip requires, in case of an unforeseen emergency such as a storm.

RACQUET SPORTS
Spike sports, which require quick starts and stops, will put strain on knees and ankles. Like bowling and fencing, these are unilateral sports and require bilateral effort to balance them out. Remember to warm up, and that goes if you have been sitting out a couple of sets as well as just starting. See the Pain Chart and give special attention to feet and legs.

ROCK CLIMBING
Rock climbers are the elite of mountaineers and this is a jealous sport. It cannot be done for a couple of weeks in summer, or just once in a while. The rock climber risks his or her own life and that of someone else on the rope, and that's a responsibility all rock climbers know about. Calisthenics, weight training, and endurance work are musts all year long. There are no "usual injuries" that can be planned for. A fall is like an auto accident: it can

result in a bruise, or death, and everything in between. Check the Pain Chart for old injuries. The price for many years of utter joy, which usually hits in the after fifty years, is hand damage. Such pain responds to Myotherapy to the arms, chest, shoulders, and upper back.

RUNNING
There are many forms of running. Cross-country is best and safest, as it works for endurance and cardiovascular improvement yet does not damage legs. Any running on cement will do damage, but then any serious competition will cause damage, too. The trick lies in taking out all old trigger points *before* running and checking to see that new ones are erased *after* the run. Warm-ups before running are essential; save your stretches until afterwards. Alternate running with calisthenics and weight work. Marathon running requires the same program, only more intensive. Running indoors must be done in alternating directions at about 10 minute intervals. Check for a long second toe.

Injuries: Feet, legs, back, and groin.

SCUBA DIVING
Scuba diving is definitely an after fifty sport. It opens up whole new worlds as does its cousin, skin diving. The ability to swim is something most of us seem to have and all of us can get. Prepare with classes in the hometown Y and then take more classes when you reach your goal, which is usually a place like the Caribbean or the waters off Greece. Good general condition is required; attain that at home with your Myotherapy and exercise program.

SKIING, CROSS-COUNTRY
Get in shape by walking and then hiking in the hills. Arms can be prepared by working with weights. Trigger points will show up in chest muscle, lower back, and calves.

SKIING, DOWNHILL
Once a skier, always a skier, but if you have stayed away from it for any reason, bought new equipment, or had an injury or an illness, begin at the bottom of the novice slope and *climb*. Better still, start with stairs and calisthenics long before the season begins. Climb mountains, hike, carry a pack. Skill is only part of any sport. Condition is the other big part, and "ski conditions" are the joker in the pack. Mount Washington has claimed lives of the unwary every month of the year. Skiing in Tuckerman's Ravine is the thrill of spring in the blazing sun and a nightmare past imagining if the weather closes in.

Usual Injuries: "Skier's thumb" (dislocation or subluxation), from ski pole straps. Twisted knees have replaced twisted ankles since the newer boots were invented, though both are still possibilities. Shoulder injuries are another possibility—usually from a mishandled T-bar. Old fractures should be remembered, and any pain in their area called by its right name—"old fracture," not "arthritis." Arthritis may well be present, but it is rarely the cause of the pain.

SOCCER
The after fifty crowd doesn't go in much for soccer or touch football, and it's just as well. Nothing wrong with the sports, but unless you have time to work out hard every day, you will be stiff and sore after every game.

SPORTS CAR RACING
These are not only within the reach of the after fifties, we are usually very good at driving them. They *can* make you feel as if you are having an angina attack. If you change cars, get a new one, or over-do the driving, check out the chest pain, but don't have a heart attack worrying over the possibility of having one: it's probably over-work on the "pecs." You need strong arms and hands to drive a sports car.

Figure 63B. SPORTS CHART

Sport	Map Figure #	Myotherapy
AEROBIC DANCING	21, 25, 36, 49, 51, 56	22, 23, 26, 27, 28, 37, 38, 39 Do all trigger points on Maps 49, 51 and 56
BADMINTON	21, 40, 44, 45	22, 24, 32, 41, 43, 46 Do all trigger points on Maps 44 and 45 Do both armpits

Usual Injuries: Low back, arm, and shoulder strains.

SWIMMING

Swimming is thought to be the perfect all-around exercise. It isn't. It's good, however, and it's *the* sport if you are recovering from injury. (See Aqua-ex, page 345.) Serious swimmers, or people who have been competing swimmers at some time, often have arm and shoulder pain. Neck pain is not unknown, and the chlorine in pools is likely to irritate eyes. You can avoid both problems by wearing goggles and snorkel gear. Fins will provide the resistance you need for strength. As in biking or skiing, once you learn how, you can always do it, but be in shape for the adventure you undertake. I used to swim regularly across Peconic Bay when I was eleven, but I'd get in condition before I tried it now.

Usual Injuries: Chest, arms, and shoulders.

WEIGHT TRAINING

This sport has blossomed in the last years and now includes women. There are two basic rules: start easy and work up, and alternate with another form of sport such as hiking or swimming. You can begin with the weight bags. You are not going to try to become "cover boy or girl," so work for definition rather than bulk. That calls for many repetitions, using lighter weights. I work out to music, which keeps the movement fluid. If movement becomes jerky, the weight is too heavy.

Usual Injuries: Shoulders, chest muscles, and knees. The knee injuries are almost always thigh and calf muscle injuries, with the knees holding the bag. Clear out the trigger points before your workout.

Check the Sports Chart and find the sport you do and the ones you want to get into. The Pain Pattern will be marked with likely trouble spots left over from another time. Check out your muscles. Then you will find the exercises that will prepare you, *and the exercises needed during the season.*

Many people think that what they are doing a *lot* of is enough. Again, there is no single sport that is a complete workout in itself, except perhaps modern dance taught by a *real* teacher.

Myotherapy Exercise	Exercise/ Preparation #	Exercise/ Concurrent #
7, 8, 10, 11, 19, 20	Floor progressions Foot exercises 117–124 31, 82, 83	Weight training Warm-ups Flexibility
13, 14, 31	Floor progressions	Weight training Warm-ups Flexibility

Sport	Map Figure #	Myotherapy
BASEBALL	Same as for BADMINTON	
BASKETBALL	Same as for BADMINTON but add the following: 49, 51	50 Do all trigger points on Maps 49 and 51
BIKING	21, 25, 36, 40, 44, 45, 49, 51	22, 23, 24, 26, 27, 28, 31, 32, 37, 38, 39, 41, 42, 44, 46, 47, 50, 53, 54, 55
BOATING	21, 25, 40, 44, 45	22, 23, 24, 26, 27, 28, 32, 41, 43, 46, 47
BOWLING	21, 36, 40, 44, 45, 49, 51	22, 23, 24, 32, 41, 43, 46, 47, 50
BOXING	21, 25, 29, 30, 36, 40, 44, 45, 49, 51, 56	22, 23, 24, 26, 27, 28, 32, 37, 38, 39, 34, 35, 41, 42, 43, 46, 47, 50, 53, 54
DANCING	21, 49, 51	22, 23, 26, 27, 28, 50, 53, 54, 55
FENCING	21, 25, 29, 36, 40, 44, 45, 49, 51	22, 23, 24, 26, 27, 28, 32, 41, 43, 46, 50, 53, 54

Myotherapy Exercise	Exercise/ Preparation #	Exercise/ Concurrent #
Same as for BADMINTON		
18, 19	Foot work 110–123	Warm-ups Flexibility Floor progressions
7, 8, 9, 10, 13, 14, 15, 18, 19, 20, 31	12, 58, 82, 83	Warm-ups Flexibility
7, 8, 9, 10, 13, 14, 15	Weight training 160– 171	Weight training Warm-ups Flexibility Floor progressions
7, 8, 9, 13, 14, 15	Weight training 160–171 31	Pulleys Warm-ups Flexibility Floor progressions
7, 8, 9, 10, 11, 13, 14, 15, 18, 19, 20	Foot massage and exercise 110–123 Floor progressions Flexibility	Same as Preparation
1, 7, 8, 9, 10, 13, 14, 15, 18, 19, 20	24, 45, 46 Foot massage and exercise 110–123 Floor progressions Flexibility	Weight training Warm-ups Floor progressions Flexibility
7, 8, 9, 10, 13, 14, 15, 18, 19, 20	Warm-ups daily 1, 2, 3, 4, 31	Floor progressions Flexibility

Sport	Map Figure #	Myotherapy
FISHING	21, 40, 44, 45	22, 23, 24, 32, 41, 43, 46, 47, 50
GARDENING	21, 25, 44, 45, 49, 51	22, 23, 24, 32
GOLFING	21, 25, 40, 44, 45	22, 23, 24, 32, 41, 43, 46, 47 Do trigger points in armpits
HIKING	21, 25, 40, 49, 51, 56	22, 23, 55 Do all trigger points on Maps 49 and 50
HOCKEY	Same as for HIKING	
HORSEBACK RIDING	21, 25, 29, 36, 40, 44, 45, 49, 51	22, 23, 24, 26, 27, 28, 41, 43, 46, 47, 53, 54
ICE SKATING	Same as for HIKING	
MARTIAL ARTS	21, 25, 40, 44, 45, 49, 51, 56	22, 23, 24, 26, 27, 28, 32, 41, 43, 46, 47, 50

Myotherapy Exercise	Exercise/ Preparation #	Exercise/ Concurrent #
7, 8, 9, 13, 14, 15, 18, 19	Weights 160–171 31	Warm-ups Flexibility Floor progressions Weight training
7, 8, 13, 14, 15	Warm-ups Floor progressions 31, 35, 47, 50, 53	Weight training Warm-ups Flexibility Pulleys
7, 8, 9, 10, 13, 14, 15, 18, 19, 20	Foot massage and exercises 110–123 Stairs 175–180	Weight training Warm-ups Flexibility
7, 8, 9, 10, 13, 14, 15, 18, 19, 20	Floor progressions 70 through 78 and 82, 83	
Same as for HIKING		
10, 13, 14, 15, 18, 19, 20	Floor progressions	Weight training Warm-ups Flexibility Stairs
Same as for HIKING		
7, 8, 9, 10, 13, 14, 15, 18, 19, 20	Weight training Flexibility Pulley	Floor progressions Warm-ups Flexibility, continuous

Sport	Map Figure #	Myotherapy
MOTORCYCLING	Same as for BIKING	
MOUNTAIN CLIMBING	Same as for HIKING	
ROCK CLIMBING	21, 25, 40, 44, 45, 49, 51, 56	22, 23, 24, 32, 41, 43, 46, 47, 50
RUNNING	21, 25, 49, 51, 56	22, 23, 26, 27, 28, 50, 55
SCUBA DIVING	40	41
SKIING, CROSSCOUNTRY	21, 25, 44, 45, 49, 51, 56	22, 23, 24, 26, 27, 28, 32
SKIING, DOWNHILL	21, 44, 45, 49, 51, 56	22, 23, 50, 55 Do all trigger points on Maps 49, 51, 56
SOCCER	21, 25, 49, 51, 56	22, 23, 26, 27, 28, 50, 55 Do all trigger points on Maps 51 and 56

Myotherapy Exercise	Exercise/ Preparation #	Exercise/ Concurrent #
Same as for BIKING		
	Same as for HIKING but add 1, 2 Weight series 160 through 171	Same as for HIKING
7, 8, 13, 14, 15	Floor progressions Flexibility Weight series	Warm-ups 14, 15, 16 Flexibility
7, 8, 10, 18, 19, 20 Foot massage series	Foot exercises Foot progressions Flexibility	Weight training Warm-ups Flexibility Stairs
13, 14, 15	Warm-ups Weight Series 31, 32, 33, 35, 36, 37, 38, 39, 40, 41, 42, 43, 44, 45, 46, 47	Warm-ups Flexibility Stairs
7, 8, 9, 10, 11, 13, 14, 15, 18, 19, 20	Foot exercises Floor progressions Flexibility	Weight training Warm-ups Stairs Flexibility
7, 8, 18, 19, 31	Floor progressions Flexibility	Warm-ups Flexibility Stairs
7, 8, 10, 18, 19	20 Floor progressions Flexibility Stairs series	Weight trainig Warm-ups Flexibility

Sport	Map Figure #	Myotherapy
SPORTS CAR RACING	21, 25, 36, 40, 44, 45	22, 26, 27, 28, 37, 38, 39, 41, 43, 46
SWIMMING	21, 25, 44, 45, 49, 51	22, 23, 24, 32, 43, 46, 50 Do arm pits
WEIGHT TRAINING	21, 25, 40, 44, 45, 49, 51, 56	22, 23, 24, 32, 41, 43, 46, 50, 55 Do arm pits

Myotherapy Exercise	Exercise/ Preparation #	Exercise/ Concurrent #
7, 8, 9, 10, 11, 13, 14, 15, 16, 17, 18, 19, 20	1, 2, 3, 4, 5, 16, 17, 32, 33, 35, 36, 37, 38, 39, 40, 41, 42, 43, 44, 45, 46	Warm-ups Flexibility Stairs
7, 8, 9, 10, 13, 14, 15, 18, 19, 20	1, 2, 3, 4, 5 Floor progressions Flexibility	Weight training Warm-ups Flexibility Stairs
7, 8, 9, 11, 13, 14, 15, 18, 19 Foot exercises and massage	Weight training Foot exercises Floor progressions Flexibility	Pulleys/stretch Warm-ups Flexibility

EXERCISE

"Exercise" is a strange word when used by Americans. Its meaning changes with the times, the occasion, the application and the sex of the user. In the forties and fifties the idea of exercise for women was anathema. Mothers were afraid that exercising daughters would become muscular, masculine, and unmarriageable. Olga and Nadia had not yet come out of the East, but pictures of muscular Russian girls putting shot and launching javelins had. In a word, "Ugh!" American girls would not be allowed to exercise, but they could take dancing lessons. That alone should tell you something about our ignorance regarding exercise. Of all the sports activities or performing arts, dance is the most difficult and requires the greatest degree of muscular expertise. Boys couldn't take dancing lessons because mothers and even fathers were sure that two weeks after they started, they would become homosexuals, Fred Astaire and Gene Kelly notwithstanding. Doctors, who had been taught absolutely nothing about exercise in medical school, told any man over thirty, "Slow down, Jack. For God's sake, do you want a heart attack?" Physical education had virtually disappeared from public schools and the excellent programs provided by German Turnvereins and Czech Sokols had gone with the war. Some lingered in small pockets here and there, but the back of organized exercise was broken.

President Eisenhower was directly responsible for the sudden interest in "fitness" starting in 1955 when he appointed the first President's Council to look into fitness in America. Even then, *exercise*, fitness, and anything remotely suggestive of sweat was suspect. The Citizen's Advisory Committee, made up almost totally of totally unfit members, decided to sidestep the word "physical" and use the words "youth fitness" as a name for the new committee. "Youth" is so all-inclusive that it means nothing at all.

President Eisenhower's heart attack was also *indirectly* responsible for the revival of interest in exercise. The typical handling of heart attacks in his day ensured that the sufferer would become a cardiac cripple. Treatment included bed rest, long months of inactivity, no sex, and large doses of fear. The recipients of such "care" were sure that each flight of stairs would be their last. Not the president; no way was that going to happen to him. He chose Dr. Paul Dudley White to be his attending physician. *Doctor White believed in exercise.* He not only believed in it, talked about it, and knew something about it (rare even today), he actually did it himself. He traveled about on a bike if it was possible and he used the stairs. Twenty flights was a breeze. To my knowledge he never ran anywhere or suggested that anyone else do so. That didn't seem to matter. The word "exercise" was being connected with the president, he had not died of his attack, and that was enough for the country. Exercise was "in."

What do you do if something is "in" and you want to get on the bandwagon? You do what you think is meant by the "in thing." The YMCAs already had gyms and running tracks; surely "exercise" now meant "run." "Run for Your Life" programs were soon instituted.

Not a single voice (other than mine) even whispered, "You wouldn't run a good horse on cement, it ruins its legs. Why would you suggest that for humans?"

But they ran . . .

In no time at all the bandwagon was loaded with "exercise." We soon had thirty *million* registered runners. A registered runner belongs to something. He (and they were mostly he's) wore the club colors, registered every mile run, and checked his pulse constantly to be sure his heart was beating properly. The media went insane with enthusiasm. Ads appeared everywhere, and everyone began to run. Thirty million pairs of expensive running shoes can't be wrong! Can't they, though! Pretty soon the expensive shoes began to fill up with even more expensive orthotics—molded splints designed to ease pain. Sometimes these devices allow the runner to go twice as far before pain overwhelms him.

Five years after the Fitness Fit attacked America, fifteen *million* runners had to stop running due to foot, leg, and back pain. Their knees, already housing trigger points from the days of high school sports, were so painful they wouldn't bend. Many had to give up tennis when the orthotics no longer prevented muscle spasm from taking over. Some were (silently) noticing the results of pelvic floor injury—impotence. How can something so masculine, so virile, so sexy as running cause something so none-of-the-above? It may take time but if you understand muscles and their clannish behavior, you can understand that insulting one set can start a vendetta with neighbors.

Large numbers of people were advised to take up biking to prevent those heart attacks. The trouble with that advice was, if leg muscles have been injured running (and biking uses those same muscles to extremes) there will soon be more pain. The precipitating pain will be blamed on the biking (as it was on running), when actually, if the victim sat down to think about it, he might recall his long-ago sprains in basketball, football, or baseball. Had he known about Myotherapy he could have done both running and cycling without pain. His best bet would have been cross-country running, where he could have strengthened his heart and lungs without breaking up his body.

This brings us to exercise for women. Now that it was publicly acknowledged that women had minds of their own, how could that market be made to pay off? Easy. Sex was in: put women in short shorts, tank tops, leotards, and wilted woolies. Fine, but what should they do in them? That brings us to the word "aerobic." "Aerobic" really means "in the presence of oxygen." I am writing this book aerobically and you will read it the same way. *Aerobic!* What a bonanza for Madison Avenue! The ad men had just about used up the words *chlorophyll* and *hormone* and here was a brand new one for them—*aerobic!* It practically guaranteed a way to prevent a heart attack or cure a heart already damaged. Women had feet too, didn't they? Surely someone would get women running! Someone did, but they called it "aerobic dance."

Physically uneducated, the American public was fair game for fleecing, and was it ever fleeced! But the bill won't come in for about ten years when the insulted muscles begin to team with increasing stress. Today the coming pain would be diagnosed as "arth-

ritis," "bursitis," discogenic disease, chondromalacia, "carpal," "cubital" or "tarsal tunnel syndrome," "spondy-something-or-other" (back pain), the aforementioned impotence and its female equivalent, spastic vagina. Those two will be considered the byproduct of mental or emotional problems and the consulted psychiatrist will have a field day.

Running on cement will ruin your legs no matter how well muscled they are or how expensive your shoes. *Get off the road.* Aerobic dance has the same propensity because most of it is done on cement under rug or tile. Running shoes or aerobic dance shoes turn a foot into a hoof, and if perchance you have a "classic Greek foot," otherwise known as "Morton's toe" or a long second toe, these shoes can cause everything from corns and calluses to a migraine headache. You do need to wear shoes while running out-of-doors, but you certainly do not need, nor should you wear, sneakers or their reasonable (though more expensive) facsimiles for dance. You have ten separate toes, each in need of exercise. Why deny them that?

And they "aerobic-danced" . . .

Aerobic dance is probably aerobic, since almost everything is. It will probably strengthen your heart, but there are far better ways to do that. It will most certainly damage muscle if for no other reason than that it isn't good exercise and it is too often done without warming up, one of the main reasons for muscle damage in both sports and dance. If there is *any* attention given to exercise before a sport, it is stretching done before sweat is raised. In aerobic dance, most of the routines that have evolved are for cheerleaders, age fourteen. Cheerleaders are already in some kind of shape, usually from dance classes, while the American public is in every shape from A to Z. The ones who are really in shape are off using their condition in sport or real dance. The others don't know any better, which is improving the business of the sports medicine specialists and orthopods and ultimately the rheumatologists. Learn the proper way to design *your* exercise class so you will get results without present or future pain.

And they pumped iron . . .

The third body-banger to drift out of the murk is weight training. When free weights were the only thing around it was called weight lifting. For a long time this "sport" was thought of as a greasy, grimy, under-the-stairs-at-the-Y activity and the Commander at West Point tore up the periodicals he found in the weight room with both rancor and vigor. Then weight-training machines were invented, and now there are weight emporia on every other corner.

What's the matter with weights? Nothing. They are like running. If you know how and where and how much, they are excellent. I have been using them since the forties, even with women and children. The trouble is, knowledge is not included with the purchase of a machine. For the novice, the outcome will be insulted muscles and future pain.

Or they joined a health club . . .

Spas we have had with us forever. The word comes from Europe and used to mean a health center near a hot mineral spring often referred to as "the Baths." People spent weeks and sometimes months at such centers. They drank "the waters," soaked in tubs of

"the waters," rested, dieted, and got into shape for "The Season." They even did some exercise and certainly they took long walks. Most of them, freed of stress and schedules, improved mightily. The upper echelons of American society did the same thing only they went to Europe or to Saratoga Springs. It was the thing to do.

With time, the "health and fitness" trend fizzled and the bath tubs turned brown from the minerals. It was no longer the "in" thing to float, be pummeled, salted, oiled, massaged, sprayed, and purged. The war interrupted "health" pilgrimages to Europe and gave the elite something else to think about. There was a hiatus until out of the West came Vic Tanney with "gyms." But these gyms were definitely "different." The new decor began with wall-to-wall-carpet and chrome machines with lots of dials on them. There were all kinds of memberships, including lifetime. Recently, one such gym announced a "Gala Reopening in Honor of Life Members." That "spa" has changed hands and closed twice since its first opening a year ago. Now a third owner has taken over. That just about describes what spas are about; they have a 75 percent attrition rate. Why? They bore people into leaving and/or get rid of them through injury.

Then came the books, records, cassettes, and exercise and yoga shows on TV. The injury level mounted with each new "method" as did sickness from each new "diet."

It has been interesting to watch all of this. It's also interesting to note that unpromising areas like the schools and the after fifty crowd have been pretty much ignored. But watch out . . . as soon as "they" figure out that we are neither poverty stricken nor decrepit, they will be on us.

Let's beat them to the punch. Fore-warned is forearmed, and the best armament is knowledge. Now that you know the negatives, let's examine the positives.

ALL ABOUT EXERCISE

There are all kinds of exercises—eye exercises, finger exercises, foot exercises, exercises to take off weight, put on muscle, move a bulge from here to there or get rid of it altogether. There are remedial exercises and there are even exercises for sex. Sport is exercise, and so is dance. There are baby exercises and women's exercises, exercises men do and some designed for oldsters. It's a confusing array, or it would be if you didn't understand that exercise merely means *an activity that requires physical or mental exertion.* There are just so many ways to move the human body; the rest is presentation. Baby exercises are exactly the same ones we use all through life. Someone moves the baby (or the handicapped person or the very old). The rest of us move ourselves, but the aim is always the same—*to put each joint through a full range of motion so it will not get "rusty."* The very same exercise is done by the housewife who wants to improve a flexibility level as is done by the gymnast, but not to the same degree. The weight lifter, striving to be cover boy or cover girl, lifts many pounds; the man who wants to improve his backhand far fewer. The marathoner runs longer than the fun runner and the person recovering from illness or injury . . . or dis-use, starts slower.

One thing is true for every exercise, even finger exercise, and that is *the muscle's need to be warmed up before being thrown into sudden action.* A perfect example of such a need is connected with police officers. They sit in their cars most of the day, then one day there is an emergency. They hop out of the car and race at top speed after a man who may have a gun. They start cold and go fast. They are also scared to death, which is a form of stress. They are so scared they are like soldiers who can go on fighting after a terrible wound and never know they have been hit. Later, when it's all over, the soldier collapses from his wound and loss of blood. The police officer often has such bad back pain that he can't get out of bed the next day.

THE WARM-UP

People have begun to hear about warm-ups, but most confuse it with stretch because they don't know what warm-ups are for or what they do. *The purpose of a warm-up is to ready the muscles for action.* A warm muscle is 20 percent more efficient than a cold one and much better protected. The system by which these qualities are obtained involves the body's pump, the heart. The heart needs to be primed a little and the motor brought to a higher level of function before exercising. This is accomplished via exercises that increase heartbeat but neither stretch nor strain cold muscles. That means there is no jumping as in jumping jacks (the warm-up standby of coaches for years). It also means that you don't warm up by jogging or doing a lay-up drill or a light contact drill as in basketball and football. A good warm-up is rhythmic, swinging exercise done to music and with feet flat on the floor. Such exercise is usually done for anywhere from 3 to 10 minutes (one band of music is usually sufficient). When you can feel your heart beating a tattoo and there is a film of sweat on your upper lip, you know that your extremities are getting the warming blood they need for whatever you are going to do next.

THE STRETCH

Stretch is totally different, but of primary importance to the after fifty crowd. Stretch improves flexibility and flexibility, unless we work for it all our lives, leaves us early. When I was using the minimum muscular fitness test on children I found seven-year-old boys who couldn't come nearer to touching their toes than a minus six inches. Since little boys are often not more than thirty six inches tall, you can see what had already started to happen: they had not really begun to work for coordination and already they were missing half of the requirements. *Strength plus flexibility in the proper timing and intensity yields coordination.* As we get older and our ways of living do not require that we put all our muscles and joints through full range of motion, our muscles shorten and the joints behave like rusty hinges. The noise the hinge makes stands for the pain we feel. Always keep this phrase in your mind (or taped to your mirror): *What you don't use, you lose.*

Light stretches may be added at the end of a warm-up session, but strong

stretches are done only when the whole body is hot and sweating. Then the muscles are soft as butter. When they are cold and you try to stretch, you tear a few fibers each time you do it. That is what you see happening when a jogger starts a workout with stretches. This sort of mistreatment can go on for a long time, and then one day when the climate is right—when he or she is under some form of stress, such as competition—the muscle will be thrown into a tearing spasm and that will mean the end of the race (or, as for Randy Gardner, the end of a chance for an Olympic medal).

YOUR EXERCISE SCHEDULE

The next thing you want to know, whether you intend to design your own class, or attend one, is the proper form for a workout. Whether you intend to spend an hour or only a half hour exercising, the schedule is the same. The design is for a full hour plus extra time for the correctives which are needed to improve your basic strength and flexibility and correct posture flaws. You'll find the correctives in Taking Stock, page 67. Your posture needs are on page 127 in the same chapter.

You will note that the first 10 minutes of your exercise schedule are given to warm-up exercises. These are done standing. The next section is given over to floor exercises. They are often called calisthenics and are essential no matter what sport interests you. If you have not yet settled on a sport, these 30 minutes should be spent on exercises with equipment and floor progressions. Most of the equipment is very inexpensive and some of it can be found around the house. Floor progressions are various forms of walks guaranteed to improve

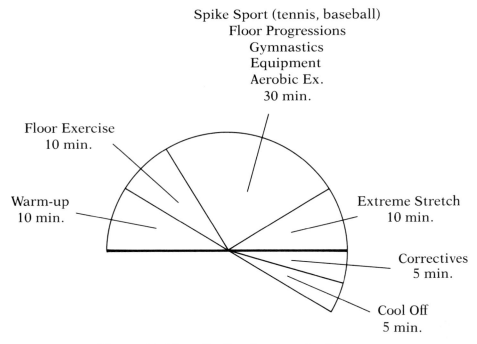

Spike Sport (tennis, baseball)
Floor Progressions
Gymnastics
Equipment
Aerobic Ex.
30 min.

Floor Exercise
10 min.

Warm-up
10 min.

Extreme Stretch
10 min.

Correctives
5 min.

Cool Off
5 min.

Figure 64. *Time Outline for Exercise Class*

posture, coordination, balance, and rhythm. They will do something else, too: they will change your self-image. By the time you reach the last segment—extreme stretch—you will be hot. Sweat will be trickling, and you will be ready for the stretch exercises. The next-to-last segment is for your correctives and the very last for a cool-off. What is a cool-off? Exactly that. The exercise will let your system slow down. The best cool-off is the one given to million-dollar race horses: walk around. Swing your arms easily, since unlike the horse, you are not four-legged.

Now that you have the structure, let's fill in the spaces with the right exercises. Make copies of the following ex-

ercises and pin them up where you can see them. Do them for 3 minutes before you do *anything* requiring physical effort. Each week these warm-ups will seem easier, as will everything else. If you have time for nothing else, do the warm-ups. Notice that every few seconds the exercises shift to include a different part of the body.

Two things you must *never* do: work through pain and "go for the burn." "Work through pain" was what the high school coach told you to do, and he probably has a number of crippled after fifties he should apologize to. The instruction about the burn is newer. It goes with the latest crop of "exercise leaders" who are frequently ill-informed about the human body. If a muscle hurts or burns, you are *injuring* it and it is trying to tell you so. Pain is a warning; in three clear little words it says, "CUT IT OUT!" Exercise gently, and always rest one part of the body while exercising another to allow the body's "exercise products" like lactic acid to be absorbed rather than to collect in the muscles. You don't have to stop; just keep changing. Exercise is cumulative and the workout mounts up even when the hour is spread over a whole day.

WARM-UP EXERCISES

Warm-up exercises have several uses, but one major purpose: to get the heart beating faster in order to pump more blood to the extremities which are about to require greater than usual action from their muscles. Warm muscles are both more efficient and safer than cold muscles.

When we are tense emotionally, our muscles respond with corresponding tightening. If we put them to the test of physical extremes we are apt to tear small fibers of those muscles. It isn't the once or twice that causes a problem, it's repetition of small tears which by now you know results in multiple micro wounds, micro scars, and a gaggle of trigger points. Warming up with easy, swinging movements is a way to bypass existing trigger points and prevent new ones. *Always* warm up with standing exercises before any real action.

If you are starting from scratch keep in mind that you have plenty of time. Use slow music at first as a control. Slow motion is always harder than fast because it forces you to complete each exercise to its full range. When the music is fast one tends to pull up short of such completion. If possible, learn your warm-ups in front of a mirror; and *do* learn them. They should be yours to do anytime, anyplace.

#21 The Swim

Your shoulders are your most versatile joints and need constant care.

- Stand with your feet apart for good balance.
- Keeping your knees straight, lean forward from the hips.
- As if you were swimming, use an overhand crawl stroke for sixteen strokes. (To make it easier, count only the *right* arm movements— eight reaches with each arm.)
- Turn your upper body to the right for eight more counts; then left.
- Finish with eight forward.

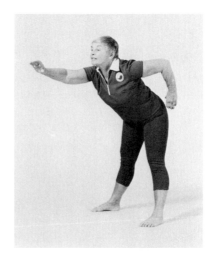

At this point your arms will be tired as you have spent roughly 30 seconds on that body area. How can you keep going without overworking the arms? You shift to the waist.

#22 Waist Twists

- Keep feet in the spread stance.
- Bend your elbows and bring fists to chest level.
- Twist the upper body as far to the right as possible, leading with the right elbow.
- Immediately twist left, leading with the left elbow.
- Repeat for eight twists (counting only those done to the right).
- Next, face the upper body to the right and holding that position, do eight more waist twists.
- Turn left and repeat.
- Finish with eight forward. That is one set and will take 30 seconds.

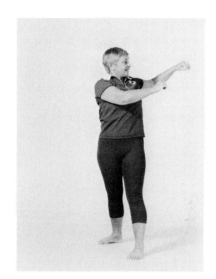

#23 Bent-Over Waist Twist

- Move without hesitation into the bent-over waist twist.
- Keeping knees straight, bend over from the hips and repeat the eight twists forward,
- right,
- left, and
- forward. Remember to keep your head still, eyes on the floor. That makes up a set and will require 30 seconds.

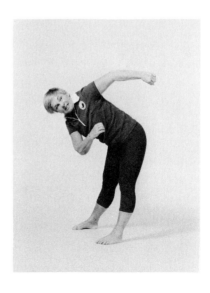

#24 Thigh Shift

To rest the arms and shoulders, switch the action to the legs.

- From the spread leg stance take one step to the left.
- Keeping the right leg straight, bend the left knee. There will be some pull felt on the inside of the extended leg.
- Keep your body erect as you shift for eight counts (counting only one leg).

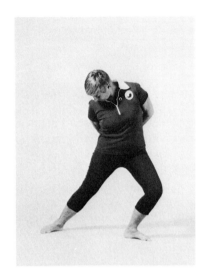

#25 Hip Twist

- Stand on the left leg and turn the right foot inward as far as possible, using only the tips of the toes.
- Bring the hip around and try to see the back of it. This will put pull on your back.

- Next, turn the foot out as far as possible, keeping the knee bent.
- Do eight twists with each leg.

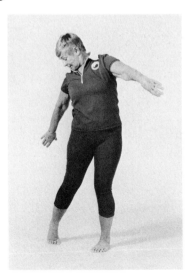

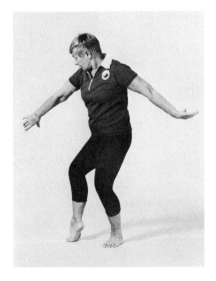

#26 Torso Shift

This exercise will keep the waist slender and flexible. It will also contribute to balance.

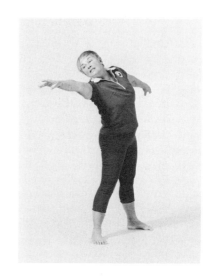

- Stand with feet apart and arms extended to the sides. Pretend you are in a closet with walls six inches beyond your reach.
- *Keeping your shoulders level,* reach with the right hand to touch the imaginary wall.
- Shift the entire upper body so you can touch the opposite imaginary wall.
- Start with eight shifts (done very slowly) and stay at this pace until you have mastered the exercise. Then pick up the speed.

#27 Pelvic Tilt, Standing

The pelvis must be brought under control. It influences balance, supports important organs, and adds to sexual pleasure.

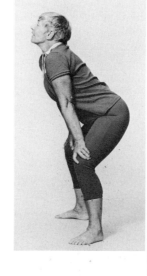
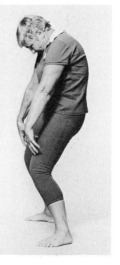

- Stand with feet about eighteen inches apart.
- Place hands on bent knees, even arching your back a little. You will resemble a small boy watching a sandlot game.
- If someone were to swat your seat with a canoe paddle and it was against the rules to run, jump, or let go of your knees, or straighten your legs, what would you do?
- You would tuck your pelvis under and tighten your unprotected rear into a hard knot.
- Hold that position for a slow count of five.
- Return to the seat-out position.
- Do this eight times.

#28 Shoulder Twist

There are two directions in which to do the shoulder twist exercise and both are important. One is primarily an arm and chest exercise in which the arm is extended *to the side,* and the second is primarily an arm and shoulder exercise in which the arm is extended *forward.* The twist shown here is forward. To do the second exercise, simply point your arm to the side and repeat the action.

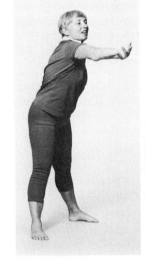

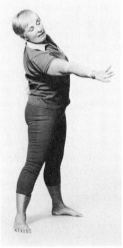

- Twist your arm counterclockwise until your thumb points to the ceiling.
- Then rotate your arm in the clockwise direction so that it points straight back. You will feel the pull throughout and especially to any muscle housing a limiting trigger point.
- Do eight twists with each arm to the side.
- Do eight twists with each arm stretched forward.

#29 Ski Shift

- Place your feet together in parallel position and bend your knees.
- Keeping the upper body absolutely still, push both knees to the left. This will force the feet over onto their left-side edges. Just pretend you're wearing skis. (This is an excellent exercise to do when preparing for skiing.)
- Next, shift the knees to the right (this will bring you onto the right-side edges).
- Shift the knees from side to side for eight counts (counting only the shifts to the right).

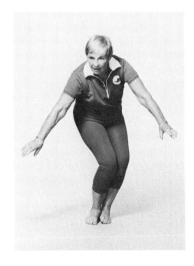

#30 Snap and Stretch

The last exercise in this warm-up series is all important for the after fifty crowd since long years of work at desks, tables, and machines, have foreshortened chest and arm muscles. These must be lengthened and made supple again. This exercise comes at the end of the warm-up because these muscles *must* be warm if they are to respond immediately and safely.

• Stand with feet apart and bend your elbows in front of you at chest level.
• To reach the starting position, cross the right arm over the left until the hand is even with the elbow.
• Snap both elbows back, keeping them at shoulder level.
• Return to crossed-arm starting position.
• Swing both arms wide, still at shoulder level.
• Return to starting position.
• Do eight.

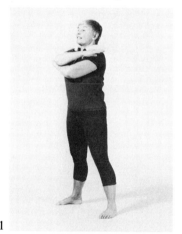

1

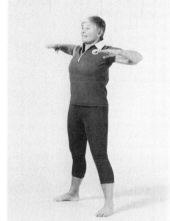

2

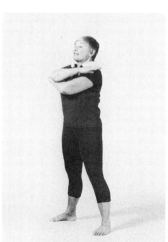

3

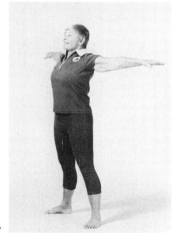

4

You now have ten exercises you can do anywhere—at home, in the club locker room, in the dressing room at the Y, or right out in front of God and everybody. Your tee-off in front of the club veranda will improve, your bowling score will rise, and you will be unlikely to pull up lame on the court or down the road. If football players did these exercises daily and before kickoff, they could cut their injury rate considerably. If they learned the flexibility exercises you will learn, they'd avoid even more injury. If they knew what you already know about Myotherapy, they could wipe out most injuries!

We're in charge!

You and I need this knowledge and these exercises for war. What war? It's our war against ignorance and prejudice and the mythmakers. If trends are to be set for us, *we* will set them. We would look silly in wilted woolies, so we won't wear them. We would damage ourselves running marathons on cement, so most of us won't run them and those who do will know how to protect themselves with Myotherapy and with warm-up exercises. We would not only feel ridiculous doing "aerobic hop-hops," we would know we were following a pied piper down a rat hole.

You want to "young" instead of "age"? Come on, let's get at it.

FLOOR EXERCISES

For some, getting down on the floor is as easy as saying, "Get down on the floor." For others it may be a problem. After my hip operations I found it very difficult. Getting down was one kind of problem and getting up another. If this kind of activity is hard for you, do the following exercise around the house.

#31 Getting Down and Up Series

Doors have two handles you can count on, and in most houses there are many doors. Each gives you many opportunities to exercise all day long.

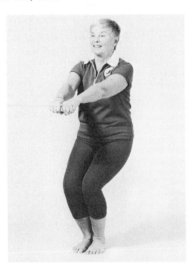
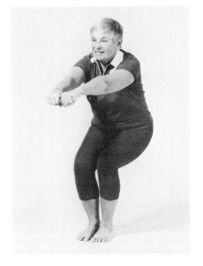

- Go to the nearest door.
- Open it halfway and facing the edge, grasp both knobs as I am grasping the rope.
- With your feet together, go down into a half-knee bend and then straighten.
- Do three of these at every door you

go through for a week. At the end of the week you will be able to drop down even further. That new gain will be good for three dips at each door all the following week.
- On the third week, go all the way down into a *deep* knee bend at each door.

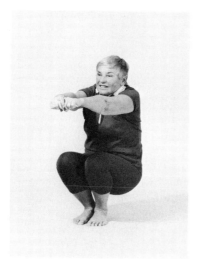

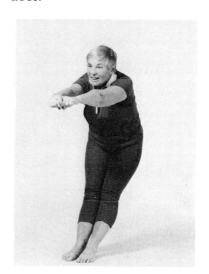

IF YOU EXPERIENCE ANY PAIN ANYWHERE AT ANY TIME CHECK WITH THE PAIN CHART AT THE END OF THE MYOTHERAPY SECTION. FIND THE TRIGGER POINTS AND GET RID OF THEM.

When you are able to squat all the way down to the floor and come back up easily you are in line for something more demanding and exciting. For this you may want a friend to stand behind you and support you with hands under your armpits. If you don't feel sure of your hand strength get going with the hand exercises on page 159.

- Drop all the way down as you have been doing.
- Then, holding tight, straighten both arms and legs. You will look like a V turned onto its side.
- Keeping the legs straight, pull yourself to the erect position.
- Do three.

ON HANDS AND KNEES

The after fifty crowd has done a lot of time in this position. We've weeded, painted, scrubbed, waxed, and crawled under cars and beds. This position is not foreign and aside from sitting in a chair, is the next level down.

At this point we divide the exercises—not by value, they are *all* valuable—by *what's possible at this point*. Everyone who's able to get down and up (though needing a door or chair as an assist) can do the exercises designated **A.** Everyone should do each exercise because each one addresses a different need. The exercises marked **B** are a little harder. Keep trying them, and begin doing them only when they do not cause you pain or stress. Take your time—you've got lots of it!!

#32 Angry-Cat-and-Tired-Horse Stretch (A)

If possible place palms flat and ankles and insteps tight to the floor. If your hands won't go flat, see the Myotherapy pattern for arms and hands on page 142, exercise #9 for inner arm stretch, and #14 for chest and armpit stretch. If there is air between ankle and floor, see Myotherapy patterns on page 144 for the lower leg and exercise #123 for the instep. Then do the foot exercise series on page 296. Keep in mind that muscle spasm, not age, keeps you from full stretch. Get rid of that spasm and reeducate your muscles.

- Dropping your head down while keeping your arms straight, push your back up into an arch.

- Push as far as you can while paying attention to any spot that is holding you back. For the after fifty crowd there is usually tightness across the shoulders.
- Hold the push for about five seconds.
- Let your back drop into a reversed arch—the back of a tired, old horse ridden too long and too hard.
- Bring your head up to stretch chest and neck muscles. Leave your mouth open. The tightness may be in the groin and probably in the neck.
- If you get dizzy while doing this check the Myotherapy pattern on page 135 for the neck, and if there

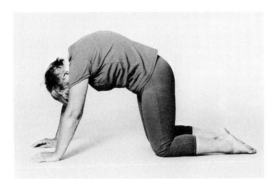
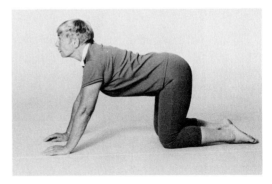

is any pull at all in the groin use Myotherapy pattern on page 129 for the groin. Remember, the groin muscles attach to the ribs. This exercise stretches both the back and abdominal muscles and *streeeeeeeeeetch* is what we need.

- To use this for sphincter control, tighten *everything* inside as you press into the Cat back.
- Relax fully as you drop into the old horse.
- Do eight for a set.

#33 Knee to Nose Stretch (A)

- Still on all fours, bring your knee as close to your nose as possible. Never mind if it's miles from the target. This stretches your back along its whole length and strengthens the abdominals.
- Next, *keeping arms straight,* extend that same leg back and up as you raise your head. This works the back, especially the *gluteus* muscles, which improves your walk and gives you a tighter, better looking seat. At the same time it stretches the abdominals and fronts of the thighs. You don't have to be perfect right from the start. If you can *aim* in the right direction, you are doing fine.
- Do eight with each leg for a set.

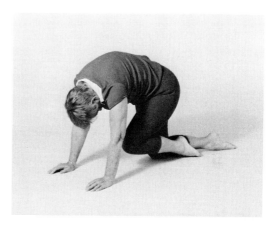
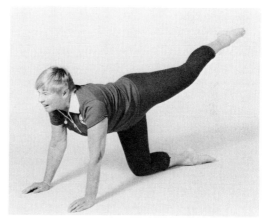

34 Corrective for Knee to Nose: Back Stretch (A)

If getting your knee to your nose feels like an impossibility check with Myotherapy pattern on page 124 for the upper and lower back and with page 89 for the backs of the legs. Spasms are preventing your stretch toward flexibility. Find the rascal trigger points and do the corrective.

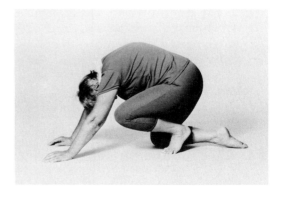

- Still on your hands and knees, place the left foot as close to the right knee as you can manage.
- Pointing your nose toward your knee as you drop your head, rock back as though you wanted to sit on your heel.
- Bounce gently several times in that way.
- Then change knees. If the knee has a tendency to turn outward, the leg is housing trigger points on its outer side. Check with myotherapy pattern on page 144 for the side of the leg and also on page 124 for the lower back.

- Tuck the knee inside of the arm on the same side and do the exercise again.
- Do a few of these correctives *every time you exercise* and it will be only a short time before your knee will reach your nose. What will that mean? You are "younging" your back!

#35 Thread Needle Stretch (A)

The purpose of this exercise is to improve the flexibility of the shoulder girdle, stretch both chest and arm muscles, stretch the upper back and all the muscles on both sides of the torso, and improve waist flexibility.

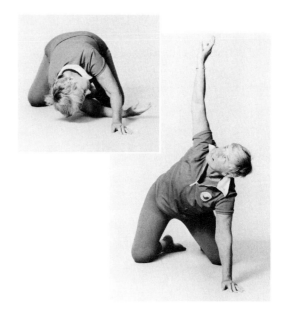

- Start on all fours and thrust one arm in the space between the other hand and the knee on the same side. *Ideally* your shoulder should lie flat on the floor. Usually it takes some practice to accomplish that and may require some work with Myotherapy patterns on pages 124 and 127.
- Swing that same arm out from the "needle's eye" and upward as if to wave to someone in a third-floor

window. (Tight chest and arm muscles will interfere with a free swing. Use Myotherapy patterns on pages 137 and 140.)

ONE OF THE PROBLEMS WITH EXERCISE WHEN OFFERED AS A "CURE" FOR A CONDITION IS SPASM. YOU CAN EXERCISE ALL DAY AND IF THE SPASM REMAINS ACTIVE, WHICH IT USUALLY DOES, YOU WILL NOT GET FULL STRETCH, FREE OF PAIN, OR RETURN OF FUNCTION. DETERMINATION ALONE DOES NOT WORK AGAINST SPASM. GET THE TRIGGER POINTS OUT.

#36 Three-Legged Foot Swing (A)

If you can move your swing-leg one foot right and left of center, you can do this exercise. *Ideally* the forward swing should bring your foot in front of your hand, and on the back swing you should be able to see the foot by looking over the opposite shoulder.

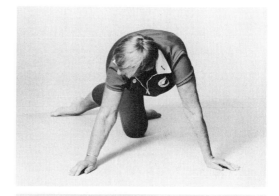

- From the all-fours position, swing a *straight* leg as far forward as you can manage. The foot should be flat to the floor.
- Next, swing that same *straight* leg around back to cross over the other foot.
- Lay the instep flat on the floor.
- Do four swings to a side. This exercise strengthens the lower back and leg and tightens up the seat. It also stretches the inside and outside of the upper leg.

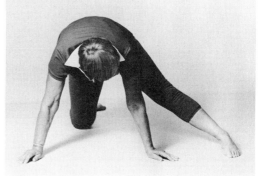

#37 Pelvic Tilt on Knees (B)

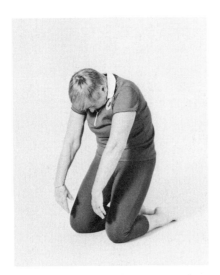 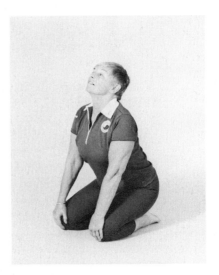

- Get down on slightly spread knees, insteps flat on the floor. (If insteps are too tight, place a rolled up washcloth in the space under the ankles, but as soon as you can, do the foot stretch exercise, #123.)
- Resting your hands on your thighs, arch your back as much as you can.
- Then, without rising more than a couple of inches, tilt the pelvis forward.

- Do eight. If this is difficult, practice the pelvic tilt standing, #27.

This is an abdominal flattener and sex-life-improver, and don't hand me that nonsense about being too old. *Nobody's* too old. Opportunity just *keeps on* knocking, and you've got to be ready to open the door!

#38 The Hydrant (B)

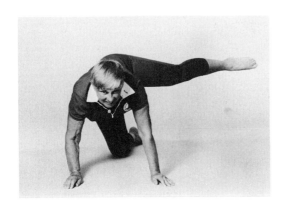 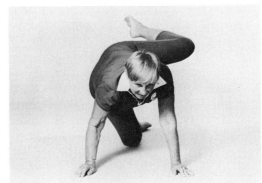

- Start on all fours.
- Raise the right leg to the side, keeping the knee bent.
- Stretch the leg straight out to the side.
- Don't change the level of the working leg, but *bend* the knee again.
- To rest the muscles and yet not stop the action, extend the working leg straight back and up. (It is the same as the second position of #33.)
- Start with two to a side, but work up to eight. When your hip feels the strain, STOP. In time it will be easy. Take that time.

The easiest and most logical direction to go from your knees is flat on your stomach, known as the prone position.

#39 Prone Gluteus Set (A)

It doesn't look like much is going on in this exercise, which is one reason it can be done almost anywhere you can lie prone—the beach, the gym, in front of TV, or in bed.

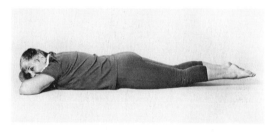

- Rest your head on folded arms and pinch the seat together as hard as you can.
- Hold for five seconds.
- Relax.
- Next, pinch the seat and pull in your abdominals.
- Hold for five.
- Pinch, pull in, and tighten the sphincters.
- Hold for five and repeat for five. As you improve you will find it easier to contract than to relax. Practice; the dividends are numerous.

#40 Seat Lift (A)

The seat lift improves back, abdominal, and groin flexibility, and back strength.

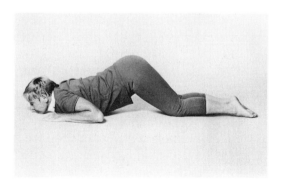

- Pretend to glue your chest to the floor.
- When the glue has set hard, raise your seat in the air. It may not go very high at first, but give it time.
- Lower, and repeat eight times.

#41 Push-ups or Let-Downs (B)

If you are male, one push-up may be no big deal unless you are recovering from an accident, have had surgery on your chest, or haven't done a push-up since you turned in your football jersey. If you are female, chances are you have never done one. On the other hand, you may do lots of them . . . wrong. The real push when your car is stalled comes when you have to shove it from inert to rolling. The real effort in a push-up is made from flat to one inch off the floor. If you watch a football team do them, they only move between all-the-way up to half-way-down. You are now going to do *real* push-ups, and if you have to start from scratch, here's how.

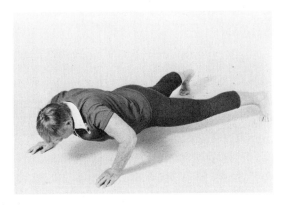

- Spread your legs wide and get to the top of the push-up position however you can. Have straight arms a shoulder-width apart.
- Now let yourself *slowly* down, *one inch at a time*. (The last six inches will be awful and you may flop down for the last three.)
- Turn your face to the side unless you want to explain a bloody nose.
- Do three slow let-downs every single day. When you can go down in ten counts and not flop the last inch or two, you will find you can push *up* at least once. Be sure not to cheat.
- *Go all the way down* between push-ups.
- Touch your hands together over your back to prove you are down.

Why do push-ups? Because they strengthen your arms, chest, shoulders, back . . . and image. You once did them? Do them again. You never could do them? That was because of bad teaching; you can do them now.

THE PRONE ARM AND LEG SERIES

This series is essential, but it will be a mix of hard and easy depending on what has happened to you. A shoulder injury, a CPA job or that of pianist, computer analyst, or secretary will make the chest tight and cause limitation of arm lift. A back injury, groin pull, or a sedentary life will limit leg lifts. Push *hard* when you find the work easy, but take it *easy* when you find it difficult. Two leg lifts would be enough if you are starting and find those two difficult. Eight would be ideal. Just clearing the floor would be great if that's all you can do today, but in a month you'll have to think higher.

#42 Prone Leg Lift, Parallel (A)

- Tuck your arms in close to your body to provide a stable base against which to work.
- Raise first one straight leg and then the other.
- Alternate for eight.

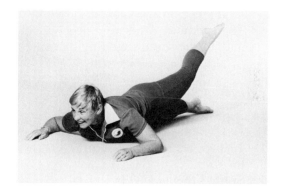

#43 Prone Arm Lift, Parallel (A)

- Extend your arms straight out in front and parallel.
- Raise one arm straight up, then lower it. DO NOT ROLL THE ENTIRE BODY FROM SIDE TO SIDE. Do the lift out of the shoulder.
- Alternate for eight.

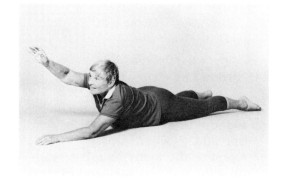

The next exercise is inserted to offset the prone lifts which put strain on the back if done for too long.

#44 Stretch-Curl-Stretch (A)

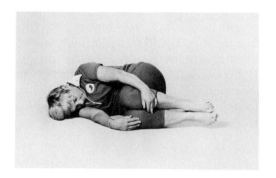
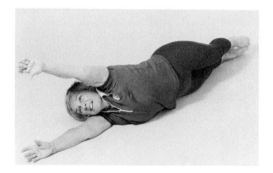

- Lie on your right side and draw your knees up to your chest in the fetal position.
- Then extend arms and legs fully, and, in the same swinging motion,

- Roll over onto the left side and curl into the fetal position.
- Repeat four times to stretch the back.
- Repeat again *after* doing the next two exercises.

#45 Spread Leg Lift (B)

- Tuck your arms closely to the body for stability.
- Spread the legs wide.
- Lift first one leg and then the other.
- Alternate for eight.

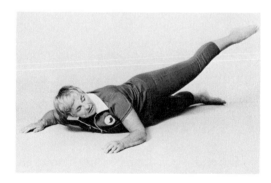

#46 Prone Leg Cross-Over (B)

- Lie prone with arms stretched out to the sides.
- Spread legs wide.
- Keeping the arms at full stretch, raise the right leg high and carry it across in back to come as close to touching the anchored left hand as possible.
- Swing it back and do the same with the left leg to the other side.
- Start with four and work up to eight.

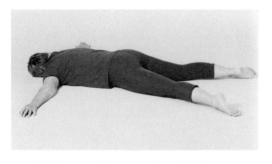 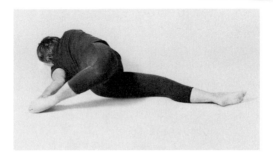

- Follow with exercise #44 to ease the back.

All of the above exercises can be done with weight bags later on.

SITTING AND LYING

Sitting and lying (supine) exercises are all of a piece since one feeds into the other. If you are out of condition, have had a hip or back operation, or have been forced to "enjoy" bed rest, sitting exercises will be harder than kneeling or prone exercises. So wherever you are on the condition scale accept this fact, and don't be discouraged.

#47 Pelvic Tilt, Sitting (A)

- Sit on the floor with knees bent.
- Clasp your hands in front of your knees and lean back as far as possible.
- Drop your head, round your back and tighten your abdominals . . . *hard.*

- Tighten the seat muscles and return to the starting upright position, hands on ankles, knees open.
- Hold the erect position for a count of five and drop back again.
- Repeat eight times.

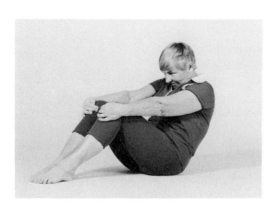 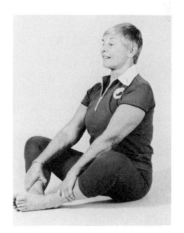

#48 Knee to Nose, Supine (A)

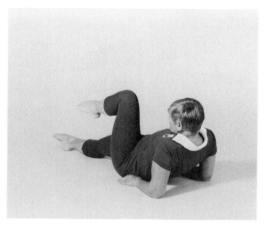

- Lean back on your elbows.
- Bring one knee as close to your nose as you can.
- Then, keeping it close, try to extend the foot straight up.

One of three things will happen: the leg will stay close to your nose and go straight up, (in which case you have flexible hamstrings); the knee will stay close, but the leg won't straighten very well; or the leg will straighten, but far from the nose. All three have happened to me. The answer, when you are not satisfied, is hamstring stretch (see exercise index at the end of this chapter).

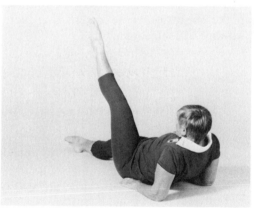

#49 Supine Leg Twist (A)

Hip rotations in any form are important for the after fifty crowd. Although we have spent years exercising our brains, our tongues, and our walking and lifting muscles, we have neglected our hip joints shamefully. That is one reason for mediocre results in hip replacements and why much older people walk oddly. So, as we wore braces on our teeth in order to have a prettier smile, let's do hip exercises so we'll always walk well.

- Lie supine, completely relaxed.
- Rotate the left foot outward until it is lying on its outer edge.
- Maintain that rotation and raise the leg at right angles to the body.
- At the peak of the raise, turn the foot in as far as you can.

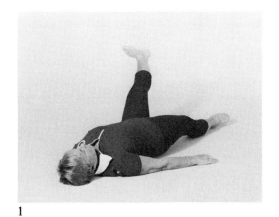

1

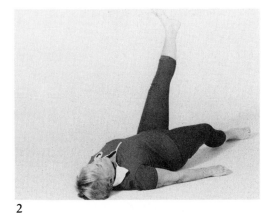

2

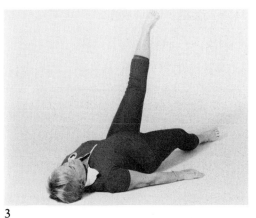

3

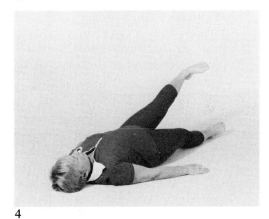

4

- Maintain that position as you lower the straight leg to the floor.
- Keep the inward rotation as you raise the leg again to the top of the lift.

- Turn the foot out and lower it to the starting position.
- Do four twists with each leg. (In Exercise #51 you will repeat this hip rotation, but in the sitting position.)

#50 Leg Walk-Up (B)

The leg walk-up exercise is not very difficult *if* your hamstring muscles are well stretched. It works the abdominals hard but if you have done the correctives on page 87, that won't worry you. It takes a lot longer to stretch shortened muscles than to strengthen them, and some men have never had a chance to lengthen hamstrings and worse still, their sports training may have worked against them. The more stretched you are, the easier *everything* will be.

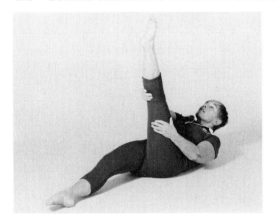

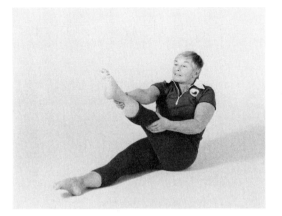

- Lie supine and raise one leg straight up.
- Using a hand-over-hand method, walk yourself up your own leg to the ankle.

- Let go at the top and lie back.
- Do four walk-ups.
- Repeat with other leg.

When you find an exercise difficult, ask yourself why. If you were asked to chin yourself and you couldn't, what could be wrong? You could have weak arms. If you were a little kid taking a test in P.E., you would be marked as a failure if you couldn't do a chin-up and sent to play baseball, where you wouldn't be very good either. If your teacher happened to be a sadist (and there are many), you could hang there squirming, but not pulling up. Now that you're an adult, you can help yourself improve. Look up "weak arms" in the index and do the *easy* exercises suggested until you are ready for harder ones. In time, you will be able to pull up.

#51 Leg Twists, Sitting (A)

- Lean back to rest on your hands or elbows. (Elbows are easier at the start).
- Spread your legs wide and turn the right foot out so that its side rests on the floor.
- Raise the leg in its everted position.
- Once off the floor, rotate the foot inward and carry it across, over the other leg, to touch the floor—as far over as it will go.

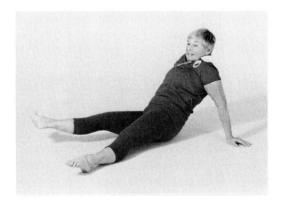

- Then, keeping the leg far over, rotate the foot *outward* and carry it across to touch the little toe to the floor.
- At that moment, rotate the foot *inward* and repeat.
- Do four to a side.

These next exercises do something for you that you will like: they take fat off the thighs.

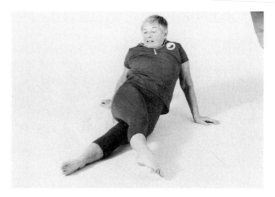

#52 Bicycle

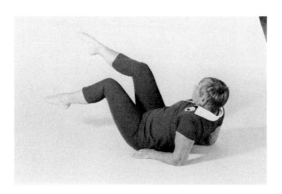

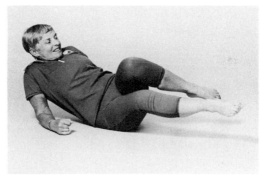

The first two parts of this exercise are **A** and the third is **B.** until the abdominals are strong.

- Rest back on your elbows and do a *slow* bicycle action with your legs for eight counts.
- Next, keeping both elbows tight to the floor, roll over onto one side and repeat the biking action to the other side.

That makes up an "A" set. As soon as it feels easy, increase the number of sets. For "Look, Ma, no hands," you will need abdominal strength.

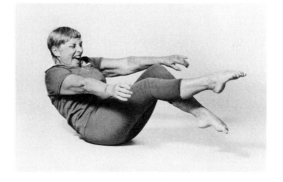

- Raise both hands and feet from the floor. Do eight forward and eight to each side for a set.

#53 Side Drops with Reach (B)

- Start in the sitting position with legs spread wide.
- Drop down to the right side, catching the fall on the right hand so as to stretch that side of the chest.

- As you recover from the drop, sweep both arms forward to touch the toes on your way to a drop to the left caught on the left hand.
- On the return reach forward again.

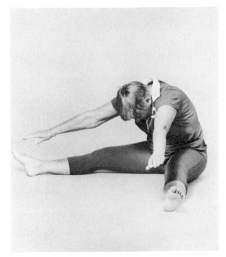

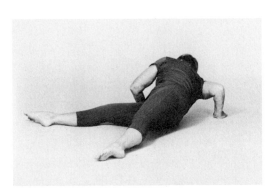

#54 Lateral Leg Lifts (A)

- Lie on one side and, if hip bones are not well padded (lovely thought), put a folded bath towel under them.
- Rest on your elbow. Be sure you are on your side and not back a little too comfortably on your hip.

- Stretch your body out long and raise the top leg.
- Lower it.
- Point your toes.
- Do four.
- Roll over to the other side and repeat for a set.

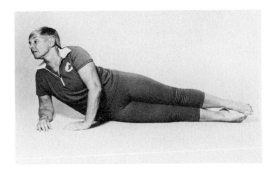

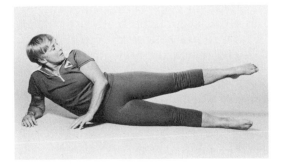

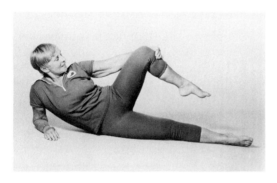

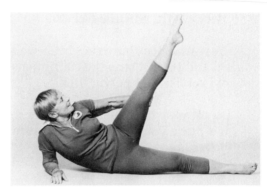

- Roll back to the starting side and draw the top knee toward your shoulder.
- Then extend the leg, trying for height.
- Lower.
- Do four to each side for a set.

- Combine the exercises for two sets.

Exercise #54 can be turned into **B** very simply by rising up from the elbow support and leaning on a straight arm.

#55 Prone-Supine Twist (B)

- Lie prone with right arm extended and left supporting, close to the body.
- Lift the left leg as high as possible.
- Keeping the leg in the air, roll the body back onto the hip, raising the leg still higher.
- Roll back to the starting position.
- Do four each side.

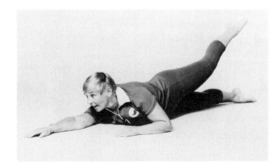

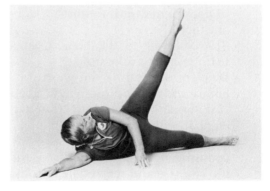

#56 Pelvic Tilt, Supine (A)

To rest muscles that have been well worked and yet not stop the continuous flow of exercise, use pelvic tilts.

- Lie on your back, bend your knees, and place your feet about eighteen inches apart.
- Keeping your hips and shoulders tight to the floor, arch your back as far as possible.
- Then, pressing your spine down to the floor, tilt the pelvis forward and tighten seat muscles and sphincters.
- Hold for five seconds.
- Relax and do four.

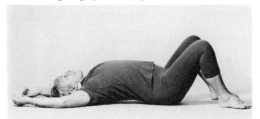 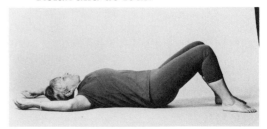

STANDING

Standing exercises can often be combined with daily tasks—toe rises and deep knee bends at the sink, hip shifts before picking something off the floor, followed by descending hip shifts.

#57 Toe Rises (A)

To improve balance and walking form, you must strengthen your feet. At first you may need to hold onto a chair or the basin in the bathroom in order to do this exercise.

- Rise *slowly* to the top of the toe rise (it doesn't matter if that rise is only one inch).
- Slowly lower to the floor. Use as little support as possible.
- Do eight every time you wash your hands, use the bathroom or kitchen sink, brush your hair, tie your tie, etc. *Use* your day to help you.
- By the end of the first week start counting eight (slowly) to get to the top of a rise and then eight to come

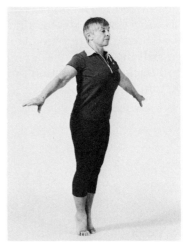

back down. If you have trouble with balance see the section on the long second toe, page 149.

#58 Knee Bends without Support (B)

Knee bends are marked as **B** exercises only because the after fifty crowd, especially the men, have so many injured knees. First, before you even think *deep* knee bend, do the door-handle knee bends on page 238. If there is a catch in the knee you will find it; check Myotherapy pattern on page 146 for knee pain. You do not need to have pain to have potential trouble in the knee; stiffness should be warning enough.

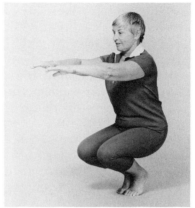

- Stand with legs together and feet parallel.
- Rise to the toes for a count of one, bringing your arms forward for balance.
- Tighten your leg, seat, and abdominal muscles. (This will prevent teetering.)
- Keep your back straight and lower yourself into a deep knee bend, *keeping the knees together.*
- Rise to the toe position.
- Lower from toes to starting position.
- Start with five and work up to fifty a day. You can take all day to do fifty; exercise is cumulative.

#59 Hip Shift: Lateral Pelvic Shift (A)

The pelvis must be moved daily in every direction. This improves everything from making love to walking down the street. Every sport demands pelvic control, strength, and flexibility. It doesn't come about by accident.

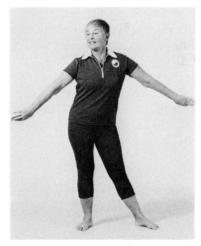

- Stand with feet apart.
- Keeping both legs straight, sit over onto the right leg. (That's the way you stood as a teenager when you had an arm full of books.)
- Shift to the other side.
- Do side-to-side hip shifts whenever you can, all day, but also make it a part of your program. You can vary it by altering the rhythm. Instead of even beats go, slow . . . slow . . . fast-fast-fast.

#60 Descending Hip Shift (A)

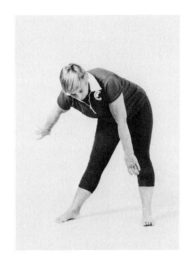

- Start by swinging your hips from side to side as you did in #59.
- When the hips are swinging freely, lower your upper body toward the floor, taking a full eight counts to get as far down as you can. (Is your back balky? See Myotherapy pattern on page 124. Is the floor light years from your fingers? See Myotherapy pattern on opage 144.) You are supposed to be able to touch the floor; spasm, not your age, is preventing it.
- Take eight swings to return to the standing position.
- Do four.

One of the worst aspects of the myth-makers' thinking is arrogance. Of course, ignorance isn't far behind. When I looked at programs provided in senior centers I was first annoyed and then furious. How dare these so-called "exercise teachers" perpetuate the idea that the over fifty crowd are feeble, inadequate, and incapable? Certainly there will be exercises too hard for some of you to do at the start and for some of you, ever. They aren't the right exercises for *you*, that's all. Do the ones you can do, and use the Myotherapy patterns to get rid of any spasm or weakness. Keep on with the correctives and the suggested Extra Exercises and then, every so often, try one of the ones you find hard today. You will be surprised. Weren't you surprised when you first understood the words on a printed page? Didn't it come as a pleasant shock when you actually understood a group of people speaking a foreign language you had labored over? Well, that's the way it will be with the exercises.

#61 Walk-Outs (B)

- Start in the standing position with legs well apart.
- Without bending your knees (hamstring flexibility), lean forward from your hips and place one hand on the floor.

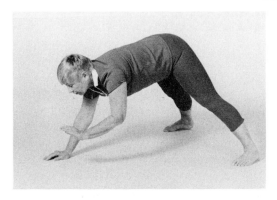

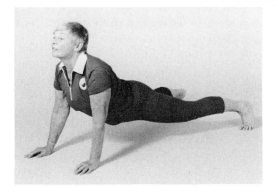

- Without moving your feet, walk your hands forward for three counts.
- On the fourth count, when your body is at full stretch, press the pelvis downward with a sharp movement. Don't bend your arms.

- Hand-walk back to the starting position, taking two counts.
- Use two counts to stand straight.
- Start with two and work up *slowly* to eight.

#62 Thread Needle, Standing (B)

This is the same as Exercise #35, only a little harder.

- Stand with feet spread very wide.
- Lean forward to take your weight onto the right hand.
- Thrust the left hand through the

space between the supporting hand and the right foot.
- Then rotate the body outward as you reach for the ceiling.
- Start with two to a side and work up to eight.
- Repeat with other hand.

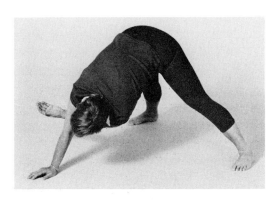

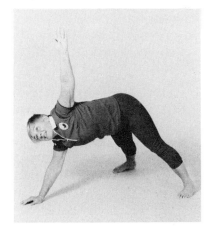

FLOOR PROGRESSIONS

The third segment in your planned program consists of floor progressions. These exercises look so easy that many people (especially those brainwashed by the current kings and queens of sweat) wonder why they should bother. The answer to that question will be found in airline or bus terminals or on any street corner: just watch other people walk for about ten minutes. Disaster!! Walking is so wonderful when it's right and so sad when it's wrong.

Vast numbers of the after fifty crowd have problems that spoil walking, problems ranging from "trick" knees to shin splints. Long before the brain learns about a problem through the medium of pain, the legs and feet know all about it. They try to compensate any way they can—by substitution. They wear down the heels and soles of shoes unevenly, they grow protecting calluses here and there. They turn in or out and wobble in high heels. Sometimes the heel cords are so tight they have to walk on tip toe to the shower. Occasionally a leg will circle out to the side instead of moving straight forward through the stride. Backs sway or flatten, one hip or shoulder may ride higher than the other. A head may tilt to the side. The individual with a poor walk may develop headaches or jaw pain. These are all ways the body calls attention to a problem. Your body now has your attention. Start learning about it.

Floor progressions are "weight-bearing exercises" and just the ticket for those who want to *prevent* osteoporosis and for those who have already seen its signs. Along with a daily dose of calcium, exercises are recommended; but which exercises? "Walk," says the doctor. I say add the following exercises; you can do them intermittently all day long.

First, walk down a hall and measure your strides with a tape measure. Take ten or twelve steps and measure the trip. Ten strides for me adds up to 260 inches. If both my left and right strides are even each will cover 26 inches. However, if one stride is longer than the other, something is holding one leg back and that something has to be a tight muscle. What I am doing is limping, although so far, imperceptibly. By the time someone asks me, "Why are you limping?" my tightness is already well established and my self-image knows all about it.

Your mind's eye never closes and it never stops spying on you. False eyelashes, a new shirt or girdle, the most expensive designer jeans and aftershave can't hide a thing from your subconscious. If you say, to yourself even, "God, I'm bushed!" Your body will immediately act as though it's worn out. The subconscious is nothing if not literal. That's one reason for not saying, "He gives me a pain in the neck." You could actually develop one. A friend of mine once told me she did say that and she did *get* that. A week later she said someone gave her a pain in the rear and she developed hemorrhoids. After that she announced to everyone who would listen that she was never going to say, "He slays me." But he or she can! Or is it you who can slay yourself? I have almost "died of people" twice. Now, when people irritate me, I take my toys and go home.

Check your strides for a match or a shortening. When you do the floor progressions, and whenever you walk, try to take longer and longer strides. When you walk out of doors take purposeful strides and use the rope exercise #10 to stretch your groin.

Do your FLOOR PROGRESSIONS catty-corner across a room, straight down a hall, or around a room in a circle. Hitting the beat is the first thing you want to accomplish; only after you have that do you think posture. Gradually pay attention to getting your head up, chin in the air, shoulders back, and arms aswing. Then add to that thoughts of a spring morning when you were ten . . . and in a parade.

#63 The Walk (A)

- Walk to brisk music and cross the room, go around the room, down the hall, or anywhere you have to go. Remember, long strides and purposeful posture.

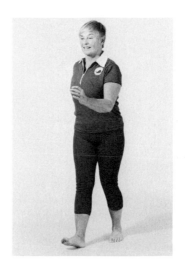

#64 Turned-In Walk (A)

- Walk with toes turned in to exercise the tibialis anterior, the muscle on the outside-front of the lower leg. That muscle must be strengthened if you have flat feet and stretched *and* strengthened if you have a long second toe. The sillier you look while doing this, the better. "Silly" means "play," and "play" means "laugh at self." When was the last time you played, were silly, and laughed at yourself?

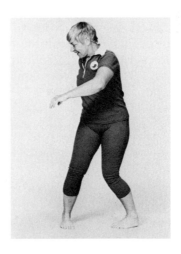

#65 Turned-Out Walk (A)

- Tilting your pelvis under, so that your seat does not stick out in back, bend your knees and turn them out as far as possible. This walk strengthens the quads (or thigh muscles), tightens thigh flab, and hardens the abdominals.

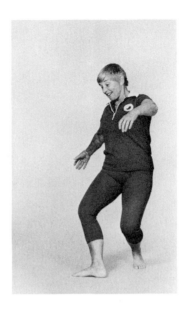

#66 Toe Walk (A)

- Rise high on your toes, tighten legs, hips, and abdominals, lift your chest and chin, but press your shoulders back and down. Relax your arms. If you are doing this exercise across a large room go one way on your toes, but come back flat-footed. The surest way to get muscle cramps is to overdo an exercise, which may lead you to think exercise isn't for you. It is, but do it right.

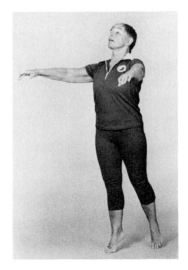

#67 Drop-Over Walk (B)

- The drop-over walk is a **B** if your back isn't very strong yet or if your hamstrings lack stretch. You can tell at once when you lean over and take the first two steps. *If it feels insecure, wait.* Do the suggested exercises (find them in the index at the end of the chapter) and in a couple of weeks, try again. If the first two steps feel OK, go across or around the room with knees bent, head and arms hanging, and your body in a low crouch as though scurrying behind your hedge, hoping to get in the house before the neighbors see you.

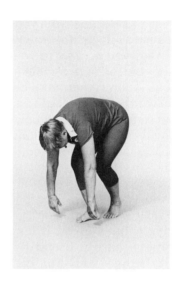

#68 Hip Twister (A)

- Take each step forward with the foot turned way in, which brings the hip around. Forget your arms except to get them out to the side and out of your way. As you improve, the arms will quite naturally move *against* the foot action to increase the twist. This is an excellent exercise for increasing flexibility of the waist, separating the upper from lower torso (essential in all sports), and increasing reach.

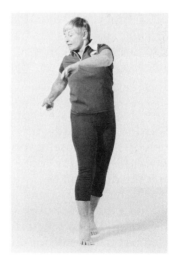

#69 Backward Walk (B)

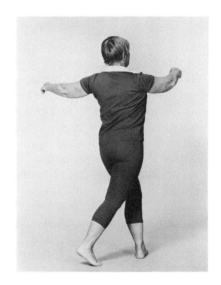

- When was the last time you walked backward? It is absolutely essential that you be *able* to walk backward and also that your subconscious *knows* that you can walk backward. If it doesn't, and you need to back up fast sometime, you won't be able to. If walking backward is a cinch for you, concentrate on reaching far back with each step, placing the toe exactly as you want it, rolling back onto the heel with definition, and keeping your body erect. If it's a scary business, have a friend (who will walk behind you) put his or her hands on your shoulders. Your subconscious will register "safe" and you'll do just fine. However you handle it, do it.

#70 Cross-Over (B)

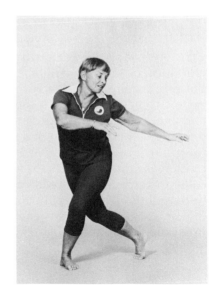

This is a **B** exercise only if you have trouble with balance or hips. If you have had a hip replacement and not done the right exercises, or have been told not to cross your legs, you need to do Myotherapy patterns on pages 124 and 144.

- Do the cross-over by walking either forward or backward with the stepping foot well across in front or in back of the standing foot, depending on the direction.
- To vary the exercise and make it even more fun, cross over with the right foot and then touch the toe of the left out to the side for one count before bringing it in to cross in

front of the right. In dance parlance this is called cross-touch-cross-touch. Purpose: to improve rhythm and balance and strength.

- A second variation would entail crossing the right foot over and bringing the left around in a wide arc before crossing in front of the right. From then on, the foot coming forward always goes through the arc.

Every new exercise assures you that your legs will be better able to aid you when and if you should need aid. Also, you will look better and better.

Look at the heels and soles of your shoes. Are they unevenly worn? If they are, the muscles are not meshing correctly. Notice what happens to the treads on tires when the wheels are misaligned. Unevenly worn shoes means *you* are misaligned. That must be corrected.

#71 Backward Reach (B)

This is another **B** exercise simply because balance may interfere with good execution and therefore discourage the subconscious. That's one entity we cannot afford to discourage.

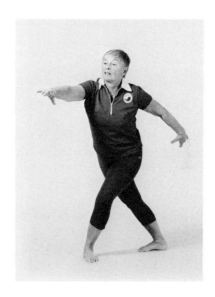

- When your balance is assured, step as far back as you can manage.
- Turn the foot out before you place it on the floor.
- In order to get a good reach you will have bent the forward knee. That puts you on a lower than full height level . . . stay there.
- As you transfer your weight from front to back, *keep the level steady.* Don't straighten up.

This exercise improves balance plus the strength of the quads or thigh muscles. It does wonders for the feet, too, and the subconscious begins to perk up.

#72 Knee Lifts (A)

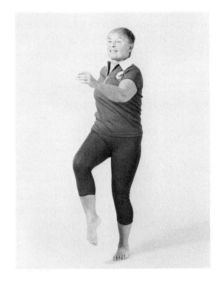

- As you cross the floor or circle the room, lift each knee until it is at right angles to the floor.
- Be sure the toe is pointed as this strengthens the muscles in the lower leg and increases the range of the ankle joint.
- The support leg should be absolutely straight and the foot flat on the floor.

Later, when you get into running, this is a good variation. To get the worst from running, just run on the straightaway. To get the best, do cross-country running; it makes you use your legs and feet in a variety of ways. If you are indoors, vary your runs as on page 343.

#73 The Goose Step (A)

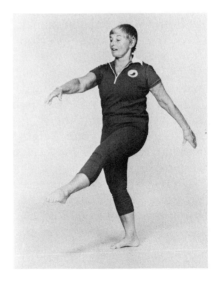

The reason the goose step is used by armies around the world is that it strengthens the legs. You want the same thing; just don't overdo it.

- Bring the straight leg forward from the hip.
- Point your toe and lift as high as is comfortable. The height and strength will improve in a complementary fashion. As the flexibility of your hamstrings gets better it will be easier to lift the leg. At the same time strength will have improved enough to provide plenty of the needed stretch.

#74 Race Walking (A)

One of the newest things to come along is race walking. (It's not really new; people have been doing it for years and calling it "heel-and-toe.") It is very fast walking—as fast as jogging but without the jarring. At no time are you in the air, as the heel of one foot must be on the ground before the toe of the following foot has left it. In order to achieve any speed, the hips must swing fast from side to side and the arms pump hard for balance. Race walking gives the walker all the cardiovascular work he or she needs, improves strength and pelvic motion, and injures nothing at all.

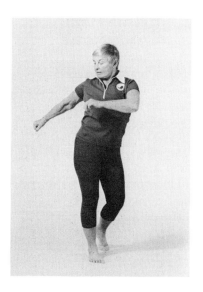

- Go back and check with Exercise #59, the hip shift. Do that in place, just to get the feel of it.
- Then step forward on the right foot as you swing your hips to the right.
- As you land on the heel of the left foot, swing your hips to the left. The swing must be exaggerated and the landing leg straight.

Don't try for speed, try for swing and rhythm. Speed always comes after basic function has produced form. Do this exercise to different speeds of music, from fast to very slow. Slow is always harder to handle than fast, but shows up flaws better.

When was the last time you took a step to the side? When was the last time you took a *big* step to the side? There is a whole dimension to be explored. Remember the "grapevine step"? Do you remember the tango? How were you at tour jetés? Remember the feel of running out for a pass? How about that fake move to the right and dodge back to the left in basketball? Sure you remember. Well, your subconscious remembers. It just needs to be nudged a bit.

#75 Side Cross-Over (A)

- Turn your right side in the direction you want to move.
- Lead out with the right foot.
- Bring the left behind the right, leading with the heel.
- Go across the room, first with the left foot crossing in back and then the right.
- Follow that with the following foot crossing in *front*.
- Finish with the "grapevine" in which you alternate first crossing in front and then in back.

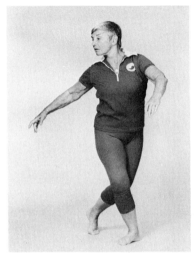

cross over with the right
Step again with the left
Lean left to listen at the door

A fine dance pattern will probably suggest itself to some of you just about now. Face front and imagine a zigzag line running across the room from corner to corner. It will take you three steps to cover each zig to the right and another three to cover each zag to the left. However, if you are using 4/4 music, you will have one extra count to use up each zig and zag. The best thing to do with it is to pretend to be listening at a door to the side. That will unweight the leg you need to step out on. This is how it "talks":

ZIG . . . Step right on the diagonal
          Going in the same direction,
          cross over with the left
          Step again with the right
          Lean right to listen at door
ZAG . . . Step left on the diagonal
          Going in the same direction,

Continue across the floor zigging and zagging. Why? It improves your rhythm, your balance, and your control, and the subconscious thinks it's wearing a high hat and tails and is swinging a silver-headed, ebony cane. Its stiff, white shirtfront was never so stiff and those diamond studs are gleaming . . . and you think I'm kidding? I'm not. The more you picture yourself as king of the mountain, belle of the ball, or whatever positive imagining pleases you, the closer you will come to being it. I need not even mention what happens if you spend a lot of time thinking "not good enough."

Next question: When was the last time you ran anywhere? If you are jogging, your answer will probably be last week, but jogging isn't running, and you may be doing yourself more harm than good. If you are landing on your heel, you are doing yourself a great deal of harm.

To develop your legs with running, you must first develop your feet. Watch most joggers; you will see the most awful form in the world. Most of them are so miserable they look as if they have to go to the bathroom . . . now!

Put on a good record, one with a nice firm rhythm, and start to jog, but landing first on your toes and *then* dropping to the heels. The best way to break old habits is to do something a very different way. To run forward correctly, run backward first.

#76 Backward Run (B)

The **B** designation is again for balance. Get the backward walk under control first.

- Run backward, landing first on your toes and then dropping to the heel with each step.
- When you are sure you know how it feels to bounce along landing on your heels *after* you have taken your weight on the ball of the foot, where it should be taken, try going forward doing the same thing. WARNING: It looks easy and feels easy. It will cost your muscles, however. Do it in short stints . . . down the hall to the bathroom, on your way to answer the phone, thirty seconds in between other exercises . . . and walk. *Walk everywhere and whenever you can.*

#77 Side-to-Side Jumps (B)

- Using the toe-catch-lower-to-heel system, pretend there is a narrow gauge railroad track running across the room. You must jump to right and to left, landing on each rail. Make your set of tracks as narrow as you like, just so you jump from side to side as you progress. This exercise will help feet, legs, hips, and groin.

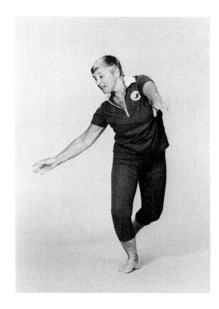

#78 Skips (A)

Why is a skip an **A** exercise? Because we all could skip once and if you ever could, you can again. What would stop you? Pain would stop you and so would weakness. Don't try the skips until you have done a lot to strengthen your legs and gotten rid of all leg, groin, and back pain. When you are out on your daily walks, find hills to climb. When you use the stairs, make an extra trip each time you have to go up for something; even if it's to go to bed. Never send someone else to get something; get it yourself. If your subconscious hears you say, "Johnny young-legs, run up to my sewing room (or out to the tool shed) and bring me my whatever," it hears three things. One: Somebody has "young" legs; mine must not be. Two: If my legs aren't young, maybe I can't get that thing for myself. Three: Hey! I'm old enough to ask favors of the younger generation, maybe I'm really getting up there and ought to act my age. You have to keep on the up and up with your subconscious all the time. You want to fulfill the gloomy prognosis of the mythmakers? Then read them to your subconscious.

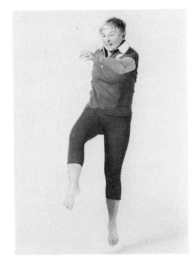

- First, skip forward for a few lifts when the music is right.
- As you improve, skip longer and try a few skips backward, to the side, and in circles—any way that pleases you. *But skip!*

Now you are warm—verging on hot—and if you have worked very hard, you are dripping with cleansing sweat. What do we do now? What are we finally ready for? Stretch.

STRETCH

#79 Snap and Stretch (A)

- Start with feet apart and bent elbows held at shoulder level, hands in front of your chest.
- On the count of "one," snap your elbows back to stretch your chest muscles.
- On the count of "two," bring your arms back to the front, crossing the

arms so your hands overreach your elbows to stretch the upper back muscles.

- On the count of "three," fling both arms wide at shoulder level to stretch chest and arm muscles.
- On the count of "four," return to the crossed-arm position.
- Do eight.

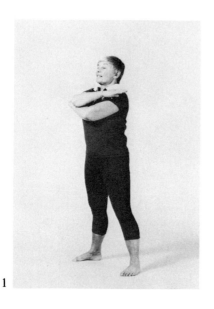

1

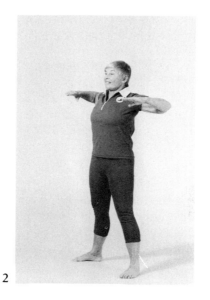

2

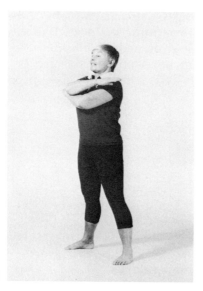

3

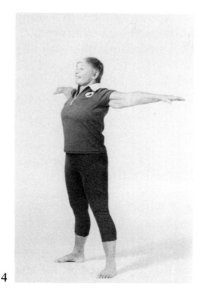

4

#80 Back Stroke (A)

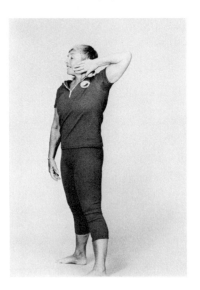
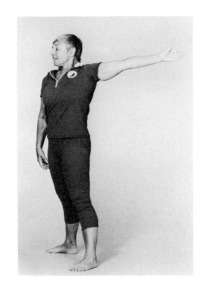

- Place the back of one hand on your cheek, and press the elbow back as far as it will go.
- Hold it there.

- Keeping the elbow anchored, circle your hand up, back, down, and around.
- Alternate four to a side.

BACK AND HAMSTRING FLEXIBILITY

Before we start let's explain a confusion wrought by exercise physiologists: they have developed something called *static stretch*. They stretch a muscle to its utmost and then hold the stretch. The results are less than good. Dancers use BALLISTIC *stretch*, which calls for gentle, rhythmic bounces. Dancers are the best-stretched athletes in the world. But whichever stretch you use, be sure to be fully warmed up before proceeding.

#81 Flexibility Bounces (A)

- Stand with feet wide apart, knees straight, and hands clasped behind your back.
- *Keeping your head up*, bend forward from the hips and bounce the upper body downward in eight easy bounces.
- Next, allow your arms, head, and torso to droop downward, completely relaxed.

- Do eight more easy bounces.
- Stand straight and turn the upper body to one side.
- With head up, do the same set of head-up bounces eight times.

- Then allow the upper body to droop downward to the side and do eight more.
- Repeat to the other side.

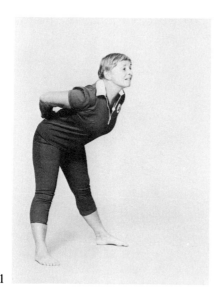

1

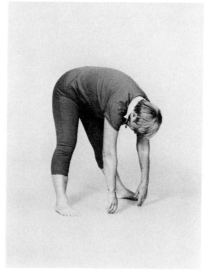

2

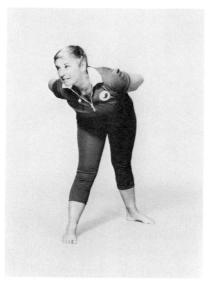

3

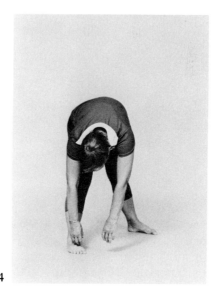

4

#82 Heel-Down Knee Bend (B)

- Stand straight with feet together, heels flat on the floor.
- The object of this exercise is to either keep your heels on the floor or work to get them there when you go down into a deep knee bend. The trigger points preventing a successful knee bend of this kind are in Myotherapy pattern on page 46; the best exercise to build up your strength is #31. You can also use weights, as in exercise #164.
- Go down into the deep knee bend, heels staying flat on the floor.
- Then, keeping your head at that level, straighten your legs.
- Start with four and work up to ten.

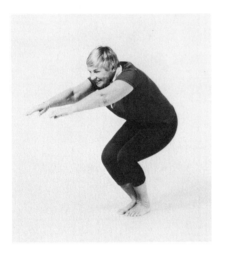
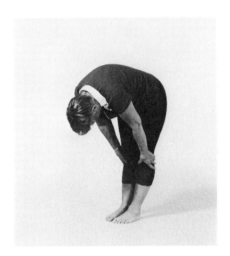

#83 Stretch-Outs (B)

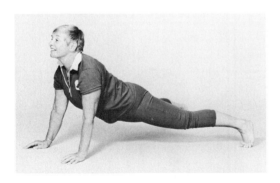
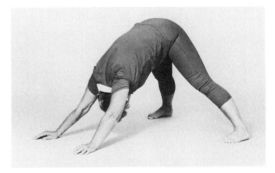

- Start by standing with feet wide apart and toes pointing straight ahead. They are to stay in that forward position throughout.
- Walk the body out to the stretched-out position on your hands.
- Then, keeping the toes forward, press the heels back flat on the floor

and drop your head between your shoulders.
- Try to bring your chin to your chest.

- Stretch forward and back eight times. This is a multiple exercise strengthening and stretching many muscles.

#84 One-Leg Stretch (B)

- Lie on one side and grasp the foot of the top leg at the instep.
- Extend and retract the leg four times to a side. If there isn't a prayer of getting that leg straight

while holding at the instep, hold at the calf or ankle. Check Myotherapy pattern on page 146 for limiting trigger points and work with flexibility bounces, #81.

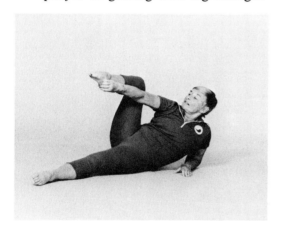
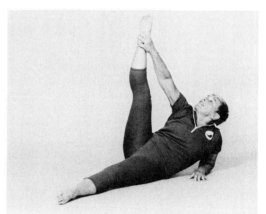

#85 Roll-Out Jackknife (B)

- Lie supine with arms overhead.
- Stretch as long as you can.
- Roll up to a sitting position and

reach the upper arms forward as far as possible. Repeat eight times.

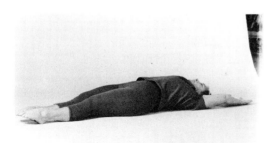
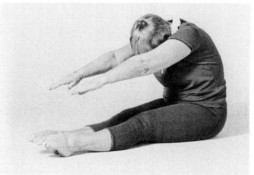

Before we start the next stretches let me remind you, again, that I have had both hips replaced, and while my limitations are few, they do exist. I can show you the direction in which to struggle but you will ultimately do better than I can. It isn't age that limits; it is disuse—or, in my case, a mechanical device that isn't quite as good as the real thing.

#86 Hamstring Stretch, Sitting (A)

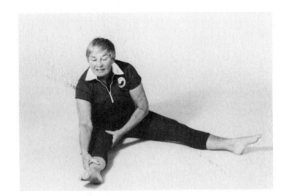

- Sit spread-legged on the floor.
- Grasp one leg at the ankle and just under the knee.
- *Keeping your head up,* back flat, and legs straight, try to pull your chest down toward your thigh in short bounces.
- Do eight right and eight left. The Myotherapy patterns to help erase limiting spasms are on page 124 for the lower back, page 129 for the groin and page 144 for the hamstrings.

#87 Back Stretch (A)

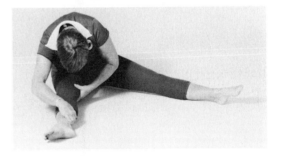

- Stay in the same position, holding the leg in the same way, but this time try to bring your *ear* close to your knee.
- Do eight bounces to each side.
- Grasping both ankles, bring your head as close to the floor as you can.

#88 Gluteus Stretch (B)

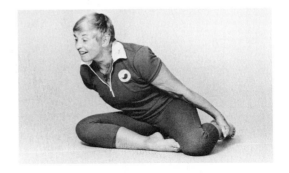

- Bring one foot close to your body, and bending the other knee, carry the foot to the back.
- Clasp both hands behind your back and try to bring your chest close to your front leg.
- Do eight bounces over each leg.

#89 Head to Insteps (B)

- Sit on the floor and bring your feet close to your body, facing sole to sole.
- Grasp your ankles and pull your head down so that its top approaches your feet.
- Using short, easy bounces, try to bring your head lower and lower.
- Start with eight and work up to fifty. While you work, try to feel where you are tight—and try to let go.

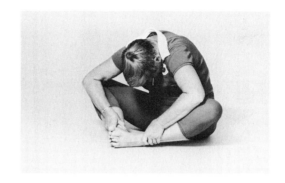

#90 Crotch Stretch (B)

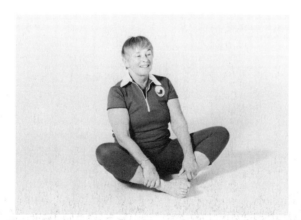

- Place the feet sole to sole as in exercise #89.
- Grasp your ankles firmly and place your elbows on your knees.
- Press the knees down as far as possible toward the floor and hold the stretch for five seconds.
- Relax and repeat eight times.

If you have been forced to spend any time in a hospital bed the next exercise is a dreadful-dreadful. Hospital beds often keep your knees bent, which is exactly the position the person with a bad hip prefers. "Hippies" usually fight against having the operation long enough to louse up every muscle connected with the hip, unless they have been ordered into water exercises. Even then, the quads have been allowed to deteriorate terribly. First, use Myotherapy pattern on page 144 for the fronts of your legs and on page 129 for the groin, then go at the next exercise slowly and carefully.

#91 Hurdler's Stretch (B)

- Sit on the floor with legs out-stretched.
- Bend one knee, pulling the foot parallel with your body.
- Lean back to stretch the front of the thigh. (Up until now we have concentrated on the back of the leg. The front is just as important.)
- Allow your body to lean back and recover in easy bounces, doing just a little, but every day.

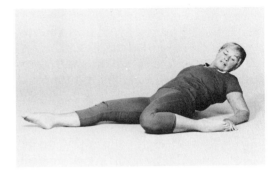

Why exercise regularly? Because this is war, and every front you retreat from is ground lost. Your enemies are the injuries you've incurred over the years, the weight you may have added, and worst of all, what you believe are your limitations. You have no limits . . . you never did. You just *thought* you did. Now you must *know* you don't, and see where that lack of limits takes you. That's what's so interesting about tomorrow.

EXTRA EXERCISE

BED BALLET

My mother-in-law was always going to write "An Ode to Bed." She never got the chance to spend much time there and even when she was very, very old, she avoided it like the plague. Bedtime is for resting and loving and if too much time is given over to either, that can be a fatal mistake. Think about it. There actually can be too much of a good thing, and boredom is only one of the results. Good loving, like good living, requires a modicum of good health and anyone who "rests" most of the day destroys health. Circulation slows; calcium leaches out of the bones and they turn brittle; unused muscles atrophy and shrink; skin loses elasticity and tone; insides go all swampy. The un-challenged body becomes weak and tired, but can't sleep. As old trigger points respond to the stress of inaction, stiffness is compounded by aches and pains which make movement unattractive at first and unacceptable later on. Medication is needed to move slowed bowels. Medication is needed to bring on even fitful sleep. Medication is given for pain and soon medication is required for depression *caused* by medication. If the medication befogs the mind and causes a fracturing fall, surgery may follow with more medication. The bed becomes a prison. Prison often provides solitary confinement, and any POW can tell you that being back on the front line is preferable to that. Even rookies can tell you how to avoid booby traps and ambushes. Bed rest is both.

"BUT . . ." I can hear the wails from every side. "Suppose," (like me, with a multiple smashed pelvis) "it has to be?" Does it? Does the sprained knee really require a cast? Are you sure? Do you know the price of inactivity? Do you know anything about your own muscles, functions, or needs? If you think you do, where did you get your information? Was your mother the source and if so, what was *hers?*

At this point in your life you are going to have to make *you* the object of serious study. I no more needed that traction and body cast for three months than I need it now. Times change and what was thought "right" even five years ago can well be "wrong" now. When I had my cesarean sections it took three weeks to get out of the hospital. Two months ago a friend of mine had one and was home in three days and she recovered much faster. If your doctor says "bed rest," ask *why?* It means one of two things: your problem is expected to go away by itself or it is hoped that it will. In either case there must be an absence of anatomical pathology. Myotherapy is in order. Ask about that as an alternative.

But suppose the order for bed rest is totally legitimate. Let's say that you, your friend, or parent has "bought it": a leg, hip, shoulder, wrist, knee, or foot is busted. Or somebody had a heart attack or a stroke. When young Mark was brought to the clinic after an auto accident, he had had all kinds of damage plus brainstem injury. When I asked what he had left that we could work with I learned that his left thumb still moved under his volition. He couldn't talk, his vision was impaired, his body was inert. As far as Mark's ability to exercise went, he was as helpless as a baby and he was almost twenty years old. Do you know why we weren't dismayed? Because we know a lot about babies. We also know that exercise

should begin as soon as possible after birth. Bed rest isn't good for babies either.

Try to imagine what the last two months before birth must have been like. You were like Alice finding yourself growing and growing as your swimming pool shrank. The provider of your natatorium could probably describe those weeks as not very comfortable for her either, as you tried to stretch, wiggle, and twist to find a spot free of her backbone. If you could have been heard you would have been saying "Lemme outta here . . . !"

Folded, collapsed, and untouched by human hands your little packaged person slid into the world needing, above all, stretch. In baby-exercise we stretch little arms and legs, rotate shoulders and hips, turn feet in and out, roll little people around, and let them *feel* different positions and *see* from different angles. Exercised babies exposed to warm water are soon swimming babies, and should they be handicapped on land, they rarely are in the water.

With people who are confined for any reason, the needs are the same as for babies. This was amply illustrated the first time Mark made a move on his own. He patted the therapist's bottom. Everyone was jubilant! He was normal! He was moving. He would get well. Where did we start? With bed ballet which, for Mark, was the first step to homeplate. For many it is merely a restful interlude. For me it would have been a God-send.

There is one condition worse than Mark's—coma. It's bad enough for the victim, but worse for those who really love the person, who for a time is nowhere at all. If you have a friend in a coma I have some interesting information you may need. Comatose patients exist at varying levels and from appearances you can't be sure just where they are—in deep sleep or just under the edge. Be cheerful and hopeful around them. I have been in a coma, and somehow I knew.

So what can you do for your friend who has been in an accident and ends up in the hospital . . . bring flowers? Plants are better; they last to go home, and the mere fact that you think your friend will, too, helps. You can't imagine what gloomy thoughts the hospitalized entertain at night! But in addition to plants, bring this book and ask the doctor if you can exercise what's OK. If only one arm is still free and uninvolved, you can do bed exercises. If you have older friends who really have nothing but stiffness and disinterest to bother them, bed ballet is just what the doctor should order.

If your friend or loved one has "hit the wall," or as some say, "bought it" and quite obviously has a broken back and you ask permission to use the BED BALLET, if the doctor is pleasant the answer will be "No." If he or she has had a rough day you will be handed your head, so use it first. A stroke or heart attack patient has to be moved very soon after stabilization (remember Eisenhower!). If a hip is broken or re-

placed, only parts can be moved, and gently. However, if an arm is broken, there's still one arm, two legs, a torso and a head calling for action. If a leg is in a cast, what about the rest?

Before you do anything, line up the music you will use. If your friend is to be exercised, choose music from his or her youth. Music seems to bypass all kinds of problems and will even make pussycats out of jamming, jerking, palsied muscles. Music reaches past the here and now and carries people to other places and other times. Notice when you are out to dinner and the conversation is lively and interesting you are suddenly moved away from everyone into another dimension. Your nostalgic mood may be well advanced before you realize that the orchestra is playing "our song." It has reached through years and layers of other lives to touch a spot long forgotten, but remembered by a deeper part of you that really forgets nothing.

The best rhythm for bed ballet is a medium-slow waltz. The ballet costume that serves best is men's pajamas. The greatest "ballet masters" are two people who care about the "student." The "masters" stand on either side of the bed and the subject, or "student," should simply close his or her eyes and go with it.

#92 Open Arms–Cross Arms (A)

- Grasp the patient's wrists and raise both arms slowly toward the ceiling.
- Keeping the pressure even and

going with the music, open the arms wide to stretch arm, chest, and upper back muscles.
- From the outward stretch, carry

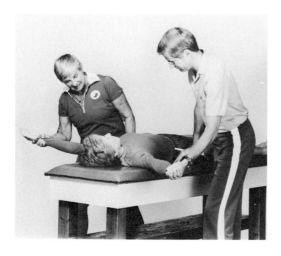

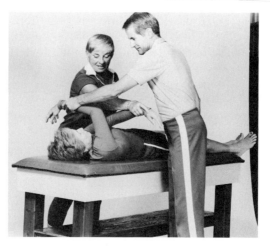

the arms back to cross over the chest to stretch the upper back.

• Do several of these exercises, listening for a change in the music.

93 Arms Over Head (A)

• Carry both arms overhead. This will open up the rib cage and improve breathing. If the subject has either emphysema or asthma, it will help if the trigger points are removed from the pectorals as in the Myotherapy pattern on page 137.
• Bring both arms down to the sides.
• Do four.
• Alternate arms, one up and one down for four.

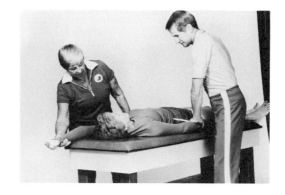

#94 Bicycle (A)

Legs that are lying around all day in an unexercised state become "rusty." They are also no help to a beleaguered heart.

• One "ballet master" bends one knee and the other keeps the second leg straight.
• Alternate for eight.

• Do four double knee bends. This will flush the blood that pools in the legs when they are not used. If care is taken to remove the trigger points from the legs as in Myotherapy pattern on page 144, there will be no "tired," "achy," "crampy" leg muscles and the feet will not be as cold.

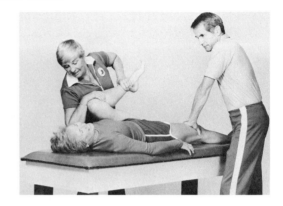

#95 High Kicks (A)

• One "master" holds a leg flat on the bed while the other raises a *straight* leg overhead. If the leg cannot be kept in the straight position during the raise it means the hamstrings are tight and must be detriggered with the help of Myotherapy pattern on page 144.
• Alternate legs for eight.

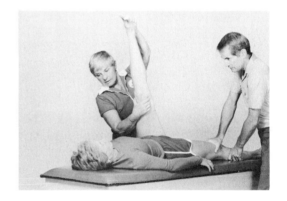

#96 Side-to-Side Rock (A)

There is nothing worse than lying supine all day and night in the same hot spot, especially if there is a rubber sheet under you. Bed baths come only once a day and *maybe* a back rub at night. Incidentally, don't let anyone come near you with the creams hospitals provide. It's bad enough to have to eat hospital food without developing a case of what I call "terminal diaper rash" . . . all over.

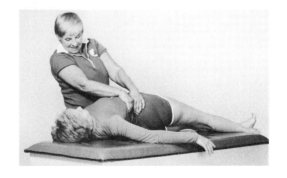

• Reach across the body, grasping at the waist and pelvis.

- One "master" rolls the body as far as it will go while basically supine.
- Then the other "master" pulls the other way.
- Rock and roll for at least eight

changes. The change of position is only one of the pluses; the pulling stretches the entire torso and relieves the pressure on the hips.

#97 Feet In . . . Feet Out Ankle Circles

Lack of circulation, as much as pressure to heels, causes both pain and sores. Propping is not the answer. Check the Myotherapy patterns on pages 124 and 144 and do the foot massage on page 291.

- Turn the feet inward and outward, bringing the edges of the feet to the bed each time.
- Do eight each direction.

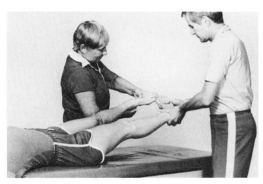
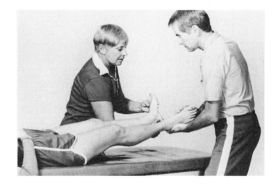

#98 Leg Crosses (A)

- Turn both feet outward and open the legs as wide as they will go.
- At the widest point, turn both feet inward and bring the legs to the crossing point. (One takes the high road and the other the low so they can cross without interference.) Be

sure that each leg gets a chance at each level, one crossing high one time and low the next.
- Do eight. Trigger points are apt to be felt in the groin and inner aspects of the thighs, try the Myotherapy patterns on pages 129 and 146.

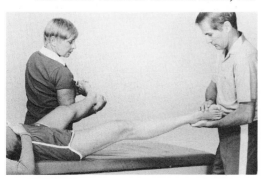
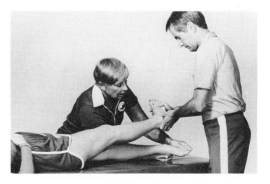

#99 Arm Circles

As is our custom with exercise, we never stay very long in any one area; but we don't stop exercising either. Moving on gives the just-worked area time to rid itself of lactic acid. Go back to the now-rested arms.

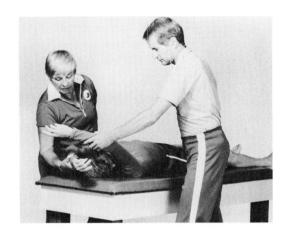

- Each "master" moves an arm in a circle, mirroring the other's movement.
- After four circles, reverse directions.
- Do two sets of eight.

With the next exercises you have to use your head. What is the state of the subject *and what is yours?* If your subject is Irma who was a gymnast/ballerina and her last exercise class was two weeks ago Thursday before she busted her ankle, no problem for either of you. However, if it's Harry from Houston who has been working overtime to grow a paunch and is as stiff as a board and his stroke has made him helpless on one side and mad as a wet hen inside . . . draw the line right here. You *can* sit him up if you and your partner are stalwarts, but you'll never get his bottom in the air. It hasn't been there since he was pitched into the trough by Ol' Trigger forty years ago.

#100 Sit-Ups (A)

- Grasp both arms (one "master" supports the upper back and the other the chin). You don't want a sprained neck for your trouble.
- Sit the person up and lean him or her forward to stretch the lower back.
- Roll back down again.
- Start with one and proceed slowly with time. If the sit-up causes dizziness, check with Myotherapy patterns on pages 131, 132, and 133.

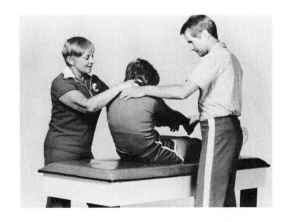

#101 Roll-Backs (B)

- Each "master" grasps a bent leg under the knee.
- Together they raise the knees and bring them toward the subject's forehead.
- When a tight ball has been achieved the subject should straighten the legs as much as possible, curl again, and sit up.
- One of these is usually enough at the start, but as flexibility and abdominal strength improve (and they will), do more.

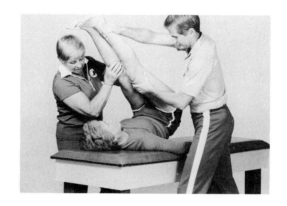

#102 Full Body Stretch (B)

Nothing feels better than stretch to the tired, bedridden body.

- One "master" takes hold of the wrists and the other the ankles, pulling gently to the music's rhythm.
- As the music comes to an end, each "master" pulls against the resistance of the other (to the extent as is wise considering the condition of the patient).
- Hold the pull steady for fifteen to twenty seconds and *slowly* release.

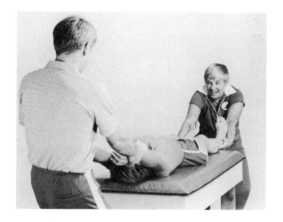

ROUND THE CLOCK

The nice thing about physical therapy is that if you are slated for it in another part of the hospital, you get to travel. Even if you are flat on your back, the scenery is different. If, by any chance, there is a warm water pool, that's lovely. Like handicapped babies in water (who become the equal of other babies in water), a handicap is greatly alleviated when you don't have to bear your own weight (see Aqua-Ex, page 345). The sad thing about physical therapy is that it usually uses up less than an hour, which leaves you lying immobile and bored for 23. In those 23 hours there are at least 120 minutes that, divided up, could be used for exercise; taken altogether, that would amount to 2 full hours of progress. If those minutes are used judiciously—say 8 minutes out of every hour from wake-up time to 10 at night—wondrous things could happen.

I have a dear friend who for years worked in cardiac rehabilitation at a YMCA and who is a fine athlete still, at seventy-five plus. After retiring to Florida he had a heart attack. Too ornery to die, he was soon slated for PT. A young gal in white appeared at his door to direct the exercise session. Being also charming and curious, he didn't tell the young person anything about his experience in the field: he just let her go ahead with it. The program consisted of shoulder shrugs (the "no-no exercise" in which you turn your head from side to side), arm and knee lifts while sitting in a chair, and short walks down the hall. He was billed $35.00 each few-minute session of that silliness. (Of course, the insurance paid for it, which makes me wonder if insurance companies really know what they are paying for.) As soon as he got out of "jail" he immediately went back to *his* post-

cardiac program, and he has just competed in the "Second-Wind Tennis Tournament for the Over Fifty." His age group, the seventy-five- to eighty-year-olds, hasn't yielded him a partner so he has been playing (successfully) in the sixty- to sixty-five-year group. Incidentally, he also has had a hip replacement plus a nitro patch.

What you need is your own program, designed by *you*, organized by *you*, conducted by *you*, and *enjoyed* by you. When you get to Aqua-Ex, it will be suggested that you purchase a tape recorder and a few tapes that have good exercise rhythm, to take with you to the pool. Since you will have such equipment at hand, you can take it to the hospital with your toothbrush if the victim is you. If it's someone you care about, instead of flowers give a recorder and a tape or two. Another valuable piece of exercise equipment is one of those cheap watches that can be set to go "ping!" every hour. You need one and if your friend doesn't have one, lend him or her yours. Two more items should go with the above: a thick rubber band and a medium/hard rubber ball.

#103 Ball Squeeze (A)

- Raise your right hand above your head and squeeze the ball as tightly as you can. That may not be enough to scare a squeek out of a mouse, but it's a start.
- Hold your squeeze for a slow count of five.
- Straight above your head is 12 o'clock on a dial: move your right arm from 12 to 6, squeezing for five seconds at each number. That will

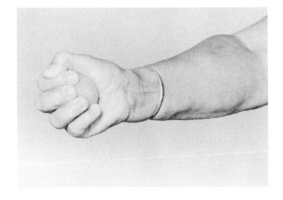

be six squeezes with the right hand or thirty seconds.
- Do the same with the left hand. That's one minute of exercise done

every hour, and if that's all you did in an eight-hour hospital day it would be eight minutes more than most patients get.

#104 Elastic Stretch (A)

On the second day, double your exercises and double the time.

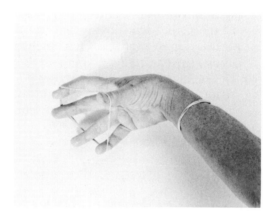

- Sliding all five fingers into an elastic band, open your fingers against its resistance.
- Hold for five seconds and relax.
- Do your hold at each number on a clock dial, as with the ball. When you have completed these two exercises, you will have exercised your arm, hand, and chest muscles.

#105 Supine Four Corners (A)

Your legs too are very important to your comfort *and to your* recovery. They need both stretching and strengthening and your blood needs to be *squeezed* back up into your torso rather than merely allowed to run down-hill when the foot of the bed is raised. When you raise the foot the heart has to push the blood uphill to your toes.

- Spread your feet about 18 inches apart and point your toes downward as hard as you can. Hold for a slow count of five.
- Rotate both feet outward and try to lay their edges flat on the bed. Hold for five.

- Pull the toes upward toward your knees and hold for five.
- Finish that circle by turning the toes inward . . . *hard,* and hold for five. Reverse the circle doing the same four stops.
- Finish the exercise by tightening the *"quads"* (thigh muscles) three times, holding for five while tight and a second five while relaxing. Do this series whenever a commercial comes on TV and after any attendant's visit. If it brings on even a whisper of a cramp in the legs or feet, check with the Myotherapy section for the legs on page 144.

THE LIMBERING SERIES

#106 Side Lying

- Lie on your right side with both knees *slightly* bent. Rest your head on your arm or a pillow and try to relax.
- Draw your top knee as close to your nose as possible. Help the stretch with one or both hands.
- Extend the leg downward to a point about eight to ten inches above the resting leg.
- Lower to the resting or starting position *on* the resting leg . . . and *relax for a count of three.* Repeat four times.

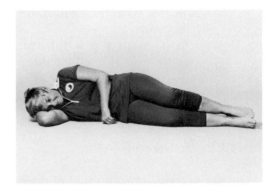

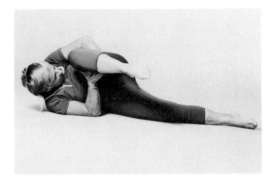

The *Limbering Series* is insurance against back pain. The side lying exercise is the most important of the five and MUST be done at least twice daily. More, if a backbone threatens or the stress level rises.

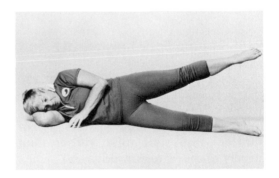

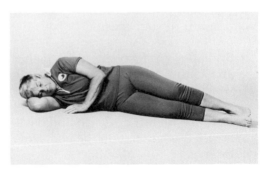

#107 Prone Gluteus Set (A)

- First, tighten the seat muscles by pinching the buttocks together.
- Hold for five seconds.
- Relax.
- Next, tighten the seat and pull in the abdominals.
- Hold for five counts.
- Relax.

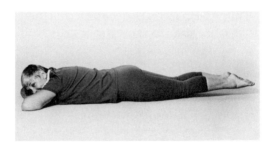

The sphincters are those muscles in the floor of the pelvis that you would tighten frantically if you had to go to the bathroom and there was someone in there already. These are the muscles that prevent incontinence and contribute to sexual pleasure.

- Tighten the buttocks, the abdominals, and then the sphincters.
- Hold tight for five seconds.
- Relax.
- Do ten, tightening everything at once.
- Roll to the other side and repeat Exercise #106 four times.
- Roll over onto your back.

#108 Supine Pelvic Tilt (A)

- Lie supine with knees bent and feet about eighteen inches apart. Arch the back as high as you can while keeping the shoulders and seat on the bed.
- Then force the spine down as you tilt the pelvis and tighten abdominals, seat, and sphincters.
- Hold for five.
- Relax.
- Do four.

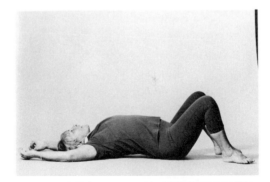

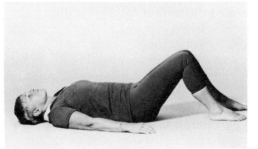

#109 Supine Knee to Nose (B)

This exercise is **B** because in a bed series it is *hard*. Everything is relative!

- Lie supine with knees bent and bring one knee as close to your nose as you can manage. (Help with your hands if you like). Don't be discouraged if all you can do is lift the foot off the bed. What counts is progress and it does *not* have to be speedy progress.)
- From the knee touch, extend the leg and return to start.
- Alternate four to a side.

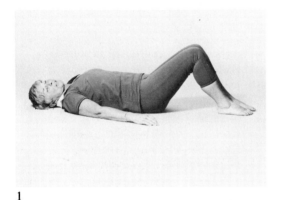

1

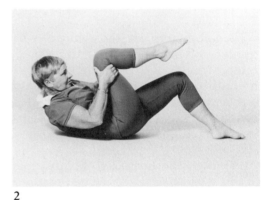

2

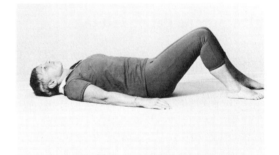

3

4

This Limbering Series will use up two to three minutes. If you did the exercises when you woke, after your bath, before your lunch, after your guests leave in the afternoon, and before lights out, you will be doing about 13 minutes of really good, very safe exercises a day *without help from anyone*. Added to your other exercises, you will be spending over a half hour a day on getting well rather than on just vegetating.

You—or your "pupil"—will heal faster due to improved circulation, and will sleep better due to the continuous workout. If you can also take some trigger points out of painful areas like the lower back and legs, you will be able to get yourself or your patient back into the world in a hurry. And you will be taking the danger out of bed rest.

FOOT MASSAGE

Feet are tellers of tales. There once was a song:

> They used to kiss my little feet,
> But they wouldn't do it now . . .

If you didn't know better you would think that age was the ruiner of pretty feet, handsome feet, strong, shapely, unmarred feet—but it isn't. I was sitting on the landing of some ancient stone stairs leading down into a market place in Mexico when a graceful, smooth, beautiful, little, brown foot was placed next to me. It didn't even seem to be dusty in that dusty land. I looked up past the long skirt and shawl expecting to see the face of a young girl. The foot was that of a woman *well over eighty*. That unmarred foot had probably never been in a shoe.

The woman was selling what looked to be some sort of nuts and still had about twenty left. If she sold them all she'd have no reason to be there gossiping with her friends, so she'd been doling them out five to a customer all day. My Spanish was limited to "Which way is the ladies room?" so my companion asked the old woman how she kept her feet so smooth and beautiful. She said she "rubbed" them. She didn't say with what, but it was probably the juice of something that grew ten feet down the path. It isn't what you rub with, it's the fact that *the feet are cared for* (so, incidentally were her hands). Brittle, yellow, unkempt toenails are a disgrace, just as disgraceful as dirty feet. They shout poor circulation, insufficient exercise, compressed flesh pressed down on chairs. In short, a swamp. It isn't fair.

Just rest a minute and start recalling where those feet of yours have taken you over the years . . . and what you owe them. To begin with, you owe them attention, real attention. Feet are as sensitive as hands.

- A dancer's feet are highly educated, *but every foot has that potential.*
- Young feet are often painless, *but every foot has that potential.*
- An athlete's feet are strong and can endure, *but every foot has that potential.*

As long as we are preparing for an exciting life up ahead, let's do something about your "base of operations."

At first, whether you are stuck in bed, a chair, or merely within the painful or limiting walls of yourself, you may need help with foot massage. *Get it.* Russian athletes are paired, and after every workout they do each other's feet. If you have started a No Pain Club, then let foot massage finish off the workout. If you are sharing your program with a friend, do the same thing. If you are caring for a friend or loved one, a foot massage could be the highlight of each day. I've been in hospitals often and confined to bed oftener, and over the years the thing I remember most vividly was having my good foot stuck into a basin of warm water and then rubbed. The leg in a sling had to make do with being wrapped in a hot, wet towel that seemed to mold itself even between my toes. Grateful is not the word. I have never forgotten, and if you want to shock your feet right out of their socks, start taking care of them.

Over half of us have a structural anomaly called the long second toe, Morton's Toe, or, more poetically, "the classic Greek foot" by Doctor Janet Travell who brought it to my attention. This condition isn't as simple as its name; you can have the problem without having a long toe. Turn to page 165 and learn why you have a callus here or there, why you have a hammertoe or the beginnings of a bunion or what has been diagnosed as a neuroma, and take the suggested steps to help your feet do the demanding and important jobs you require.

If you have a long second toe, pigeon toes, turned-out or flat feet, you have been substituting secondary muscles all your life. You have been asking muscles not designed for certain functions, but useful in others, to do both. The strain has been terrible. Your leg muscles, starting in both seat and groin, are in spasm, especially the tibialis anterior on the outside of the lower leg. Your tendinitis is probably due to that continuous strain as were your "growing pains" which shortly will be called "arthritis." Have your seat, groin, and legs detriggered at least once a week. Then do the following.

#110 Arch

- Place the fingers of your left hand flat over the toes of your right foot. Your thumb goes under your instep.
- Press your toes down to increase the arch of the foot.
- Alternate with #111. If it throws your foot into a spasm check Myotherapy pattern on page 148 for the foot and on page 144 for the lower legs.

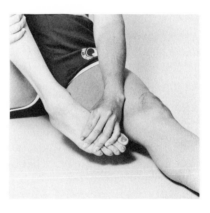

#111 Press-Up

- Place both hands under the ball of your foot and pull up as far as possible to stretch the sole of the foot and the heel cords.
- Alternate with #110.

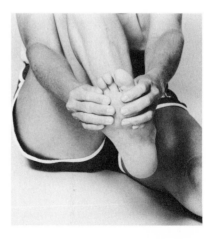

#112 Twist-Out

- Draw the right foot up close to your body and twist it, so that the sole faces up.
- With the heel of your right hand on the ball of the foot and the fingers of the left hand under the instep, press *down* with the right and pull *up* with the left.
- Alternate with #113.

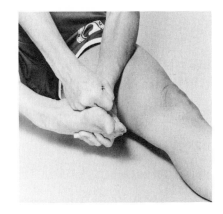

#113 Twist-In

- Place the heel of your left hand on the inside edge of your foot, just back of your big toe.
- Grasp the outside of the foot at the level of your little toe.
- Press *down* with the left hand and pull *up* with the right to twist the foot inward.
- Alternate with #112.

The above exercises will improve the flexibility of the foot and ankle and, should it be needed, reduce swelling. The swelling will remain, however, if you don't detrigger the entire leg.

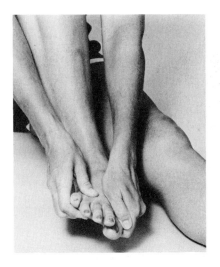

These exercises and massage are very important for anyone with diabetes, multiple sclerosis, or lupus. Look ahead: Always keep in mind that if there is a disease ahead the state you are in when you contract it can determine how fast, and to what extent, you will recover. Have *all* parts of yourself functioning well, all the time, so you always have the advantage on your side.

#114 Toe Spread

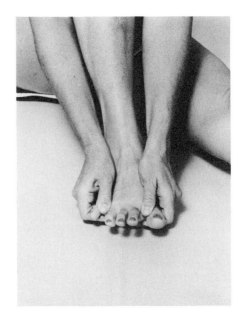

- Grasp the foot in both hands, placing the thumbs on top of the instep and the fingers underneath the metatarsal arch.
- First, spread the toes wide and then, as if your toes were webbed, try to continue the separation between the toes by pressing your thumbs to meet your fingers through the flesh of the foot between the bones of the toes.
- Spend a minute on each foot.

#115 Ball Press

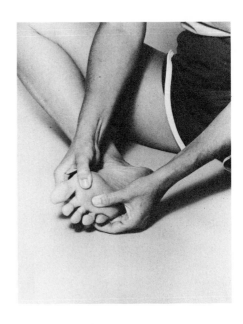

- Place your fingers on the upper surface of your foot and your thumbs on the ball.
- Press your thumbs hard against your sole and make small circles as though you were trying to loosen the foot bones (which you are).
- Spend at least one, or even two minutes on each foot. If you have a callus in the middle of the metatarsal arch, you have a long second toe, see page 149. DO NOT CUT OFF THE CALLUS; get rid of the cause for it. DO NOT PUT A "PROTECTIVE" PAD OVER THE CALLUS IN THE MIDDLE OF THE ARCH. IT MAKES THE CONDITION MUCH WORSE.

#116 Heel Cord Relaxer

Before you think of relaxing your heel cord or Achilles tendon, take out the trigger points in your calf muscles, Myotherapy pattern on page 144. Spasmed calf muscles lead to both pain and fatigue and an "old" walk.

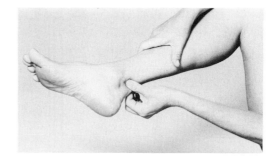

- Place your fingers on one side of your heel cord and the thumb on the other.
- Start at the heel and move the tendon back and forth from side to side as you move up the leg.
- At each stopping place, squeeze the cord, hunting for overlooked trigger points.

- Repeat the side-to-side action three or four times but the squeeze trip only once.

Feet need exercise. HOWL! "Mine get enough trotting around all day cleaning up after my busy family." "Mine are dog-tired when I get home from the plant; what do you think they've been doing all day, snoring?" "Exercise my feet, that's the *last* thing I want to do. I run them around the track five miles a day, that's exercise enough." Rubbish! Those offerings are not "foot exercises." Those are mobilization exercises; they get you from here to there and they use the muscles of feet and legs exactly the same way with every step. A few muscles are overworked; the rest, neglected. A few set up the spasms that limit circulation to the rest. A few grow shorter and shorter while the others, like passengers in a plane flown by a pilot with a dinner date in Samaria, are just as doomed. Foot exercise includes all the foot muscles. It stretches, twists, turns, and strengthens. It makes feet

feel alive. It makes feet *come alive.* It will make your day, whatever your age.

Once you have completed the foot massage, your feet are warm and ready for action, whether that action be Four Corners Bed Exercise, a game of tennis, a dance class, or a walk in the Black Forest. If you have had an illness or accident and are just getting your pins under you, these are as important to you as the marathoner (who probably thinks he or she doesn't need them, more's the pity). If you are still in the bed or chair phase, look at the pictures and see yourself doing them. Go through every one of them with your mind's eye. That's what every Olympian does with his or her skill before performing. Visualize yourself doing the foot exercise first; then, every day, take another exercise from the entire book and spend some time with it. Read the instructions over and over as you look at the picture. Inform, teach, badger, pester, and push your subconscious into knowing you can do what you see. Humans, except for Olympians, don't even begin to tap their physical potential at any age, but you have the jump on anyone under forty-five. Keep that in mind. *What you had you can have again.*

#117 Roll-Out–Toe Lift

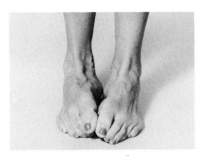
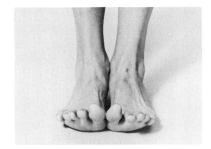

- Start with feet parallel and flat on the floor.
- Roll onto the outer edges of the feet and curl your toes under . . . *tight.* Be sure your toes touch in front and your heels in back. This exercise is also known as The Mouse Trap.
- Next, return to the flat-foot position. Keeping the balls of your feet on the floor, raise your toes as high as you can. The other name for this exercise is Hot Pennies; if you can imagine those pennies under your feet, those toes will come up!
- Alternate Roll-Out with Toe Lift, eight times.

#118 Heel Cord Stretch

Two muscles, the *gastrocnemius* and the *soleus* attach to the *Achilles tendon* or heel cord. If either is tight, leg cramps result. If you have run a lot or have worn high heels more than flat ones, the heel cords are usually tight. If you have ever had polio, same thing. If your job kept you sitting most of the time and you didn't know how to counteract the resulting foreshortening with walking or stretch exercise, same tightening. It must be counteracted *now.*

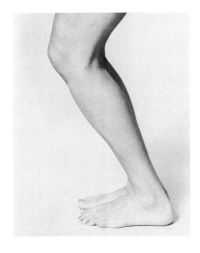

- Stand with feet close together, heels flat on the floor.
- Keeping your seat tucked under, bend your knees as far as they will go while the heels are still down.

#119 Advanced Heel Cord Stretch

- Holding onto a wall, chair, or someone else, place the balls of your feet on a telephone book (later you will use the stairs).
- Bounce your heels down toward the floor. Because your legs are straight, this is an entirely different stretch.
- Rise to the toes and lower slowly.
- At the bottom of the stretch, do eight bounces.
- Do four sets.

120 Heel Lift

Feet that are not exercised lose the ability to move in all the wonderful ways feet are supposed to move. One of those losses is flexibility in the front part of the foot where the toes attach. The foot refuses to bend and the result is something between a waddle and a bilateral limp. Stairs are no fun and your rear sticks out like a bustle.

- Stand with feet close together and heels on the floor.
- Push one knee and instep forward as you stand very tall and tighten the other leg all the way from buttock to instep.
- Stretch your groin by advancing your pelvis.
- Hold for four counts.
- *Slowly* change legs.
- Alternate for eight, feeling your

- At that point, use a short, easy bounce rhythm.
- Eight bounces make a set.
- Do four sets.

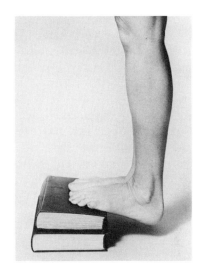

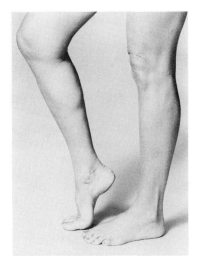

way from one leg to the other, aware of what the tightening is doing. This is a foot exercise, but like most of what the feet do, it affects many other muscles.

#121 Toe Rises

Rising to the toes is also a multimuscle exercise which can be done sloppily or well. *Think* and *feel* as you do it.

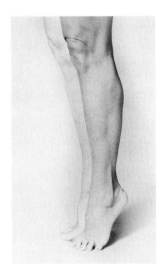

- Rise to the toes, tightening every leg muscle and your seat. (At first, just get to the top and lower. When you feel a little surer, take four seconds to reach the top and four to lower.)
- Work up to eight each way and then work back down to four. In time start with one up, one down, two up, two down, etc. When you are up and about (which may be now) do this exercise every time you find yourself at a sink.

#122 Edging

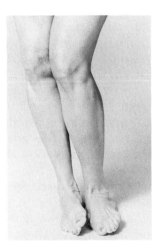

- Start with feet parallel and flat to the floor.
- Bend both knees, keeping the pelvis tucked under.
- Shift both knees to the right so that your feet will roll onto their right edges.
- Without straightening your legs or changing the level of your head, shift your knees to the left.
- Alternate sides for eight, to make up a set.
- Do three sets.

#123 Instep Stretch

If you can get down on the floor, fine. If you can't, then wait till you can before trying this exercise.

- Rest on hands and knees with insteps flat on the floor.
- Rise up onto the top surface of the

toes/instep area, stretching the front of the foot and increasing the arch at the same time. A cramp at this point calls for Myotherapy pattern on page 148 for the foot and on page 145 for the front of the lower leg.

- When this becomes easy to do, add bounces.
- Do four and rest.
- Repeat twice more.

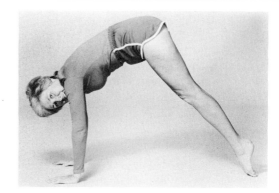

Every part of you suffers when condemned to bed or chair, but the feet, which are at the end of the line, are apt to make the most noise. When your feet feel cold your body is saying, "Trigger points in my hips, groin, and legs are limiting circulation, and therefore nutrition! If my leg is fractured, it will be slow to heal! If I get bed sores on my heels (shame on everybody), they won't heal either! If I have a tired or damaged heart, it is having to overwork getting blood through spasmed muscles, and it isn't doing that great a job of it. If I have diabetes, feet *must* have good circulation; mine are lacking in circulation, nutrition . . . and attention. *Somebody could lose me at this rate.*

"But I *always* had cold feet" is no excuse; it merely means you always had poor circulation to those poor feet and now is the time to improve that situation.

Self-image takes a beating every time you look down at ugly, yellow, brittle, broken nails. Suppose you were wearing the telltale sign of poor grooming on the end of your nose . . . you wouldn't, would you? Do you think hid-

ing it in shoes is the answer? No. Care and grooming are. If you can't get down to groom your toes, go for a pedicure. You owe those feet. It's time to pay them back.

GYM IN A CHAIR

"Dangle," he says. If you've never been hospitalized the word "dangle" won't mean much. If you have, you know it means that someone—it used to be a nurse, but now it's a physical therapist whose time will go on your bill—helps you sit up and put your legs over the side of the bed. I'd always beat them out. If the therapist said, "Dangle tomorrow," one of my best friends would arrive before breakfast (nothing pleasant happens in hospitals before breakfast) and I'd be already dangling when breakfast came in.

Whether at home or in a hospital, your body will accept "dangling" in various ways. "I can't, I'll fall apart"; that's predictable. "Great, tomorrow I can go home" is also predictable.

Take your subconscious aside and tell it that "dangling" is a piece of cake. If there's that awful whispering going on, the kind that says, "I'm safe here. What will happen when I get home? I'll be all alone like last time. I'm afraid if I 'dangle' they'll make me go home . . ." *Make* you go home? Is that what scares you? Just being in a hospital should scare you. You can't do what you want to do and what you want to do is rebuild your life with a whole set of new tools. Hospitals are for *very* sick people; you are no longer very sick and you have work to do. It isn't going to be like the last time. It's *never* going to be like the last time. *You* are going to take charge of you. *You* are the boss and your body is your staff and *you* are going to tell it what to do . . . so "dangle" with joy and expectation. "What's going to happen now?" said the child as the doors to Toyland opened. Now comes Gym in a Chair.

"Now you may sit up for a couple of hours." To someone who has been staring at the ceiling hearing this is cause for unbounded joy. Don't let it throw you. It will be incredible for a couple of days and then (thank heaven) you will want something new. "New" should be thought about before you are even ready to dangle. Sitting in a chair will be different for you than for anybody else. *You* know more than most, including the people who take care of you. Bottoms are as sensitive as feet. When you were a little kid, a baby even, you knew one lap from another. Dad's legs were hard and long and his shin was for horseback riding. Mom's lap was warm and soft and it was for loving and listening to stories. Aunt Lulu's was bony,

cousin Agatha could never keep hers even, and you were always in danger of sliding off. What told you all that? Your bottom. Now go around the house and sit in a half dozen chairs with your eyes closed. The easy chair will envelop you. The dining room chair will insist that you sit up straight, while the director's chair will give your sitting posture a slightly rakish look. What will deliver the messages to your brain? Your bottom. What is the most important part of you once the doctor says "Sit"? Your bottom.

If you are at home, no problem; there are lots of different chairs that can be brought to your room, and if you have a rocking chair you are ahead of the game. If you know you will have to do a lot of sitting for a while, buy, borrow, or rent one. A rocking chair is a friend to bottoms as much as a rocking cradle is a friend to babies. If you are in a hospital you will be more limited unless you have made a friend along the way. There may be an easy chair, there is a straightbacked "visitors" chair, and you will want a wheelchair. All else failing, tell three friends to forget the flowers and spring for a director's chair.

On the first chair day, take what you get and be glad; on the second day, divide whatever time has been allotted by the number of chairs you have available. Get your tape recorder going with some foot-tapping music and tap in all three, or perhaps four chairs. On the third day, line up your chosen exercise chair and begin.

#124 Toe Lifter (A)

- Place your feet about ten inches apart.

- Keeping your heels on the floor, slide your feet to the turned-in position and then to the turned-out position. Just that little action worked the lower legs, which are usually the last places to be considered in bed rest unless they cramp (and then some medication will be ordered).

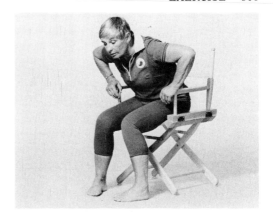

As soon as you feel a bit stronger—which may be right away—do Toe Lifts.

- Pick the fronts of the feet off the floor and rotate them inward.
- If you do it slowly, taking four counts to reach the end of the rotation, you will feel it in the tibialis anterior, the muscle so overworked by a long second toe.
- Do four slides and then four lifts with each foot.
- Then let them your feet rest for a few minutes while you work something else.

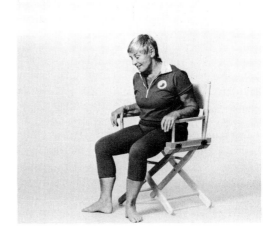

#125 Neck Rest (A)

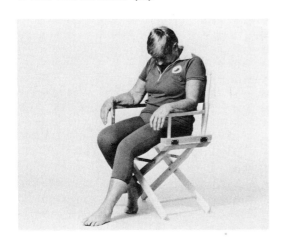

- Resting your arms on the chair arms, drop your head onto your chest.
- Let it hang there while you act the detective and hunt for spots in your upper back that seem to pull. (Check with Myotherapy pattern on page 123 for the upper back. There will be at least two points under the circles numbered 18 in Figure 21 that will be ouch-spots.)
- Next, roll your head onto one shoulder and let it rest there while

you feel for a tight spot on the other side. You won't need any help with those points; you can reach them with your own fingers or a bodo.

- Pinch, squeeze, and press all the spots, holding for five seconds each time.
- Then roll your head backward. As you will expect, there will be trigger points in your chest, so check with Myotherapy pattern on page 137. You can find and dispense with these points yourself.
- Then roll onto the other shoulder and repeat the hunt for a tight muscle.
- Once you have "cleaned out" the muscles supporting your head do three slow rolls to the left and then three to the right. If you find it the least bit difficult to turn your head to the left or right through full range, turn to page 135 and take care of your stiff neck. Being confined to a chair may turn out to be a blessing in disguise if it forces you to pay attention to your body and its aches.

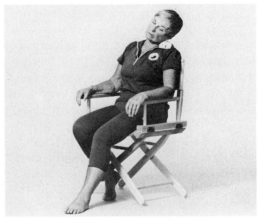

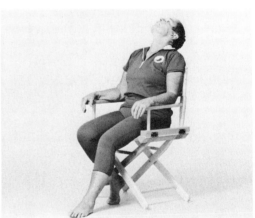

#126 Knee Lift (A)

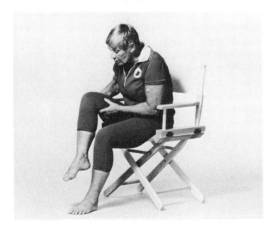

While you have been lying in bed getting weaker, your back muscles and hamstrings were getting tighter.

- Place both hands under your upper leg and lift it as high as possible. This strengthens your arms and stretches your back, and oddly enough, the thigh muscles in front as well as in back.
- Replace the leg, and do the other. If there is any pull in the groin, check with Myotherapy pattern on page 129.

- Do four on each side.
- In a couple of days, when you lift your leg, remove your supporting hands and try to maintain the hold for a few seconds before you lower it, unsupported, to the chair.

#127 Heel Lift (A)

Many feet have been trapped in shoes for years—shoes that limit normal walking. Many feet have never been properly exercised. If you want to see examples of what would be called cruelty to animals if feet were dogs, go to an airport and watch people waddle by. Age doesn't count at all; the young ones and even children are crippled already. The foot is supposed to bend into a right angle where it attaches to the toes. Do yours? If yes, be determined to keep them like that. If not, what better time than now to start working on them?

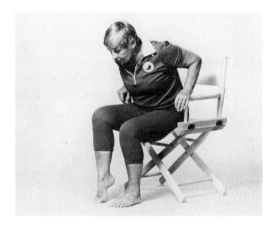

- Place feet parallel, with heels flat on the floor.
- Keep the toes and ball of one foot firmly attached to the floor and raise your heel.
- Try to push the instep forward when you are at full raise.
- Lower.
- Repeat four times with each foot. This is a good exercise to tie in with reading a book. When you come to the end of two pages, do four heel lifts. It will become automatic.

Later, when you are home again and looking at yourself in the bathroom mirror or standing in the kitchen waiting for the coffee pot to deliver, hold onto the sink or counter and do heel lifts *slowly.* Add them to your warm-ups and floor progressions. You had wonderful little feet as a child. They are still there and they still respond, no matter what you did to them or neglected to do for them. Treat your feet to regular massage and if they ache, get rid of the trigger points. They are your transportation to the world.

#128 Four Corners with Feet (A)

This exercise is the most important one we have for feet and ankles. It is also the one we use on athletes who have sprained ankles. (You need not be an athlete to sprain an ankle, but it helps.) If you have sprained yours, get someone to do the immediate mobilization described on page 166, and then do this exercise many times a day. If you have an old sprain that still swells and sometimes aches, do the same immediate mobilization. If you have a tendency to turn your ankle, see the section on long second toe (page 149).

- Slide forward until your seat is at the very edge of your chair.
- Lean back to rest your shoulders and stretch your legs out full length. (If any part of you hurts, go

no further. Check with the appropriate Myotherapy patterns for the area that hurts and then you can continue, painless.)
- Keeping your feet parallel, press the soles flat to the floor.
- With heels still resting on the floor, pull your toes up toward your body as far as possible.
- Point down and pull up four times.
- Then turn the toes first inward, and then outward, four times.
- Finish with circles, first one way and then the other. Do this exercise while watching TV.

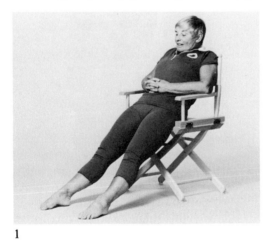

1

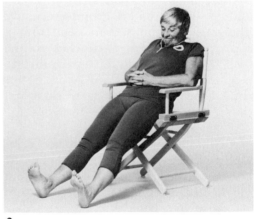

2

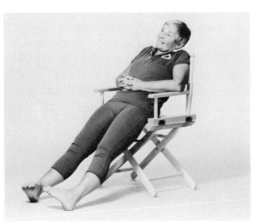

3

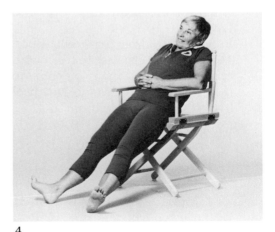

4

#129 Back Stretch (A)

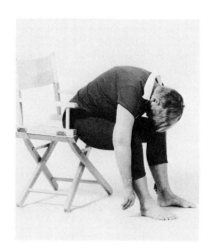

- Sit forward in your chair with legs wide apart and feet flat on the floor.
- Lean forward to drop your head between your knees (or at least in that general direction). The limiting trigger points will be in your seat muscles and at the waist. You golfers will not get your form back until those muscles are freed. Check the Myotherapy pattern on page 125.
- Once you have located the trigger points and are looser do gentle bounces, trying to drop your head a little lower each day.

#130 Waist Twists (A)

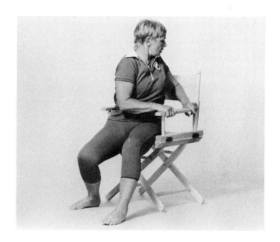

- Keeping your feet well apart and flat on the floor, twist your upper body around to the left, bringing both hands as close to the back of the chair arm as possible.
- At the same time turn your head to look over your shoulder.
- Swing to the right and repeat the action.
- (Did you feel a "glitch" anywhere? If so, check your Myotherapy Patterns)
- *Then* alternate for eight swings. You may have to start with two or four. That's fine, just *start*. This exercise will slim the waist, improve your walk, and keep that golf score in mind. This is another prep for sport.

All sports call for preparation. Once you are well again, go over the sports list and see which ones interest you.

#131 Shoulder Reach (A)

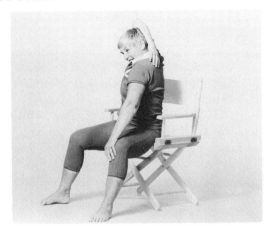

- Place your left hand on your left knee as an anchor, and in the same motion place the right hand as far down your back as possible as you twist your upper body to the right.
- Change direction and repeat to the left. This is the start of exercises for shoulder flexibility.
- Do four for a start and increase as you become stronger.

#132 Arm Circles (A)

- Sit forward in your chair and place your feet apart and flat on the floor.
- Lean forward from your hips, stretching your arms straight out in front.
- Sit erect and raise your hands straight overhead, pressing your shoulders back.
- Open your arms wide and press them back and down in wide arcs.
- Grasp the backs of the chair arms, lift chest and head.

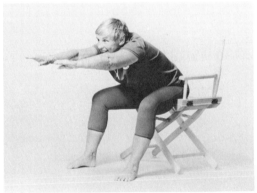

1

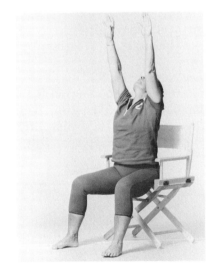

2

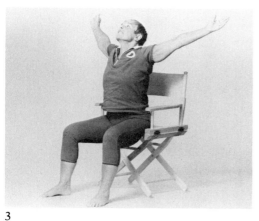

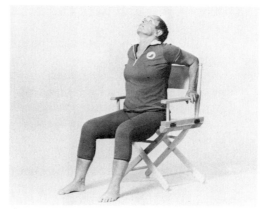

3   4

#133 Knee Kiss (A)

- Bend upper torso forward, head down.
- Raise bent right leg.
- Try to touch knee with your nose.
- Alternate legs four bends to a side.

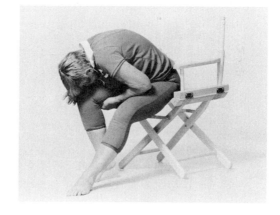

#134 Knee Cross (A)

The Knee Cross is supposed to be beyond the reach of the "hippie" (person with a total hip replacement), as is everything except walking straight forward. If the operation has been done right and the muscles cleared of trigger points, the legs are just fine.

- Simply cross one leg over the other.
- Alternate crosses.
- Start with four and add as you improve.

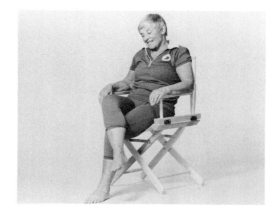

#135 Knee Cross and Kick (B)

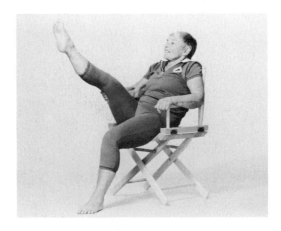

- Keep the same body position with seat forward.
- Cross your knee and then kick up.
- You can then put the leg down or, if you are feeling stronger, drape it over the chair arm as in exercise #136.
- From the drape position kick up, and bring the leg back to the knee cross.
- Start with two to a leg and slowly add week by week.

#136 Knee Cross–Pull Up–Open (B)

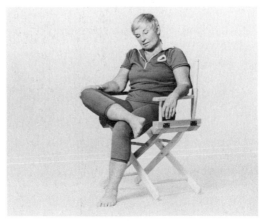

- Lean back in your chair and rest one foot on the other knee.
- Grasp the foot firmly and pull it toward your body in gentle short bounces. This will stretch your seat muscles and those running down the outside of the leg.
- Then swing the leg wide to drape it over the arm of the chair.
- Replace the foot on the floor and repeat with the other leg.
- Alternate for four. If there is pull on the outer side of the leg check the Myotherapy pattern for sciatica, on page 124.

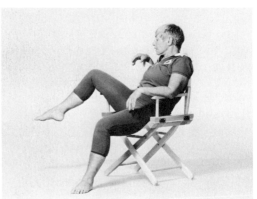

#137 Seat Lift (A)

- Place your hands on the fronts of the chair arms and straighten your arms to lift your seat into the air.
- *Lower slowly,* taking five seconds to complete the descent.
- Start with two and work up to six. You can help improve your arm strength by using the weights shown on page 322. If you find tightness in your arms or hands, see Myotherapy pattern on page 140. Right about now the chair exercises start to get a little harder; if you are not quite ready, you will become discouraged. Try a few of them and if you find them too much, stay with the first exercises until you have fixed most of the limiting trigger points. Strength will follow. Flexibility will come as you work. Remember, it will take longer to become flexible than to become strong, but you need both flexibility and strength for coordination.

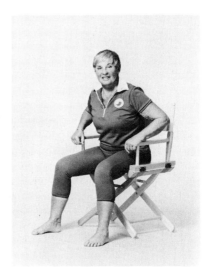

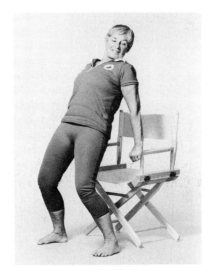

#138 Upper Torso Twist (B)

- Lean down and reach around to grasp the outside of the left ankle with the right hand.
- Return to the erect position.
- Do this same movement to the other side.
- Then reach down between the feet to grasp the outside of the left ankle with the right hand.

- Return to the erect position and repeat to the other side. These two movements improve flexibility of the lower back, upper torso, arms, and shoulders.
- Repeat the series three times.

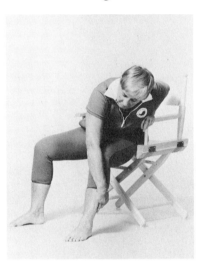 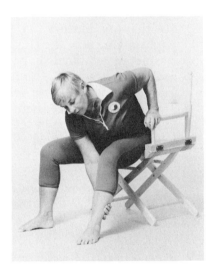

#139 Body Lift (B)

- Move your seat forward in the chair and grasp the forward ends of the chair arms.
- Stretch your legs straight out in front, pressing your feet flat on the floor.
- Keeping your legs straight, raise your entire body, arch your back as much as you can, and let your head fall backward.
- Hold the arched position for a slow count of three.

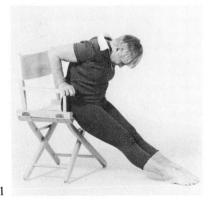

1

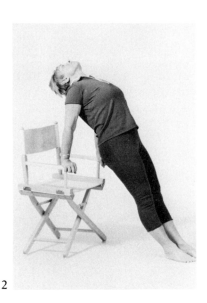

- Return *slowly* to the sitting position. This exercise stretches the chest and abdominal muscles and strengthens the arms, upper back, and shoulders.
- Start with two and work up to six.

2

#140 Pelvic Tilt, Assisted (A)

- Stand with feet flat and with hands resting on chair arms.
- Keeping your head down *and your seat tucked under,* do a half knee bend with abdominals and sphincters tight.

- As you bring your head up, return to the straight leg flat-foot position.
- Do four. In the future, when you are up and about, make a habit of doing this exercise whenever you leave your chair.

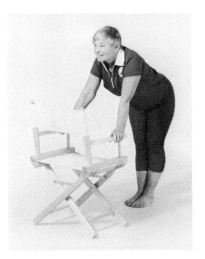

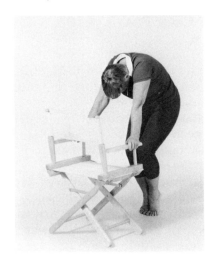

#141 Knee In–Leg Out (A)

- Start by standing in front of your chair, grasping arms for support.
- Swing the leg up to rest your foot on the chair seat.
- Then swing the leg back, and at the same time lift your head. It doesn't matter if you have to lift the leg to the chair and it doesn't matter if your lift to stern is unremarkable; it is a start.
- Do four with each leg.

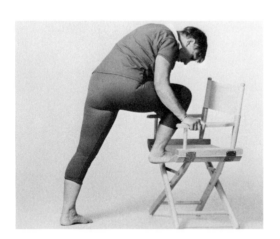
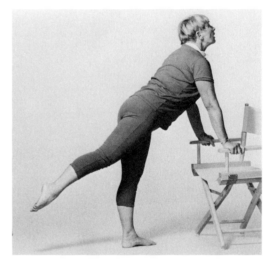

#142 Chair Push-Ups (B)

- Be sure your chair is anchored so that it cannot slip (and also that your feet are secure so that *you* cannot slip.)
- Stand back from the chair (the distance will be greater as your strength and self-assurance improve).
- Start with feet wide apart at first, as this makes the work easier.
- Grasp the chair arms firmly and *slowly* lower yourself toward the chair by doing the same let-down

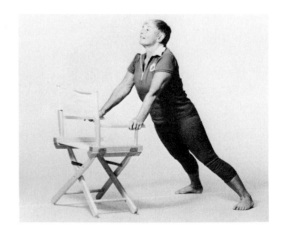

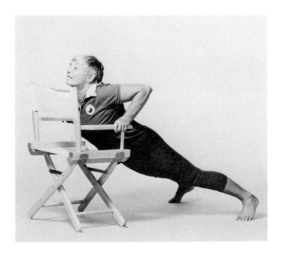 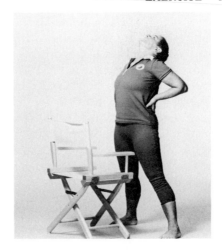

suggested on page 85. (It doesn't matter if all you can accomplish is an inch or two of descent. In time it will be better. Use the weight bag work for arms on page 324 and the pulley, page 339 before you undertake standing push-ups. Check out Doorway Gym on page 335 and designate corners in your house and office as your exercise area.

Jack Kelly, Sr., used to hang into doorways to stretch his chest muscles that had been foreshortened by rowing. Doorways make a great in-house gym.
- Start with one or two push-ups and partial let-downs.
- Then stand erect, arching your back, to rest.

HUGGING SERIES

One day, a long time ago, I learned a very valuable lesson. My troupe of teachers, graduates, and students were doing a Fitness Day at the Laconia State School for the Handicapped. I had been working with the handicapped since the fifties and was sure of my ground. There were about twenty-five of us and forty in each class that was brought into the gym. We started with the highest-functioning students, who took one look at our circus-colored ramps, sawhorses, hoops, Frisbees, ladders, and mats and were joyously off to the races. We proceeded through the day with groups in a descending order of function. We had just about had it and were gathering our "toys" to go home, when twenty wheelchairs were pushed into the gym. In each chair was a person who could not see or hear or talk. They just *were*. "Oh my God! What do I do now?" I thought.

I stood behind the nearest chair. I'm sure my crew thought I knew what I was doing because in seconds they each stood behind a chair. I leaned down and picked up two limp hands, and every other pair of hands in that strange brigade were picked up too. The music I asked for was "Nadia's Theme" because it is slow and gentle and haunting. I just did the lovely baby-exercises we have done for years with babies. These "babies" were just as new to rhythmic movement, just older and bigger. They were certainly no stronger. At the end of the piece I put the hands back and discovered that they were no longer limp—they were holding fast to mine. Far more exciting, however, was the realization that *every one of those people was smiling.* The attendants were amazed. They didn't expect their patients to react to anything and this was not only reaction, it was a happy reaction. It meant that someone lived behind each closed face. A boat had been missed, but not any more.

"Hugging" became part of the day's routine along with washing, dressing, and eating. People can die without food; they also die without loving. Being held in someone's arms is often *more* important than warm clothes and enough to eat.

We got the message and took it right to a bunch of nursing homes. What a blast! We, they, and the nurses soon discovered the value of "hugging" and every year, the first field work my students get is done in nursing homes in our area.

"Hugging" worked so well in the nursing homes that we decided to try it in a nursery school. Maybe little kids didn't get enough "hugging" either. After the very first "hugging" session, no little kid would go home unless "hugged." Then we came up with a real winner. One of my students had taken her little boy with her to the nursing home where she worked. All the would-be grandparents spoiled him delightfully, as he did them. Why, we wondered, couldn't we mix them and form a "Grandkids Anonymous"? So we did. We trained a group of five-year-olds to "hug" and to do the friend–walking Exercise. (see page 339) Then we all charged off like a bunch of scientists about to pour X into Y to see what would come out. What came out was unbelievable. Everybody loved everybody. They "hugged" and exercised and those who could, danced. Everyone swore undying fealty till the next visit, the nurses cried all over themselves, "It's so beautiful . . ." And it was. Try some of these exercises with a friend. It certainly beats a drive in the country.

#143 Arms Out and Across (A)

This is the same as the one in the BED BALLET, Exercise #92.

- Take both hands in yours and, staying with slow rhythmic music, open the arms wide.
- Then cross back to stretch the upper back.
- Vary by making full arm circles—one arm up, one down, arms pulled close, and then stretched forward.

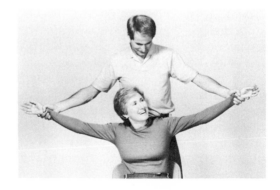

#144 Getting to Know You (A)

- Rock the person's body from side to side as you place his or her hands on the sides of your head, your chin resting on his or her head.
- Hold the head close within the circle of your arms.
- Open the arms wide to signify a change of action.
- Place your faces cheek to cheek as you rock.

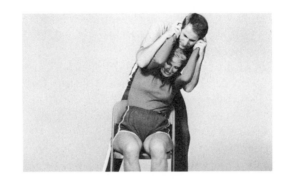

#145 Push-Down (A)

- Deposit your partner's hands in lap.
- Press gently forward on the shoulders to stretch the entire back.
- Do four and then vary by turning the torso to the left and pressing down four times.
- Same to right, and finish with four forward.

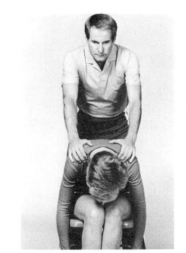

#146 Push-Down with Twist (B)

The **B** designation is to remind you to take it easy with this one.

- Let your partner's arms hang free.
- Twist the body as far to the left as is comfortable, and press down for four.
- Four to the other side. Return to #143.

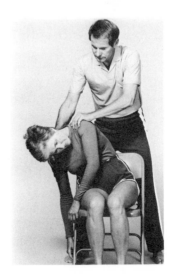

#147 Hugging (A)

- Picking up your partner's hands again, place your face cheek to cheek as before.
- Holding him or her in a close embrace, rock from side to side for several measures.
- Change your head to the other side and repeat.

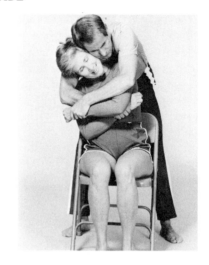

#148 Knee Lift (A)

- Pick up the bent leg, holding it just above the knee.
- Put it down.
- Repeat four times with each leg.

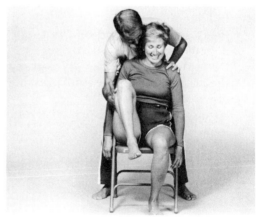

#149 Straight Leg Lift with Rotations (B)

- Grasping the leg at the ankle, lift the straight leg as high as it will go.
- Rotate the foot, first in and then out, for eight.
- Do the same with the other leg.
- Finish with more hugging.

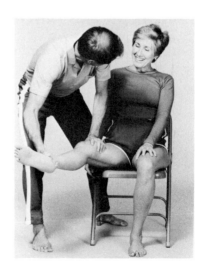

WALKER EXERCISE

Most people think of a walker as either a bridge from bed to crutches or as the end of the line. I've always thought of a walker as a fairly inexpensive piece of equipment. Two walkers, tied to some pipes, make an ideal ballet barre, especially in a place where several non-walkers are recovering in the same area. The person using a walker really needs a friend to do the following exercises. My friend is "Beanie" Whittaker, who saw me through my second hip replacement.

#150 Knee Bends (A)

- Stand behind the exerciser and clasp at the waist.
- Both you and your friend should bend and straighten the knees for eight.
- Do toe rises slowly, four counts up and four down.

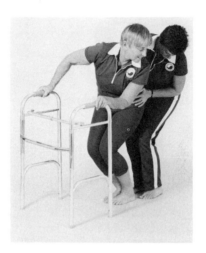

#151 Snowplow (B)

- Stand with feet apart, turned in, *both* knees slightly bent.
- Sit over to the right as you advance the right shoulder.
- Shift to the left and advance the right shoulder.
- Alternate for eight.

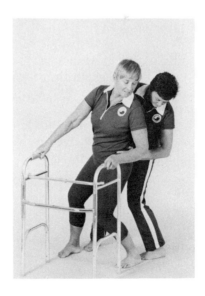

#152 Knee Lifts (B)

(You may have to lift the exerciser's knee at first.)

- Place the foot on the cross bar and do very small bends with the other leg.
- Do eight to a side.

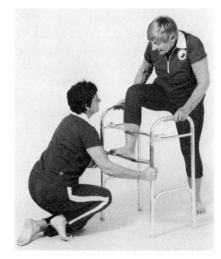

#153 Hamstring Stretch (A)

- Step back from the walker. (The friend stands on the opposite side to stabilize it.)
- With feet apart, bend forward from the hips and bounce the body downward in eight easy bounces.
- Let your upper body drop down between the arms.
- Stand straight to relax.
- Do three sets of eight.

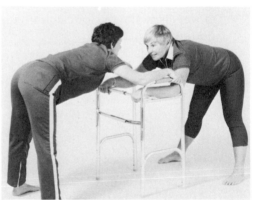

#154 Hip Wags (A)

- Stand with feet apart.
- Keeping the legs straight, wag the seat from side to side.
- Variation:
- Do the hip wags while doing #153.
- Take eight wags to get down and eight to get back up.
- Do three sets.

Then go walking with your walker. You will *feel* 100 percent more secure and you will *be* more secure.

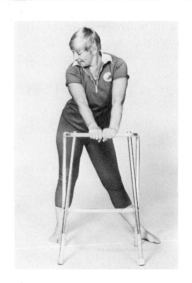

FRIEND-WALKING

For this exercise you should have two friends. Supported walking is a great help for a stroke patient who isn't all that sure what the other leg is going to do next. Along with two friends you need music, of course, and a broomstick. By this time the exerciser (and friends) should be in warm-up suits, even if you are still in the hospital. Have you ever noticed the way people look as they limp down hospital corridors, slippers flopping, night gowns dragging, unshaven and in general disarray? *Don't you look like that.* It's time friends brought you your warm-up suit, and if you don't have one, order one. Slippers aren't safe even if you are in great shape. Order your "running" shoes sent over and wear them. Don't hand me, "At *my* age?" Of course at your age and at any age. Young, messy people don't look any better than older, messy people.

Ideally, you need a mirror for this one because eyes, like the subconscious, believe what they see. They see the friends moving well and they tell the brain that your legs are doing the same thing. Pretty soon your legs will be!

#155 Friend-Walking–Cross-Overs (A)

- Stand between your friends and do the Cross-over (Exercise #70)
- Step first one foot across, and return.
- Cross the other foot.
- Cross first in front; then in back.
- For greater support, hold onto a lightweight pole with both hands. The pole should be long enough for the three of you to move freely.
- Next, turn to page 160 and do as many floor progressions as possible.

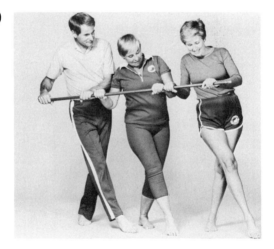

SMALL EQUIPMENT

I have always found that exercise done with something in one's hands is more fun, just as exercise without music is no fun at all; it's work.

The following treasure chest of exercise equipment can be had for very little money if you are interested in working with a group. These pieces give direction and form to exercise, and are delightful to use. All of these are demonstrated with friends in the hope that you will take networking to heart and get a bunch together, even if only to exercise and stay free of pain.

#156 Blocks (A)

Blocks are made from two-by-fours. Cut them in 6- to 7-inch lengths, then sand and and enamel them.

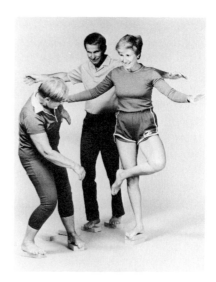

- Lay the blocks end-to-end in a line.
- The exerciser travels the length of the blocks with support from friends, walking frontward, backward, and sideways.

Why do this? To improve balance. When I used to teach teenaged girls to wear high heels, I had them walk on sawhorses. After that, what was walking across a dance floor! If the exerciser can't stay on the "beam," look for trigger points in the legs, seat, and groin. Variations:

- Lay the blocks crosswise.
- Walk on them as you would ladder rungs. That's good exercise for foot muscles.
- Set a pair under your feet while doing Walker Exercise #151.

#157 Frisbees (A)

- Hold Frisbees in your hands when you do many of the warm-up exercises. Frisbees can be used sitting or standing. They have the advantage of making you reach farther, twist harder, and stay with it longer. See how many of the foregoing exercises work with Frisbees.

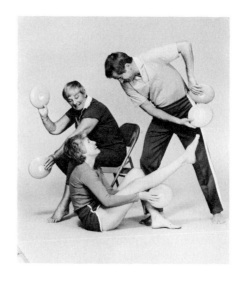

#158 Elastics (A)

- Elastics are made from ¾-inch waist-elastic strips 24 inches long. They are used to strengthen hands, arms, and legs by providing resistance. Mostly we use them in chair exercises either solo or with friends. They are also useful for bed exercises.

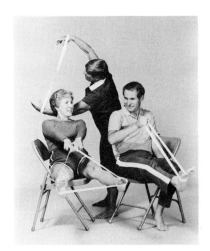

#159 Wand or Cane (A)

Wands are usually dowels 36 inches long and ¾ inch thick. Canes will do as well.
- First, be sure your chair is far enough from your friend's to prevent jabbing.
- Raise them, reach, paddle, turn, whatever you can think of. Stay with the music for eight beats before you change. If you are all alone with your program, just take up a piece of equipment, put on a good record, and start. Coordination is all there inside you. Now you can give it the chance to come out.

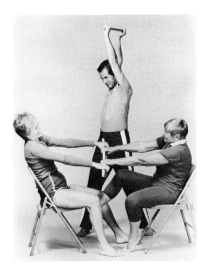

THE SELF CENTER

A Self Center is exactly that—a center for yourself. By this time you know what can be done and even how to do a lot of it; but where? "At home" is what we've been saying. You need not buy a membership at a spa or a health club. Just look what you can get together at home: weight bags, stairs, towels, chinning bar, rope climb, basketballs, and pulleys. There are many other types of exercise equipment you can get, of course; it's only a question of room. If you do have the room, I'd add an indoor bike and a rowing machine.

WEIGHT BAGS

The advantages of weight bags over barbells, dumbbells, and machines are many. Free weights are superior to machines in that they are far more versatile. There are just so many directions a machine can provide. Dumbbells are better than barbells: while the latter demand more control than machines, the former offer still more freedom. Weight bags are best of all. They are less expensive and can be stored in a small space; they also won't break your toes if you happen to drop them on your foot. Best of all, they're portable. When I go on tour I carry ten pounds' worth in my backpack, along with my current reading and toilet articles. It's a small pack and throws my host into a quandary when he offers to carry it for me!

To make weight bags, use strong, durable material (denim or sailcloth coverings look attractive and wear well) and either sand or lead shot (see Figure 65). The latter is more expensive (it can be purchased at a hardware store), but it's easier to handle and stow. In order to differentiate the weights of the bags, use coverings of different colors. I use yellow for one-pounders, red for two-pounders, and blue for five-pounders. To make up a set use two of each weight. The covering material should be cut into rectangles: 7 × 12 inches for one-pound weights, 10 × 12 inches for twos, and 10 × 13 inches for fives.

When you start using weights with any of the exercises you have already done "free," you will want to use slower music *and begin with the one-pounders.* If you sew a strip of Velcro* at each end, the bags will stay on your ankles for leg exercises. When you sit down to read or watch television, fasten a pair (or even two pair!) to your ankles and do leg exercises to the music provided by the commercials . . . or every time you come to the end of a chapter in your book. Put one next to your phone and do shoulder rotations while you talk. *Don't forget to use both arms!* When you get to STAIRS, put them in your pack. The same for WALKING.

To use weight bags like a barbell, hang them on either end of a wand, cane, or broomstick. The following exercises show you how to correctly use your homemade barbell.

*(If you use Velcro, add two inches in length to each bag.)

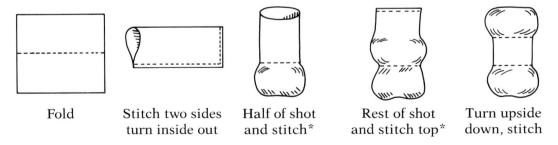

| Fold | Stitch two sides turn inside out | Half of shot and stitch* | Rest of shot and stitch top* | Turn upside down, stitch |

Figure 65. *Weight Bags*   *Use pins to hold shot while stitching

#160 Clean to Chest and Press (A)

- Lean down, with relaxed knees, and grasp the bar at shoulder width, palms facing toward you.
- Keeping your back rounded and pelvis tucked under, stand erect, bringing the bar to your chest. (That's the clean to chest movement.)
- Press the bar overhead and return it to chest level.

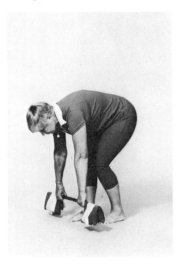 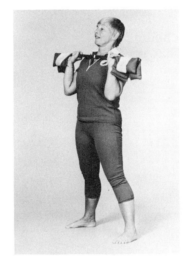 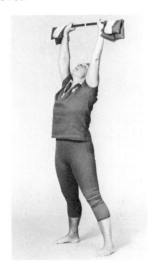

#161 Reverse Curl (A)

- From the above position, drop the bar to hang at full arm length.
- Return the bar to chest level (a reverse curl).
- Do three such curls and place the bar and weights on the floor.

#162 Curls (A)

- Reverse your hands so the palms face away.
- Stand, allowing the bar to hang at full arms' length in front of your thighs.
- Bring the bar to chest level, being sure to keep your arms close to your sides.
- Do three.

These three exercises comprise a set. Do three sets.

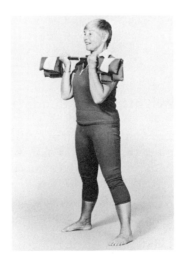

#163 Bent-Over Row (A)

- Start with feet flat and legs spread.
- Lean over from the hips and, keeping your knees straight, grasp the bar.
- Keeping that exact bend, bring the bar to your chest and lower to the floor five times.
- Work up to ten. (If you find it hard, use lighter weights. That goes for all weight bag exercises.)

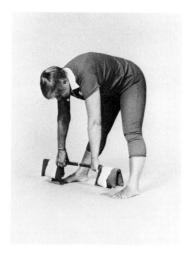

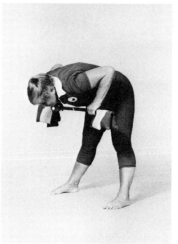

#164 Weighted Knee Bends (B)

It goes without saying that you shouldn't even think of doing weighted knee bends until you can successfully do Exercise #31 and the Ten Penny Series.

- Place the bar behind your neck and, rising to your toes, drop *slowly* into a deep knee bend.
- Rise, and return to the flat-foot starting position.
- Try to keep your back straight and begin with two, working up to ten.

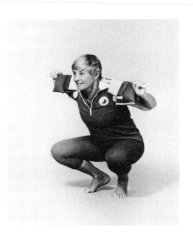

Take the weights off the bar and, starting with very light weights, lie down on a bench. If you don't have a bench, use a board supported at either end by boxes or by piles of books. You need enough leeway between you and the floor to allow your hands to drop below the supporting surface. Make sure that whatever you use is sturdy and able to support your weight.

#165 Pull-Over (A)

- Lie supine, raising both weights straight above your face.
- Then carry the arms back to hang bent over the edge of your bench (the edge of your bed would do as well).
- Bring the arms to the overhead starting position, then lower to a point just above your thighs. You will feel this in the abdominals and at the backs of your arms in the triceps.
- Do ten.

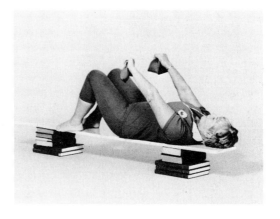

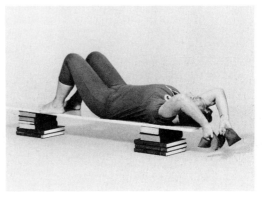

#166 Supine Press Plus Pectoral Press (A)

The Pull-over is quite hard, and the Lateral Stretch to follow is even harder. It is important to do an easy exercise between them. You should find this one easy.
- Lie supine, weights held close to your shoulders.
- Raise the weights straight above your face, and lower.
- Do eight, then, switch to PECTORAL PRESS.

- Raise the weights straight overhead, not pushing the arms past the normal lift.
- Press the weights as high as they will go as you thrust your arms upward, taking the outsides of the shoulders with them.
- Keep your arms straight as you drop the sides of the shoulders back to the bench.
- Do eight.

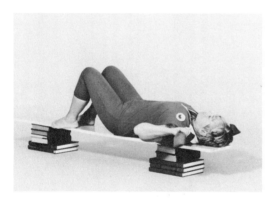
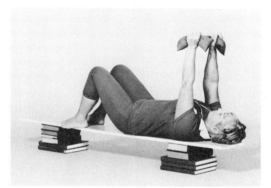

#167 Lateral Press (A)

- Lie supine with weights extended to the sides, arms drooping over the bench.
- Keeping your arms straight, bring the hands together overhead and on down to cross over the chest. Open and cross 8 times.
- "Rest" by doing #166.

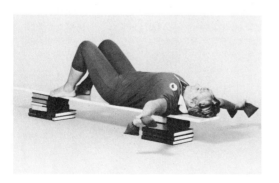
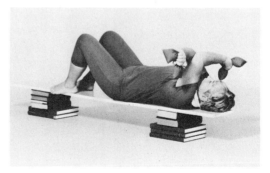

#168 Prone Arm Lift (A)

- Lie prone with weights held in your hands.
- Raise first one arm and then the other, alternating for eight (counting only the right arm).

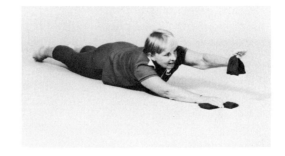

#169 Prone Leg Lift (A)

- Transfer the weights to your ankles.
- In the prone position, alternate leg lifts eight times (counting only the right leg).

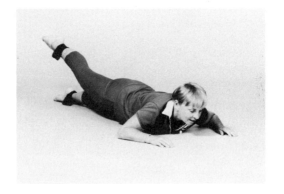

#170 Side-Lying Arm Lift (A)

- Lie on one side and rest your head on one arm.
- Take the weight bag in your free hand.
- Rest the weight on your thigh and then, keeping your arm straight, raise it over your head to hang down at the end of the lift.
- Inhale as deeply as you can during the lift.
- Keeping the arm straight, return it to the starting position, exhaling as you go.
- Do eight to a side and transfer the weight to your ankle.

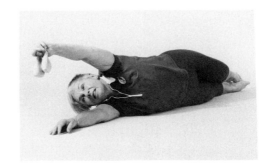

#171 Side-Lying Leg Lift (A)

- Still on your side (*not resting back on your hip*), raise the weighted leg as far as you can without twisting.
- Do eight with each leg.

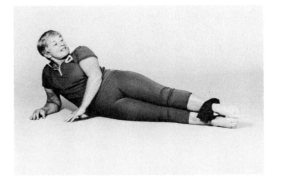

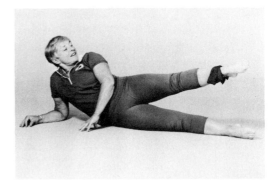

> If you do weights on Monday, you should rest from them on Tuesday and replace them with the running series (page 343). Alternate lifting with running, but *always* do calisthenics.

TOWELS

Surely your Self Center has either a bath or a shower! That means you have an exercise session waiting for you every time you bathe. Your towel can afford you plenty of resistance.

#172 Diagonal Towel Pull (A)

- As you finish drying your back, take a short hold on your towel with both hands.
- Pull upwards with one hand and note the tightness in the other shoulder. (Make a note of where you should hunt for trigger points.)
- Then, using the hand that was just pulled up, pull down. (You will probably feel it at the back of the arm in the triceps.)
- Do three or four pulls, holding the pull about five seconds.
- Reverse the hands and do the same on the other side.

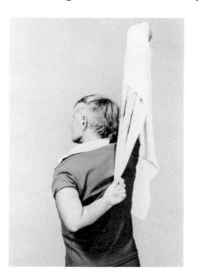 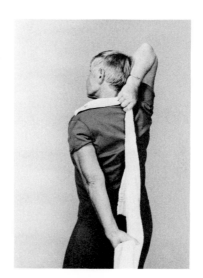

#173 Leg Pull (A)

- Sit on your bench and place one foot in your doubled towel.
- Start with the knee bent and slowly straighten your leg as you resist with plenty of power. Even resist after you have straightened the leg and are bending the knee again.
- Do four with each leg.

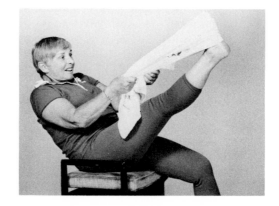

#174 Chest and Arm Stretch (A)

- Stand with feet apart for balance and take the ends of your towel in both hands.
- Raise straight arms overhead and press the arms back in easy pushes (to stretch the pectorals and also the arm muscles which tend to foreshorten without giving us much warning). If by any evil chance you have had to use a wheelchair for a long time, this towel exercise is a must. If you are in one now, hang your towel over the back and do this exercise every hour. I have seen wheelchair victims (that wasn't an error—whatever their other problems, the wheelchair itself is a danger) who

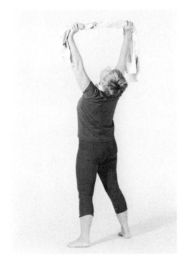

can no longer stretch their arms out straight, particularly children.

STAIRS

Most of us live in our own homes. The average home owned by After Fifties is about twenty-seven years old. Lots of people think that's bad, and I have had the misfortune to be sucked into the lectures given by such people. When they mention a house with more than one level they speak of "barriers." Barriers are supposed to keep a person from getting from one place to another. *Most* barriers are self-imposed and that's what's wrong with people who tell children not to put beans up their noses. Certainly they are right. If a child put beans up its nose they will get stuck and cause all kinds of commotion including a trip to the Emergency Room. There they could see almost anything. When I went to get my hand stitched up I saw a child whose grandmother had told him not to try and wear his potty as a hat! The doom-predicters who moan about slippery floors, loose rugs, waxed stairs, light cords that can't be found in the dark, and chairs used as ladders are right, but they should be giving house maintenance courses rather than pointing a finger at older people. A chair used as a ladder *will* slip, and down will come whoever is stupid (or lazy) enough to use it, but *as an injunction to the after fifties as a group, it is insulting.*

The same dangers face everyone in a house and most accidents happen in houses. So look around. John Glenn once all but brained himself by slipping in the shower, poor old coot of thirty-something! Have you got some handle-rails or safety grips in your shower or tub? If not, attend to it. Motels don't put those things in for "oldsters"; they put them in for traveling salespeople and conventioneers. They do it because they don't want to be sued. Do it for yourself and your family because you love all of them and should love yourself even if your mother told you self-love was a sin. If you can't love the person you are, you can't really love anyone else.

And your bathroom floor: is it cold tile covered in spots by a bath mat? Don't you know how cozy-comfy a nice, deep pile feels to bare feet on a cold November morning? Have the room carpeted if for no other reason than you have decided to live sybaritically.

As for night lights, I have them in the kitchen and in the bathroom. In a hall I'd have the same thing my father had for us when we were little—a dimmer on the regular light. He didn't do that for us because we were elderly; he knew sleepy kids could head for the stairs as easily as the john and disturb the sleeping household. If you are on drugs, you are a "sleepy kid" and it doesn't matter whether those drugs came from dear old Doctor Quinn, the neighborhood drug pusher, the pharmacy, or if it's a little pink pill Aunt Jessie uses when she can't sleep. You are a sleepy kid with all the potential that accompanies that condition . . . no matter how old or young you are.

Stairs are challenges, not barriers. They are the best piece of athletic equipment around and they won't cost you a cent except to carpet them (and I don't care if they are solid oak and an heirloom). Don't leave everything you have collected all day on the bottom stair; use every errand that might take you upstairs as a heaven-sent call. Stair risers are usually seven inches high. My house is built on seven levels on the side

of a hill. From the pool level to the gym is fifty feet. From gym to front hall is eighteen. From hall to living room, down three feet, from hall to bedroom wing, up two feet. From kitchen level to garage, down three feet. Let's see what that adds up to. If you lift a body from level A to level B and the distance between them is ten feet, you will have lifted that body ten times its own weight, or X foot pounds. You do the same as you come down, which is often harder. Suppose you weigh 150 pounds. That means 150 times 10 feet or 1,500 foot pounds. Divide that in half and your left leg has lifted 750 pounds in a matter of seconds. Go up and down your stairs ten times a day. That would be 15,000 foot pounds a day lifted by the muscles designed to help your heart. You'll also lower that same number of foot pounds!

That's only the beginning. Buy a day pack. (A day pack is a small pack designed to be used on day trips, to carry your lunch, weatherproof parka, first-aid supplies, and water bottle. You can get one in a sports or department store.) Walk up and down stairs with the day pack and added weight strapped to your back.

The following stair exercises have a purpose—as do you: you want *never* to walk upstairs the way most of those people in air terminals do. They are incensed if there isn't an escalator because they *can't* walk upstairs. Oh, they get there, but watch: feet will be flat, bottoms will be out, and they will heave like beached whales.

If they are wearing bifocals they may come down too fast, tumbling. At best they look half-blind and what the mythmakers call "old." Most of them, however, are under forty.

#175 Bent Forward with Pack (A)

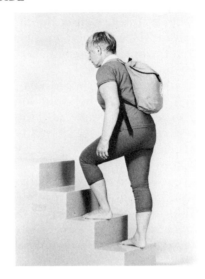

- Put a sheet of paper on the wall at the foot of your stairs as a score sheet, so your program will not be hit or miss.
- Measure the height of the risers and multiply by the number of stairs. Compute to feet so you will know the foot poundage.
- If several of you will be doing this exercise, make several score cards, as each weight will be different and so will dedication. This exercise could turn into a competition.
- Until your legs are stronger, just walk that beat, keeping track.
- When it is easier, put two weight bags in your pack (or a quart can of tomato juice). That's your "added weight" for a week.
- Double it the following week.

- *Gradually* work your way up to ten pounds.
- If you are losing weight through the program, add the lost poundage to your pack.

#176 Turned-in Feet (A)

#177 Turned-out Feet (A)

#178 Heelcord Stretch (A)

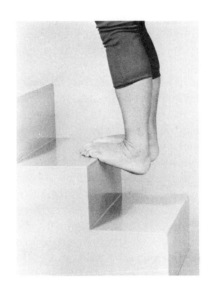

- Do the same type movement you did in floor progressions #64 and #65 and do it to music.
- Go up the stairs with feet turned in and come down with them turned out.
- Then go up with feet turned out and down with them turned in.
- On the bottom and top stairs, as you go up, do eight bounces as you did in #118.

#179 Cross-Over and Grapevine (B)

- Turn sideways to go both up and down the stairs.
- Hold onto the banister at first (and maybe always, depending on how you feel).
- Step up with the lead foot and then cross the following foot in front.
- Come down, using the banister.
- After you have mastered this, do the foot cross in back. Finally, do the grapevine, alternating the cross-over forward and back.

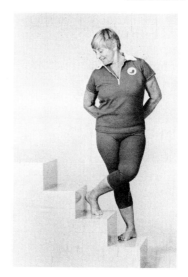

#180 Wide Cross (B)

When my hips were replaced I could reach across one foot with the other to a distance of twelve inches. When I wrote *Pain Erasure* in 1979 I had increased that spread to eighteen inches. When I wrote *Myotherapy* in 1984 I had increased the stretch to twenty-two inches, with only eight more inches to go before I reached what I could do before pain took over, eighteen years earlier. Now I can reach to twenty-four inches with only six inches left to go. What's wrong with this story? Aren't we supposed to lose flexibility, strength, balance, coordination, and control as we age? Who said? The mythmakers said. What should be one of our prime jobs? To make mincemeat out of mythmakers.

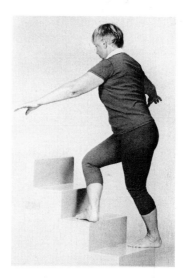

- Place your left foot on the bottom stair along the right side.
- Reach across to place the right foot as far to the left on the second step as you can manage.
- Alternate feet and zigzag your way up the stairs.
- Use the banister for extra stretch and support.
- Be sure to turn the foot out and notice where the muscles pull. Check

with the desired Myotherapy pattern. Pain is not the only indication of muscles in need of attention. It is mere the loud one. Don't wait that long. PREVENT IT. As you descend, come down straight, using every quarter inch of the muscle, not step-plop.

#181 Seat Climb (A)

When did you last sit on the bottom stair? You haven't forgotten how and you'd better not. The less you ask of your body, the less it will give.

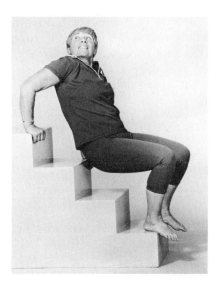

- Sit on the bottom stair and place both hands on the stair above.
- Lift your seat to that stair and continue that way, one step at a time, to the top.
- Then come back down the same way. I've had patients with busted legs and strokes go up and down this way for a while, then graduate to help-plus-the-banister, then just the banister, then no banister. It isn't where you start, it's where you intend to *go* and it shouldn't be into slippers.
- When the one-step seat lift is easy,

do two at a time. This exercise will strengthen your arms, shoulders, upper back, and chest muscles.

Now you need a set of index cards. On each card, write a way of going up and coming down your stairs. Post the cards by the stairs. Use each method for a week.

One foot at a time: Go up like a little kid, one foot at a time, but don't forget to change feet the next day. That's the way you go up and down all day for the whole week.

Sideways: Turn sideways, mount one foot at a time and bring the following foot to the same stair. It's like edging up a ski slope. Remember the other leg.

Backward: Going upstairs backward is totally different from forward and uses very different muscles. Come down the same way and hold on to the banister.

Two at a time: That's the only way I knew how to go upstairs as a kid, and when I saw Katherine Hepburn take the entire flight that way in *Coco* I thought, "Where have I been all these years?" How about you?

When I opened my first institute I had about a thousand people coming each week, and each week there was a different sign at the foot of the stairs and at the top. Suddenly stairs weren't just stairs—they were adventure. Your stairs must become adventures to get you ready for what is to come. And come it will . . . a different way of life.

DOORWAY GYM

You need a doorway gym and there are a couple of ways to put one together. The simplest is to trot down to a sports store and buy a chinning bar, which you install in your bedroom doorway. You can't trust the darned things, however, and you will need a couple of angle irons screwed in under each side to support the bar and yourself. That poses another problem: the doors in new apartment houses are often made of steel. Screwing or nailing aren't possible. In that case, you will need a much better arrangement—a frame for the whole door. It is very simple for a carpenter to throw one together and it can provide you with many possibilities. You will need a pair of wooden braces to support a piece of one-inch pipe the width of your frame. The same carpen-

ter can make you four pairs of supports which can be screwed in at various levels:

- The pair at two inches from the floor can be used to hold your feet down while you do sit-ups. They should be put in horizontally.
- The ones at twenty inches can be used to support a slant board, which in turn can be used for resting head-down.
- The ones at thirty-six inches can be used to support that same board at a sharper incline, and you can lean against it for weight bag work.
- The top bar, of course, would be for the let-downs suggested on page 86, but there are many other ways to use that top bar: The first one is to tie a length of rope to the middle and allow it to hit you in the face. Get a nice new piece of ¾-inch nylon rope about twelve feet long, double it, and fasten it to your bar. *Put it in the middle of the bar and let it hang there.* Every time you go through that door it will remind you to hang onto it and do a slow, deep knee bend. In time you will want to do two, then three knee bends. Soon enough you won't need the support but you will *always* need the reminder.

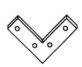

Figure 66. *Angle Iron*

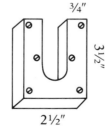
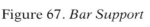

Figure 67. *Bar Support*

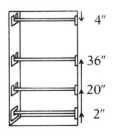

Figure 68. *Door Frame*

#182 Knee Bend, with Rope (A)

- Keep your knees together.
- Do slow knee bends.

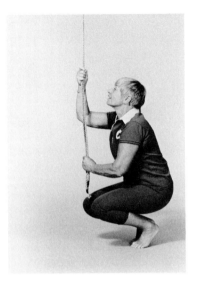

#183 Chest Stretch (A)

This exercise is important in preventing loss of height as well as a "dowager's hump."

- Place your feet apart and grasp one rope in each hand.
- Lean over from the waist and do flexibility bounces, first with the head up and then with the head and torso down.

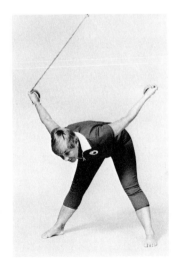

#184 Rope Climb (B)

You climbed a rope back in gym days, but only a lucky few do today.

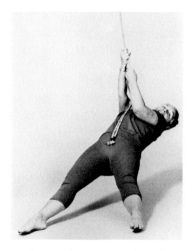

- Lie down on the floor in such a way as to have the rope hanging at pelvis level.
- Keeping your body straight, try to pull up and lift off the floor.
- One inch is a start. If you're really a beginner, pulling youself to a sit-up is a start.
- When you have gained enough strength, walk your hands up the rope to bring you to a standing position. If you can do that already, fine. Maintain it. If the mind is willing but the hands hurt, check Myotherapy pattern on page 140 and don't blame it on "arthritis." If

you have rheumatoid arthritis, use weight bags to strengthen your arms after the pain has been controlled.

Some people spend precious energy thinking up ways to avoid anything difficult. That's not you. You are more like the ones who are ingenious when it comes to outwitting a problem and somehow getting the job done.

The abdominal and groin muscles must not only be "watched", they must be worked constantly. The surest image-buster offered the subconscious, which isn't any brighter than it needs to be, are the words "bent over, poor thing." Anyone who has been an athlete, or has had to spend years sitting, or has had menstrual cramps, can suffer from the "bent-overs." Muscles injured long ago are just waiting for an excuse to go into spasm and turn you into a product of The Brothers Grimm. Don't let that

happen. First, check your standing posture with a friend. Are you the least bit bent? Next, check your walking posture; does it give a "hurry up" impression or do you look as though you are heading into the wind? If so, then the groin stretch is an imperative. Have you had a hip replaced? Same thing. Have you been told your spine is turning to stone? There are fancy names for all of these things, but what's in a name? The important question is, what form is the function causing and what function must I control.

No bone moves without a muscle to pull it and if your bones are being tugged hither and yon, *you* are the one to change it.

#185 Abdominal and Groin Stretch (B)

This exercise is labeled **B** only because you must take it easy at first. Persistance is better than over-doing which will only slow you down.

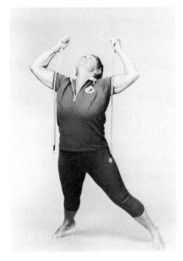

- Holding the two ropes, one in each hand, and standing with feet well apart and toes pointed forward, lean into the ropes, keeping bent arms close to the body. The pull will be felt in the abdominal line, the groin, and the backs of your legs just below your knees. If you don't feel it there, check your toes to make sure they're pointing straight ahead.
- Release the pressure by leaning back in the ropes and repeat.
- Lean in and recover five times every time you go through that doorway. As your arms gain strength, you can open them further to the sides, a very little at a time.
- Release the pressure by leaning back in the ropes and repeat.

#186 The Tuck (B)

The abdominals need work more than any other part of your body. Hanging in the ropes will help, as will sit-ups, but more work is needed, and all the time. If you don't believe me, look around. A paunch is a sign of weak abdominals.

- Stand sideways in your doorway with your back up against the doorjamb.
- Grasp your chinning bar and try to bring your knees to your chest. (Of course I'm dreaming. I tried it after my last bout with surgery.) Question: How high did the feet come off the floor? Two inches held for two seconds? That's the first step in the journey of a thousand miles. Next week, make it two inches held for five seconds.
- If you are pretty good, however, walk with your feet up the other side of the doorway and then see if you can keep them up there at whatever height you manage, for five seconds.
- Lower slowly.
- Keep lowering slowly and pretty soon you will be lifting. One knee lift through the door will help flatten your front into the youthful lines few youths have today.

PULLEY

A pulley is another inexpensive piece of equipment that will make doing an exercise more fun and also give it direction. Buy a 4-inch plastic pulley at your hardware store. At the same time get about eleven feet of ¼-inch nylon rope. Cut off ten inches of the rope (tape the "wounded" ends or they will ravel) and thread this piece through the top side of the pulley. Tie the pulley to the chinning bar. Thread the remainder of the rope through the pulley and fasten two three or four inch dowels or pieces of broomstick to each end. You now have an ideal stretcher and strengthener for hands, arms, chest, shoulder, and upper back muscles.

If you're recuperating from an illness or an accident and are bedridden, you can hook up a similar pulley system to the frame of your bed. Just shorten the rope to meet the distance from frame to bed. Add the following exercises to your recovery program.

#187 Overhead Pulley (A)

- This is no big deal. Shorten your rope ends to meet the required distance from frame to bed.
- Pull first one arm up and then the other. At first it will be like lifting a bale of hay, but strength will improve.
- Use music and it will be a happy part of your day. Be "happy" often!

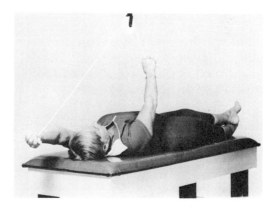

Remember, while you lie in bed doing nothing, calcium is leaving your lovely, serviceable bones. Muscles are shrinking, muscle mass (which gives you curves) is being absorbed, and you are deteriorating before your very eyes. *Do* something.

#188 Lateral Pulley (A)

- Stretch your arms out to the side and, keeping them straight, pull first one up and then the other. You need not make it easy on yourself.
- Give a little resistance with the arm being lifted.

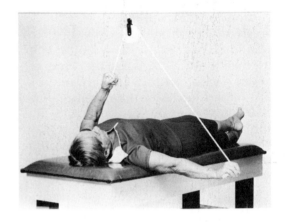

#189 Prone Pulley (A)

Later, when they have turned you over and given your ever sensitive bottom a rest, add a dimension to Prone Arm Lift with Weights.

- Shorten up on the rope ends and, without lifting your head, pull first one arm off the bed and then the other. Each pull will add to chest and arm flexibility and undo some of the harm that bed rest or confinement to a chair contribute to whatever problem you have.
- As soon as you feel stronger, raise your head and stretch further. Just a few lifts at a time will be a good start, readying you for whatever comes next.

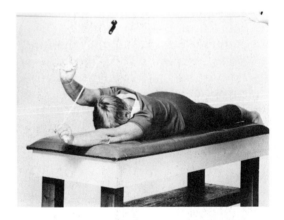

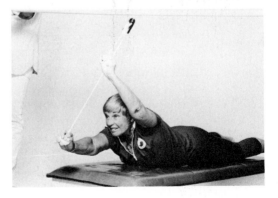

#190 Pulley in a Chair (A)

- When you graduate to a chair have the chair placed under your bar and do forward and lateral pulls.

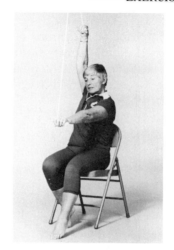

#191 Pulley, Standing (A)

- Stand facing the pulley with legs spread wide for balance.
- Lean forward and keep arms straight as you pull down with first one hand and then the other.

To do this for *stretch*, pull the arm up as far as possible. If you are working to improve *strength*, then give resistance to the pulling arm with the other arm.

- Lean over from the hips and, alternating arms, pull each for flexibility and resisting for strength.
- Make a quarter turn to the right and pull straight down with the left arm to raise the right arm overhead and stretch the side and the axilla.
- Reverse to do the other side.
- Finish by turning your back to the pulley and repeating the pulls both *overhead* and to the *sides*. If you are using one band of a record, this series will take about three minutes.

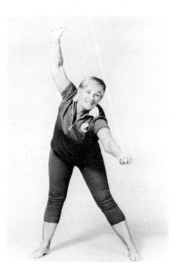
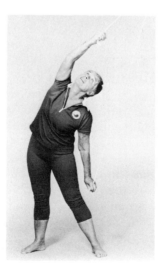
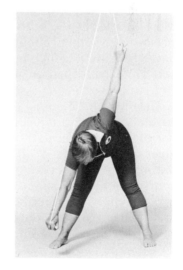

BASKETBALL

There's only one sound more satisfying than a basketball being bounced to rhythm; that's a bunch of basketballs bouncing to really good rock music.

When you ask yourself what you ought to do to get your husband, brother, father or buddy moving again, the answer is, *basketballs.*

#192 Ball Bouncing

- There are a thousand ways to bounce a basketball—alone, in pairs, in groups.
- You can do it sitting, standing up straight, bent over, or lying down, and you will probably think of ways I have missed.
- The key is rhythm. HIT THE BEAT. Just what this does for the psyche is hard to pinpoint, but whatever state you are in (including marvelous), do at least five minutes' worth of ball bouncing.

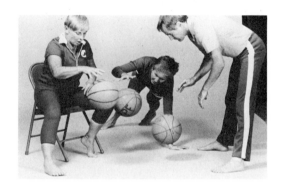

TEN PENNY EXERCISE

Ten Penny Exercise involves the bathroom and intermittent interruptions. Most people hit the bathroom, for one reason or another, about ten times a day. If you are a camel, maybe seven. If you are a face checker, maybe twelve. But ten is average.

Get two little cups together; saki cups are ideal. Put ten shiny pennies in one of them and see to it that a drinking glass is handy. Keep all this in your bathroom. Then, every time you find yourself in the bathroom, do the following exercises. The numbers of repeats are starters for the out-of-shape. Set your own pace but remember—start

easy and increase with time and muscle.

- Holding onto the sink, do three deep knee bends.
- Step back and do twenty-five waist twists (page 233) erect.
- Do twenty-five waist twists bent over.
- Do sixteen swim moves forward, sixteen right and sixteen left (page 232).
- Do eight shoulder rotations each arm (page 142).
- Do eight hip rotations each leg (page 234).

Then drink a glass of water. That will ensure your return in about two hours. One can defer almost anything but nature. Take a penny from cup A and drop it into cup B as your score. At the end of the day you owe as many exercises as there are pennies left in cup A. A promise: you will improve and never miss the minutes.

INDOOR RUNNING

There's nothing the matter with running except the way we do it, where we do it, how we do it, with whom we do it, *and why we do it*. Running cross-country, as a small part of a program that included weight training and calisthenics, would be great. If we developed strong feet *before* we took off down the road and were capable of landing on the balls of our feet instead of heels, great. If we did it with people who were not neurotic about accumulating miles, but just enjoyed the motion and surroundings, great. And if we didn't do it because we had been brainwashed into believing that if we didn't do it sooner or later we would have a heart attack, great. One more thing: if we didn't believe it was our amulet against those heart attacks, greatest of all.

You do *not* have to run to be healthy. You *do* have to exercise to be healthy. Millions have ruined their feet, legs, and backs trying to conform to what a few men have decreed. One of those men, Jim Fixx, died of the very condition he was running to escape . . . a heart attack. My friend Jack Kelly, whose father took me to President Eisenhower, died of such an attack and so did his brother-in-law. Running isn't the answer. There are many answers. Watch your diet, quit smoking, drink in moderation, and above all, keep your stress level under control. Do you think straining every sinew is keeping stress down? Walking in the woods, biking, climbing, canoeing, rowing, cross-country skiing, skin diving, and scuba are much better at that. Try to remember: you don't *have* to be "iron man." You don't *have* to win. You don't *have* to keep pushing your heart day after day to get a pulse beat that some human being has set as your level without knowing diddley-squat about you— what your background was, your genetic heritage or what has happened to you in your life. He doesn't know anything about the stresses you endure and yet he has laid a point system, a pulse system, and a competitive burden on you.

You no longer have to prove who you are . . . you know.

CROSS-COUNTRY RUNNING— IN THE LIVING ROOM

If you run on the road each foot hits the same way with the same muscle action every time for thousands of landings. If you run across fields and ditches, up and down hills, through woods and marshlands, your feet and legs must adjust to many different angles and weights. A running step forward is very different from a two-foot catch in a ditch.

You can run "cross-country" at home. Put on a good brisk record or tape. On my record *Keep Fit . . . Be Happy,* Volume I, there are two bands devoted to running. One has voice over and the other is the same music, but free of directions. If you prefer other music, here is what you can do to it.

#193 Indoor Running Sets of Counts

Eight beats to a set
Important: do not run on cement.

Relaxed running in place	4
Eight hops on the left foot, eight on the right	4
Jump feet apart and together	5
Jump feet apart and keep them open	2
Jump both feet together from left to right, to left, etc.	3
Open	1
Repeat both feet together left and right	3
Run again as in the beginning	5
Eight hops on the left foot, eight on the right	4
Open	1
Run with the upper body bent forward, kicking legs up behind	4
Run with body erect and kick straight legs out in front, point toes	4
High kicks, bring bent knees up as high as possible	6

These directions are not written in stone. Fit your movements to the music you select. There are other actions such as jumping both feet from side to side, doing the scissors, or jumping both feet forward and back. What you do is not important, as long as you hit the beat and enjoy yourself. Be sure you warm up first.

A helpful (and fun) piece of equipment to use for indoor running is a rebounder. A rebounder is basically a small, portable trampoline. The purists who are solely concerned with cardiovascular conditioning do not think much of rebounders. We who are interested in developing a better, more enduring, more resiliant, more coordinated body, think they are wonderful. To begin with they are fun. You don't have to win or push yourself or count your heart beats; you just need good music.

#194 Rebounder

- If at first you are afraid of falling, put your rebounder near your doorway gym and hold onto the rope.

- Run, jump with feet apart, do scissors, twists, bounces, anything you can think of—just do it. If you keep

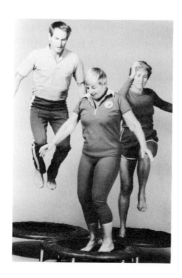

a stopwatch nearby you can time the minutes spent jumping. My rebounder stands between my typewriter and the door. When I have to leave, I leave via a minute of jumping, and when I return, I do it again.

AQUA-EX

Water exercise is wonderful fun, wonderful for you, and leads to really wonderful adventures. If you have to recover from anything or prepare for anything (like an operation), water is a great place to do it. I have a Japanese bath in my house. It is six feet deep and I can drop it down to four feet if I want to exercise. It is five feet across and seven feet long. The water can be any temperature. You can have the same thing if you have a cellar with a floor drain. Get the smallest backyard pool that will allow you to stand up in shoulder-depth water. Drain six inches out of it night and morning and replace with hot, hot water. It will stay warm enough to be pleasant.

Next, you need your tape recorder and the music you enjoy. One tape is usually twenty minutes to a side, and twenty minutes is what you want. Then come the toys: mask, snorkel, fins, and a short paddle. Wearing your fins, turn your back to the edge of the pool and hold on. Stretch your body out in the water and do slow, full-range-of-motion scissor kicks. I have worked up to 100, counting only my right leg. When I need to rest my legs I take the paddle and with all of it under water, I paddle fifty strokes to the left side and then fifty to the right. Remember, I have worked up to this; I started around ten. Next, wearing my mask and snorkel, I lie face down in the water and do scissor kicks again counting my right leg's kicks only. Then I do fifty back strokes with my paddle on each side. Then I get rid of the toys and do floor progressions for the remainder of the time. It's never boring the way swimming laps can be, but if you like doing laps, then you should do them.

Take your fins, mask, snorkel, paddle, and tape recorder to the local Y or town pool. Swim your laps wearing your gear and you'll never get a stiff neck or red-rimmed eyes. You can cover the distance faster and get a better workout using the fin's resistance. Take your Frisbees along. Underwater arm exercises are better done with the resistance they afford. Do floor exercises next to the edge of the pool at the shallow end where you can hear your tape recorder. Then what? Go to scuba school if you don't mind deep water and want new adventures. Scuba school will prepare you for scuba diving in the Caribbean.

That's what this book has been about: adventure ... *your* adventure. Get the body ready and the mind will go along. When the two of them get together you will be off to see the world as you have never seen it before. Why?

Because it's a different world and you are different, too. This time you are captain of the ship. See to it that the charts you use carry you to far-off, exciting places.

The key to getting into shape is *determination*. The key to staying in shape is *enjoyment*. As soon as your body responds and you begin to feel new waves of energy, put it to use with a sport. If you have begun by walking, then where could you walk that would be exciting? Join a walking club. You have been using an indoor bike? Then join a biking group. You enjoy your rowing machine, how about a canoe trip? Remember, you will soon be painless and have more coordination.

DON'T JUST SIT THERE ... USE IT.

EXERCISE INDEX

Index By Area

(Exercise number follows area)

Abdominals

1, 2, 8, 23, 27, 32, 37, 39, 41, 47, 48, 49, 50, 51, 52, 55, 56, 61, 72, 85, 91, 98, 101, 107, 126, 130, 133, 134; 135, 136, 140, 141, 142, 152, 165, 175, 183, 184, 185, 186

Ankles

31, 61, 64, 65, 67, 69, 71, 74, 76, 82, 97, 110, 111, 112, 113, 116, 118, 119, 120, 122, 123, 127, 128, 155, 156, 175, 176, 177, 178, 193, 194

Arms

6, 12, 14, 23, 31, 40, 41, 43, 60, 61, 80, 92, 99, 102, 131, 132, 139, 142, 143, 157, 158, 159, 160, 161, 162, 165, 167, 168, 170, 172, 173, 174, 181, 183, 184, 187, 188, 189, 190, 191, 192

Back

3, 4, 5, 8, 19, 23, 27, 31, 32, 33, 34, 36, 37, 39, 42, 43; 45, 46, 47, 48, 55, 56, 60, 61, 67, 81, 86, 87, 88, 89, 95, 102, 106, 107, 126, 133, 140, 141, 145, 152, 153, 160, 164, 168, 169, 173, 184

Balance

31, 57, 64, 65, 66, 67, 69, 112, 113, 121, 152, 153, 155, 156, 173, 176, 177, 178, 179, 180

Chest

12, 14, 23, 26, 32, 40, 41, 43, 48, 50, 52, 61, 80, 92, 93, 130, 132, 139, 142, 157, 159, 160, 161, 162, 165, 167, 170, 172, 173, 174, 175, 181, 183, 184, 187, 188, 189, 190, 191

Circulation

18, 25, 31, 33, 38, 48, 51, 52, 57, 58, 59, 60, 64, 65, 66, 67, 68, 69, 70, 71, 72, 76, 82, 88, 94, 95, 97, 102, 112, 113, 116, 117, 118, 119, 120, 121, 122, 124, 126, 127, 128, 133, 134, 135, 136, 141, 150, 152, 154, 155, 164, 175, 176, 177, 178, 179, 180, 182, 188, 193

Coordination

26, 31, 38, 46, 59, 60, 67, 69, 70, 74, 76, 88, 142, 152, 153, 155, 159, 160, 179, 180, 184, 192, 194

Feet

20, 57, 60, 61, 63, 64, 65, 67, 69, 70, 71, 74, 76, 82, 88, 97, 110, 111, 112, 113, 114, 116, 117, 118, 119, 120, 121, 122, 123, 124, 127, 128, 155, 156, 177, 179, 180, 194

Groin

2, 10, 25, 27, 32, 33, 36, 37, 38, 39, 46, 47, 49, 51, 52, 55, 56, 59, 60, 61, 68, 70, 71, 72, 88, 89, 90, 91, 98, 106, 107, 126, 133, 134, 135, 136, 137, 140, 141, 142, 154, 179, 180, 184, 185

Hands

6, 14, 23, 26, 31, 40, 41, 43; 50, 61, 80, 92, 102, 130, 131, 139, 142, 151, 157, 160, 161, 165, 167, 168, 172, 173, 174, 175, 181, 183, 184, 187, 188, 189, 190, 191

Hips

19, 25, 27, 33, 36, 37, 38, 39, 42, 45, 46, 47, 48, 55, 56, 58, 59, 60, 61, 64, 65, 68, 72, 76, 82, 88, 95, 98, 106, 107, 112, 113, 126, 133, 134, 135, 136, 140, 141, 150, 152, 153, 154, 164, 169, 173, 176, 177, 180, 182, 193

Legs

2, 5, 10, 18, 19, 20, 25, 33, 34, 36, 38, 42, 45, 46, 49, 50, 51, 52, 54, 55, 57, 58, 60, 61, 63, 64, 65, 66, 67, 68, 69, 70, 71, 72, 74, 76, 81, 82, 84, 86, 88, 90, 91, 94, 95, 97, 98, 111, 112, 113, 116, 117, 118, 119, 121, 122, 123, 126, 127, 128, 133, 134, 135, 136, 141, 150, 151, 153, 155, 156, 164, 169, 173, 176 177, 178, 179, 180, 182, 185, 193, 194

Neck

11, 125

Stretch

5, 8, 10, 11, 18, 19, 23, 26, 31, 32, 33, 34, 46, 48, 55, 60, 61, 67, 70, 72, 80, 81, 82, 86, 87, 89, 90, 91, 95, 97, 98

Waist

22, 23, 26, 46, 55, 112, 130, 159

Warm-Ups

21–35

PART THREE
WHAT SHALL WE BE WHEN WE GROW UP?

Would you like to know what it was like to grow old nearly four hundred years ago? Listen to one of Shakespeare's most famous soliloquies. (With asides by yours truly):

All the world's a stage
And all the men and women merely
    players:
They have their exits and their
    entrances;
And one man in his time plays many
    parts,
His acts being seven ages. At first
    the infant,
Mewling and puking in the nurse's
    arms.

(Few have nurses anymore, but the
    rest is right)

And then the whining school-boy,
    with his satchel,
And shining morning face, creeping
    like snail
Unwillingly to school.

(His face isn't all that shining
    anymore; he stayed up to watch the
    late show. And now it's the school
    bus that creeps)

And then the lover
Sighing like a furnace, with woeful
    ballad
Made to his mistress' eyebrow

(Now it's to whatever wiggles)

Then a soldier,
Full of strange oaths, and bearded
    like the pard,

Jealous in honor, sudden and quick
   in quarrel,
Seeking the bubble reputation even
   in the cannon's mouth

*(The beard still goes, the oaths aren't
strange to anyone over five, and the cannon's mouth is set up at the end of Wall
Street, Main Street, or the Street of Coke
Dreams)*

And then the justice,
In fair round belly with good capon
   lined,

*(It was steak for about 100 years;
   now we too are back to capon)*

With eyes severe and beard of
   formal cut,
Full of wise saws and modern
   instances;

*(The same today, unless he tries
   either in front of his wife)*

And so he plays his part. The sixth
   age shifts
Into lean and slippered pantaloon,
With spectacles on nose and pouch
   on side,

*(And here we part company with Will. To-
day's sixth age has contact lenses and a
designer wallet.)*

His youthful hose well sav'd, a world
   too wide
For his shrunk shank;

*(This fellow's stockings don't fit because
the styles have changed and he's wearing
designer jeans. If his shank has shrunk
it's because he's on a diet. It's far more
likely that his biceps are bulging from
rowing and lifting weights)*

And his big manly voice,
Turning again towards treble, pipes
And whistles in his sound.
That ends this strange eventful
   history,
In second childishness, and mere
   oblivion,
Sans teeth, sans eyes, sans taste,
   sans everything.

Poor Will Shakespeare; he did live in doleful times. That old fellow he describes is probably the same age as Whistler's mother. Did you know she was forty-three when she posed for that famous picture? The only whistling pipers I know are well up in their eighties—an age which practically none of Will's contemporaries ever reached *and* they were either cigar smokers or three-pack-a-day men. Will was an accurate observer of the human scene, so we can assume from his portrait of the seven ages of man that he lived before our lucky time, aged rapidly, and missed some of the best parts. In those days men didn't live much past forty-six and women had to make do until forty-eight. Holy mackerel! When I was forty-eight I was just getting started, and by no stretch of the imagination was I grown up! How about you?

The only doctors available to Will's friend were barber-surgeons, and it wasn't taste that was missing from the mouth, it was teeth. It's darned hard to gum a capon. Eyesight didn't stand up too well to vegetables cooked until dead. Candlelight may have made ancient women of forty look better, but it did little to preserve their vision, and when it comes to "sans everything" I imagine Will was referring to sex. He, like today's myth-makers, must have thought that sex, like sense, flies away with the approach of sixty. Poor Will, never got to fifty-three, so how was he to know? That says something about today's savants as well.

But Will Shakespeare was such a great poet he kept millions from thinking for themselves. One of the jobs our generation could take on is that of getting people off trains of thought clanking out of the past. Too many ride on them just because they are there. The world has seen more changes since we graduated from high school than in the hundreds of years between Will Shakespeare's day and our own. Not the least of those changes has to do with how long we will live—and that includes smokers, drinkers, even the drug addicted. Average life expectancy is now seventy for men and seventy-eight for women. Most people didn't even reach the after fifty crowd in Elizabethan times, and those who did were a mess. You are not a mess. Most women reach and get through menopause (which used to be a big deal), and discover they have thirty good years ahead of them. Men who approach Shakespeare's "seventh stage" are usually virile, vital, and aware (by this time) that *if* they take care of themselves, they can live longer, better, and sans nothing. "Then what?" you ask. The answer is that you then slip your cables and sail away to find something exciting to do, something you always wanted to do when you grew up.

Well, here you are—all grown up. Note, I didn't say you were old; I said grown up.

Let's start with understanding the difference between grown up and grown old. How did we ever settle on sixty-five as that moment in time when we would give up our place at the table and move to the chimney corner? Who was responsible and how did he, she, or they settle on that magic number? The decision was made in Germany in the nineteenth century in a welfare move to help the aged and infirm. That was probably reasonable at the time, but was it so smart in 1934 when we adopted it? Perhaps nobody consulted the census bureau to see how many Americans would make it to that age. That was almost twenty-five years before the studies were made in the almshouses and charity wards. No, a different attitude was taken. The government decided that we were old at sixty-five and we jolly well better act it; and we did. We (or rather our elders) were told to pick up their gold watches and move over; youth must be served. Well, there have been some changes.

Government did us no favors. In 1900 two out of every three people aged sixty-five still worked; in those days a lot of people owned their own businesses. The self-employed rarely quit because they liked what they were doing and got satisfaction, pride, and a good self-image from it. Today, how many have that satisfaction? I can hear some of you: "Satisfaction, my foot! I hated my job." That brings me to John Galbraith and the subject of work. He calls what he does, "nonwork." The people who do "real" work do the hard, useful, repetitive, boring, uninteresting, unsatisfying tasks. The people who do "nonwork" do something they enjoy. He's right. An interviewer once asked me if I'd ever considered retiring and I said I never did. I am self-employed (so to speak), I work a lot harder than most of my employees, most of whom are half my age. I've started a lot of new things ranging from fitness in America to the recent discovery of Myotherapy, but I haven't noticed any slowing down, but then, it isn't "real" work that I do . . . it's fun.

Galbraith feels that the tired workers who have done the "real" stuff have the right to sit down and put their feet up. There are a lot of them down in Florida now and they seem to be doing just that. I'd last about a month at retirement and then I'd have to find something exciting to do. Most people who have worked all their lives doing "nonwork" feel the same way.

Then, of course, there was force. One of the reasons many older people are no longer working is because they were forced by their companies to retire. Many companies are still offering bonuses to older employees if they'll get out and let the younger employees take over. That may sound altruistic—unless you've been around. At many major corporations an executive can climb rapidly, as does his salary. Shortly after he moves to Greenwich, Connecticut, buys a house commensurate with his title, gets the kids into private schools and his wife and himself accepted at the country club, he's given an assistant. Not too long after that he's gone, and the assistant has his job (at half the salary). Don't think altruism. Most things boil down to money and that's one of the problems of retirement at any age.

For most people income is cut in half at retirement, but there are a few rays of sunshine: look for them, find them, and lie in them, and you will be tanned, healthy, and worthy of our generation. We've pushed forced retirement to seventy which is great for those who do "nonwork." There are a lot of bright, experienced men and women who already have a wristwatch and no desire to occupy a shelf. They are willing to *adapt* . . . and that's the key word for us. Some will work part-time. Some smart companies are replacing temporary absentees with fully experienced, tried-and-true, "partially retired" persons. These older workers know a great deal about every aspect of the business because they have been with the business a long time and probably helped build it. This system works out well for everyone.

There are still 4.4 million after fifties who did not retire by choice. Most Americans don't like being told what they can and cannot do. They know full well that people are not all cut from the same piece of cloth. I knew girls at Horace Mann High School who were *born* old and went older from there. I also know octogenarians who are younger than springtime and will *never* be old. The only time chronological age serves a purpose is on a birth certificate. Other than that it doesn't have much value. What does have value is health, freedom from pain, maintenance of strength, flexibility, coordination, endurance, balance, and a sense of humor. Lets see how that applies.

TRUTH—AND MYTH—IN THE WORKPLACE

The American Medical Association says that there is a direct relationship between retirement and health. One study concludes that retired persons have a much higher risk of dying of heart disease than do people of the same chronological age who have not retired. When a group of retired persons was asked why they weren't working, 58 percent said it was because they suffered from poor health. My guess is that *some* of them were right, but many of them used "poor health" as an excuse because they didn't want to think of themselves as "through."

Any number of studies have shown that older working people do better than young ones when it comes to health. They don't have as many acute diseases, for one thing, and while they do have more of the chronic variety, these don't interfere too much. Annoying they are; interfering, no. They miss far fewer work days than their younger colleagues. Of one group of retirees surveyed, 18 percent said there was no work available; maybe there wasn't. Older people make up our largest group of minorities and suffer the usual discrimination against minority groups.

Myth: Poor old Pop, he's slowed down a lot.

Fact: Has he? If he's between fifty-five and sixty-four and he does piecework, he makes $5.30 an hour compared to $3.75 for the spry young blades and lasses. Have you heard that practice makes if not perfect, at least faster? Pop isn't only faster, he makes fewer mistakes and is less likely to quit.

Every study says that he and his female counterpart have fewer accidents, and that should be important to the compensation board. When older people do get sick, their recovery is quicker. In general, for all causes, their absenteeism is much lower. And here's a good one: they have a much better safety record, which may be due in part to the fact that they have fewer emotional upsets, fewer admittances to mental hospitals, and use fewer psychogenic drugs. They also have a lower rate of alcoholism, which is one of the scourges of American business from the lowest to the highest echelons. It's not surprising that older workers take fewer long weekends, but it *is* surprising that they are more stable. After all, aren't they supposed to have left their marbles on the other side of fifty?!

Myth: Hell! They're slower than molasses in Alaska!

Fact: That depends. It may be true if you are talking about reaction time pulling a lever, but older workers more than balance that with experience, wisdom, and endurance. When it comes to small muscle speed, there is no difference between young and old. The pluses are many. Menstrual cramps don't keep them home any more; the alcoholics have mostly died off, as have the heavy smokers. The stresses that surround the young have been left behind. The kids are out of school. The house is paid for, as are the braces for teeth and the piano, dance, riding, and karate lessons. All the older worker really has to worry about is staying healthy and painless . . . which now can be done. A good thing too, because the supply of young workers is drying up, especially in the high tech field. We will soon be retraining older people. As far as work goes, we are in pretty good shape . . . *if we want to work.*

WE WANT TO WORK—BUT HOW?

That phrase "want to work," is loaded with variables having to do with individual situations: what do we mean by "work" and "want"?

No two of us are exactly alike, but some situations can give us much in common. For example, let's examine the word "want." "Want" can mean desire or need and the bottom line in retirement is money. Two questions arise: Will there be enough for our essentials? Will there be enough left over to give what each of us considers "The Good Life"? Right away those questions make a major decision necessary . . . should our future work be voluntary or paid?

The first task: deciding what work to do. First, decide what sort of work you *want* to do. That decision could occupy many hours of thought, planning, and investigation. According to Galbraith, those who have done life's "real" work—the repetitive, boring, heavy, hard, unsatisfying work of any kind—deserve to retire, rest and put their feet up. Fine for those who choose that route, but what about the others, the ones who don't *want* to rest and put their feet up, the ones who want to stay active, but doing something entirely different?

A LATE BLOOMER

I know a charming lady who had three jobs: wife, mother, and housewife. (Wife and housewife are not always the same by any means, but both are jobs.) This woman stayed home, raised her kids, was always there when they came home, had dinner on the table at six. Nobody ever lacked a clean shirt or had mismated socks, and no kid wore a doorkey on a ribbon around his or her neck. For her, "Woman's work was never done." When her children grew up and moved away and her husband died, she found herself alone with no track record of work done in the work place and her only title, "Housewife," the lowest on the pay scale. For starters she didn't want to do that work anymore. She wasn't really suited for anything else but she knew she could learn.

She joined a group called The Green Thumb, an organization that places people in nonprofit organizations at a minimum wage, which The Green Thumb pays. She started off answering the phone, stuffing envelopes, doing simple filing, and learning the ropes. She also went to night school to learn how to type and to program a computer. In no time she learned how to operate the office machines and became invaluable. As a Green Thumb employee she can only work twenty hours a week, but if her employers see what she has become while costing them nothing, they may take her on as a full-time employee. Green Thumb will then use her slot for another person wanting to enter the work force.

LOOKING AHEAD

Then there are the people Galbraith says do no "real" work—and he gives himself as an example. By his standards I don't do "real" work either; but this non-real work that I do can consume up to eighteen hours a day with not even a weekend off for months on end. It's exciting and I love it. In fact, I couldn't *not* do it! The major problem for people like us lies in deciding just how much time we want to give to our "nonwork." Finding companies that have a need for "experts" part time can be full-time work in itself but it's worth doing. We have patterns we want for our work and the various companies we approach will have patterns of *want*, translated to *need*. Getting the two in sync is a major undertaking, involving months if not years of effort. Don't jump at the first offer and don't get discouraged when you discover that few things of value "just happen." If you can make yourself consider "Retirement" as a time of "Freedom and Options," and if you can start that process as you take up your membership in the after fifty crowd, you will have done the groundwork. With time to spare you can prepare your company to make use of your unique qualities at the price and in the time pattern that suits you both.

BEWARE OF ISOLATION!

If you are one of those "People Who Need People," being cut off from the workplace where you have spent most of your life will be deadly. I'm one of those people who needs people. Even if I decide to retire from some of my tasks, I would need to keep others that will continue to bring me into the company of my peers. I know that about myself; do you know that about you? Please try to realize that friends will not be enough; sharing work is another real need for most of us.

BEWARE OF BORES!

I once flew from Hartford to San Francisco with two "retired" executives in the seat behind me. One was involved in work he enjoyed, the other had moved to a retirement community and was miserable. "All the women look alike. God! They even wear the same things," he groaned. Well, I thought, they did that in school, too. Unless you wore saddle shoes, an angora sweater, and pearls you didn't belong. "The guys aren't bad, but there aren't enough of them," the grumbler continued. "The problem is, all the women start right off telling you what doctor they see and for what, for God's sake! Then they tell you what their husbands have in the way of aches and pains and who the hell cares?" What that man does not realize is that those are the same women who talked your ear off about their babies, the number of diapers used, toilet training, weaning, and first teeth. People don't really change all that much. There are interesting women, and there are boring older men, too, the ones whose conversation used to be about mileage, baseball scores, the Dow Averages, "that babe who moved in down the street." Those boring people didn't become boring over night—they were always boring. If you aren't, and if you want better company, start seeking it out now.

RESTLESSNESS—A REAL FACTOR

There are people who "have to get away." They can work nonstop for nine or ten months then suddenly—that's it! They've had it and need a complete change. The wise employer who has such a worker on the staff usually makes arrangements for that cycle. It's the rare person who will work full-out for months at a time, and companies usually appreciate him or her. When it comes to retirement, that sort of person should look for work that has a time limit—a single major project or a series of lesser ones. This is where a track record comes in. If you have done "big" things during your working life, you are still capable and the capable employer knows it just by reading your resumé. Look for such an employer and start now, even if you haven't attained the magic age of fifty.

GRADUAL RETIREMENT

Some companies are offering to help prepare the retiring employee with "gradual retirement." Koll-Morgan Corporation, an optical instrument company in Massachusetts, has such a plan. It works like this: an employee who is due to retire scouts around for a nonprofit, nonpolitical, and nonreligious group that he or she would like to join as a volunteer. The company then checks out the selection and agrees to keep up both salary and benefits of that employee during three stages of the period of severance. During the first stage, one day a week goes to volunteer work and the other four to the company. During the second, two days are allotted to volunteer work; and during the third, three days out of five. In a few years the final transition can be made . . . if desired. In that year the soon-to-be retired person ought to know whether or not that particular volunteer work is suitable. If not, there has been time to try others.

LATE—AND LATER— RETIREMENT

The trend to date has been toward early retirement, but for many reasons that trend is changing. Not the least of these reasons is the increasing need for trained employees. If Koll-Morgan had given me the opportunity to "find myself" during the retirement process, you can bet that if they called me later and said, "Hey! We're in a bind. Can you give us a hand on a part-time basis?" I'd be there.

Some companies are already looking to the future, aware that there is a time coming when there will be fewer young people joining the work force; many of those young workers will lack basic reading, writing, spelling, and business skills.

THE VALUE OF EXPERIENCE

In our Myotherapy clinics the first contact with the public is the telephone. If you are a caller in pain who has tried everything for your condition and yet you still hurt, you want some reassuring information. You need a warm and sympathetic voice coming over the wire, but warmth and sympathy won't be enough when you start asking questions. For that you want someone with experience who knows the answers and can explain them so that you understand. It takes years to develop that sort of experience, and very often the best person has reached the age of retirement. What do we do? Arrange the hours to suit both the business and the retiree. If necessary, team up a couple of people to share a job; two part-time pros are far better than one full-time neophyte. Travelers Companies has sixteen retirees sharing four positions in its Office of Consumer Information. In an article in *Modern Maturity* (June 1985), Georgina Lucas, the administrator of The Travelers' Older Americans Program said, "They (retirees) know our products and services, understand the company and have excellent interpersonal skills on the telephone." Why shouldn't they? Think a minute . . . as each product came along and the company grew, those employees grew with it. Telephone skill is only one example of the value of experience. Recognize and consider your strengths when you are looking for an option.

PART-TIME WORK

Aerospace Corporation, a high-tech engineering firm in California, makes it possible to work and still keep retirement benefits by classifying retirees as "casual employees." Federal pension law says that employees working more than 1,000 hours must be considered full time, but how about 999½? How much is that, really?

There are 365 days in a year, but if you knock off Saturdays and Sundays, as most sane people do, you whittle the year down to 261 days. There are at least 10 legitimate holidays which brings the work year down to 251 days. Everybody gets two weeks off and even though that's two weeks too few for a really restful and relaxing vacation, it's still 14 days less, bringing the work year to 237 days in which to tuck a little less than 1,000 working hours. At 20 hours a week (which is what our Green Thumb lady works), it would take 50 weeks at 4 hours a day to accumulate 1,000 hours. That's what she signed on for, but suppose she wanted to work longer on some days and not at all on others? That would be up to her and her employer. If you manage to make a "thousand-hour agreement" with an employer, you may want to discuss all the options for how to budget that time. It's like getting married; everything depends on making the right match.

KEEP UP WITH DEVELOPMENTS

One of the problems older workers face is keeping up with technological change. Often a short sighted employer

will deny older employees (forty is considered "older") the opportunity to participate in training sessions. The implication is that the old dog can't learn new tricks and the forty-year-old is an old dog. That's wrong to begin with, but there's more: The employer thinks that if he trains his people young, he will have them longer and that's the better investment. The employer who thinks that way doesn't know much about life. The "older" employee may stay a lot longer than the youngster for several reasons. The younger one still lacks roots and has an eye out for greener pastures. Young women are likely to take maternity leave, and many don't come back. In addition, if either partner in a working couple is offered a really good job in another state, the thought of a swelling joint checking account at that age will win and they'll be off. After all, the training their employers gave them can be used as well in one place as in another. Few people sign onto anything for more than thirty days.

The "older" worker is different. He or she has a house and it may even be owned free and clear. The kids are either in schools where their friends are, or off at college, or settled in homes of their own. That means grandchildren, and no "Grand" gives up the joy of grandkids lightly. Train the "older" worker and you can probably count on fifteen years instead of two or three. That's cost effective. Incidentally, the old dog learns just as well as the young one, sometimes better. In learning there is always the question of motivation.

One huge company, General Electric, has started to bring back its veteran engineers for retraining. They are doing that rather than hiring young engineers who have known nothing else but high tech. A broad base of information used for many years becomes part of the fiber, a lot like being able to swim, ride a bike, or ski . . . it's second nature. Such a broad base is a good foundation for new information. Building on a secure base is a lot better than starting from scratch. This is especially true in our rapidly changing world where what was effects what is and what will be.

DEVELOP AN INFORMATION NETWORK

There are many sources of information which are keeping up (or at least are trying to) with the occupational changes of the after fifty crowd; now is the time to make your contacts. If you were planning a trip you'd have brochures and circulars all over the table so you could pick and choose and wouldn't miss anything through ignorance. Well, your life is a different journey, and you want to know its destination. Some good sources (found in *Modern Maturity*, the magazine of the American Association for Retired Persons) follow:

The AARP itself is located at 1909 K Street NW, Washington, DC 20006. It was formed to promote wider employment opportunities for older workers and at the same time to break down barriers to their legitimate career goals. Write to Worker Equity Initiative Department, same address.

Networking is essential, and if you are in the Midwest check out an organization called OPERATION ABLE. It coordinates a network of many groups. 36 S. Wabash Ave., Suite 1133, Chicago, IL 60603.

And there's more!

OFFICE OF NATIONAL PROGRAMS FOR OLDER WORKERS, U.S. Department of Labor, Employment Training Administration, 601 D St. Room 6122, Washington, DC 20213.

U.S. HOUSE OF REPRESENTATIVES, SELECT COMMITTEE ON AGING, Room 712 HOB Annex 1, Washington, DC 20515. Remember, a vote is a vote. As a matter of fact, you may have time now to get together a number of voters with similar questions and complaints. In numbers there is attention!!

U.S. SENATE SPECIAL COMMITTEE ON AGING, Room G-ss DSOB, Washington, DC 20510.

WORK IN AMERICA INSTITUTE, 700 White Plains Rd., Scarsdale, NY 10583.

NATIONAL ASSOCIATION OF AREA AGENCIES ON AGING, 600 Maryland Ave. SW, Washington, DC 20024.

EQUAL EMPLOYMENT OPPORTUNITY COMMISSION, 201 E St. NW, Washington, DC 20507.

If you make a project of your retirement options, you will find many more sources of information, but you have to start somewhere. A warning should go here: Don't believe everything on any printed page. Always use common sense along with your glasses and a healthy share of "prove it."

WHAT IF YOU DON'T WANT (OR NEED) TO WORK?

Suppose you don't have to work for an

income. That would be a lovely thought for a lot of people and not so impossible as you might think. Expenses change with the years and we don't need as much money as we used to when we supported children and paid off loans and liens. I can't say a word to my extravagant daughter who goes shopping and if it's gorgeous, expensive, and fits, buys it. I did the same thing. That would bore me now. Not long ago I helped support the Bureau of Motor Vehicles with licenses for a sports car, a station wagon, a trailer, and a truck. The sports car and a little help from my friends are enough for today.

If we keep our health (which we now have a good chance of doing) and *if* we stay painless (which we now have almost *every* chance of doing), life without deadlines, alarm clocks, parking tickets, train and plane schedules, business luncheons, hotel and motel accommodations, lost luggage and "withholding" is perfectly possible. But how do you make the transition from paid to unpaid? What would suit you best at this time? What can you give time to that has value? How much real value does a volunteer worker have? How can you get the best returns in self-satisfaction?

TAKE A GOOD LOOK AT YOURSELF

I recently read a good book, *Retirement, You're in Charge* by Eleanor Furman. It is one that should be read, if possible, *before* retiring. Mrs. Furman herself is now "retired" (sort of), but before entering what turned out to be an interesting and satisfying way of life, she was an active business woman working in the field of placement and career counseling. That should tell you that she knows how to help you discover what you want to be when you grow up. Her book begins by telling the reader she was contemplating retirement, but not yet talking to anyone about it. We all seem to do that occasionally, especially on rainy, sleety, humid, miserable Monday mornings when there is an unpleasant task waiting in the office. In letter form, she writes about her experiences to her daughter—day-by-day accounts of the wonders of retirement. She wanders around in fairyland for about nine months, (the fateful nine months needed for gestating a baby or getting a book through from manuscript to bookstore shelf!) Suddenly there's a rainstorm on her parade and she is faced with depression. What can she *do?* The question she asks herself and her daughter are exactly what others face in the same situation: Should I get another job? Should I take courses? Should I write? What should I do? She notices the similarity between her plight and that of the adolescent who is trying to "find herself" . . . (or just as poignant, "find himself").

Sometimes we forget that we are constantly trying to "find" ourselves. We disguise the search with, "I'm trying out a new career," or "We're getting married next Sunday," or "I really want a baby," or "I've just joined the ranks of the divorced." No matter what we call it, we are always hunting for ourselves; one reason we do it is because we are different people all the time and it takes a long time to "find" all those selves. Try to remember what you were like at age eleven. Compare that child with yourself at seventeen. What were the similarities and differences that came with experience and learning? Some of the differences were great; you began to have some control over your life. Some weren't so great as you developed prejudices and unexpected fears. Let's hope you grew out of those.

Compare yourself at twenty-one with that same self at thirty-five. If you are a woman those were fateful years, dangerous years. What happened to the plans you made? Were they the right plans? Compare forty-five with fifty-five, the fateful years for a man. What about your plans? Did you realize the first ones or go off on an entirely different track? What were you like before marriage as compared to after? What were you like before having children—and after? Do you like yourself better now?

I do. Heavens! All those years wasted trying to please others. That's an exercise in futility. My friend Joan Grant, the writer, says that pleasing people is like the sounds you hear in an English railway carriage. The wheels on the rails keep repeating "It's-never-enough-it's-never-enough-it's-never-enough . . ." Now I have a few select friends I'd do anything for, and they reciprocate. The others will have to fend for themselves. Is that better or is it selfish? For me it's better. Ayn Rand calls selfishness a virtue. If you keep on giving and never getting, you turn bitter. You've seen it in people's faces: "After all I did for him . . ." Wherever you are on the scale of giving and/or getting, now is the time for *you*. Nobody is likely to fix your life for you, so do it for yourself.

Retirement often takes more initiative than working, and for many it may be the first real initiative taken in a lifetime. Those who fell into a "life-work"

by accident, inheritance, or influences beyond their control come under this heading. Many such people had decided to become lawyers or doctors, teachers or soldiers before they were really sure what any of those professions were all about. The surge of education then carried them along. The serendipitous folk haven't taken much initiative either; for them the winds of change and chance have always decided.

Don't be surprised if, while you are trying to find out what you will be when you grow up, you suffer depression, lack of confidence, and a new uncertainty. These are allowed.

A SUCCESS STORY

I first heard about the National Executive Service Corporation from a man I knew many, many years ago. We had both delighted in "projects," and when life moved us around and we didn't meet anymore, I often wondered what "projects" he had taken on. Then I heard he had retired and I wondered again. One of two things would happen to a man like him: he would find "projects" or he would not survive. When I started to write this book I wrote to ask what he was up to and he told me about the NESC.

NESC was founded about eight years ago by Frank Pace, the ex-Secretary of the Army and an executive at General Dynamics. It is made up of retired managers and executives who handle problems for nonprofit organizations like the Boy Scouts, Head Start, museums, and hospitals around the world. This super gang of high-powered people cover most business disciplines—finance, marketing, manufacturing, legal, administrative, and what was once called "employee relations" but is now called "human resources." These are the "retired" who can consult for free (with all expenses paid) but cannot afford to be mothballed.

What I wanted to know from my friend was what he actually got out of membership in that organization. I learned long ago that anyone who does anything has to get something out of it, even if it's only a promise of an hour in heaven. So I will share his response to my question:

Dear Bonnie:
In answer to your question, "How do you feel about what you are doing . . . ?" I speak for myself, but I know many others share my views. NESC wants us motivated and we are motivated because we feel good about what we are doing.

Now, "motivated" is a key word when you come to deciding what you'll do now that you're grown up. Without motivation we can't even get out of bed in the morning. One of the things that is wrong with so many "senior citizen" programs is lack of motivation. Who with the brains to come in out of the wet, can be motivated by a game of tiddledy-winks? Who can feel good about making pot holders? I once moved a huge hill with one small wheelbarrow and a shovel. What was the motivation? I wanted the cliff that was under it. It is now part of the background for a swimming pool and was a rewarding experience. "Rewarding" is another key word when you decide on your future.

The key thing is, there are real and difficult problems out there with organiza-

tions trying to cope in a world that gets ever more complicated, without being able to pay for the proper tools, i.e., experienced managers. The people who seek help are bright professionals, but they are swamped, drowning in some cases, or desperately trying to innovate without having time to do so. I may have overstated the case of some projects, but certainly not for ours.

My friend had been recruited for a project involving several New York hospitals and if ever there was a time when hospitals need experience and smarts, it's now.

You would think none of us had ever retired.

And there is your main thought for the day. No matter what your work, no man and no woman should ever "retire." Even the word suggests giving up. The first ten of the after fifty years should be spent preparing the body, the mind, and the world for when you will be grown up and free to work at something else even if it masquerades as "play."

To a man we are motivated, interested, frustrated, and hard working . . ."

Is that any different from the foregoing years? Yes, very. When my friend was the head of his firm, all the responsibility was his. Others went home with time to play. He went home with the day's worries. Now he shares that responsibility with three others as qualified as himself. Eight shoulders and four minds are better than just two and one. But there's more: he doesn't sit there alone in the office twisting and turning the problem, knowing that if he makes the wrong decision, he and he alone is to blame. Now he has the whole edifice of the NESC behind him and both praise and responsibility can be shared.

We can put in as much time as we want to . . . more than one project or just enough to satisfy whatever it is we are satisfying.

That's a profound statement and gives you one of the reasons top executives become top executives. While too many people working in the geriatrics field seem to think that all people are alike—look alike, dress alike, think alike and have the same needs—NESC knows there is variability. Let's try that one more time.

. . . enough to satisfy whatever it is we are satisfying . . .

You know what you need to be satisfied right now. Well, you aren't going to change too many of those basic needs ten years from now. You will be pretty much as you are now. You will be enthusiastic, energetic, serious, fun loving, straightforward, complicated, interested, thorough, or whatever else you are now when you are sixty, seventy, eighty, or ninety, so long as you are healthy. You will want basically the same things you want now but with a difference: you will have more time in which to get them.

The peer group contact is very satisfying. I'm associated with two ex-competitors of mine! I consider some kind of effort

related to a retiree's background as vital. You just can't turn the switch off, at least as it relates to successful lifetime managers.

There in one short paragraph are the answers to three problems that are probably rattling around in your mind:

1. You need your peers; they know a lot of the same things and working with them will give you a chance to use, again, those skills that have been honed so fine in all of you.

2. Doing something to which you can bring all your past experience is very satisfying.

3. Knowing right now that there is no way to turn yourself *off* should be motivation enough!

Start looking and planning now, just as you did in school when you said, "When I get out of here . . ." or earlier and more to the point, "When I grow up . . ."

The NESC offers a spectacular opportunity. Working with nonprofit organizations is particularly difficult for all of us "bottom liners" where profit and time are essentials. But we learn to cope and press harder on elements that produce income for nonprofit organizations, for . . . productivity or efficiency. . . .

Here again is an example of myths being confounded. If these hard-driving dollars-and-cents people can rearrange themselves to rearrange businesses that have never had to face a bottom line and win . . . well, that's a monumental trick at any age. The young often have nervous breakdowns over less.

Do you think I don't like what I'm doing?

Let me give you a list of keys to success:
1. THE PROJECT MUST BE REAL, NOT SYNTHETIC.

Leave it to business people to understand that. In the business world it's do what has to be done and do it now. If it doesn't work, do something else that does. Providing the after fifty crowd with busywork is not only foolish, it's destructive. Where do you suppose erstwhile busy, productive men and women get the idea that they are washed up? They get it from do-gooders who have either never met deadlines or have worked in the real world.

2. THE PARTICIPANTS MUST BE QUALIFIED AND MOTIVATED . . . AND SO MANY ARE.

Notice, he said "qualified." Well, what are you qualified for right now? Do you enjoy doing what you are "qualified for"? Can you think of any way those qualifications might be used when you no longer do what you are doing now? If you can't, perhaps you should start looking for something you *do* like to do. It certainly doesn't have to be anything you ever did before. It won't be like it was when you were starting out, when you appeared hat in hand saying, "Can you use me?" You've got several months or years in which to become proficient in something that motivates you. If you are already assured of a welcome because of who you are and what you know, don't rest on it. Everyone should learn one new thing a year. You may want to drop it at the end of a term or study period as you used to drop classes that turned boring. That's fine. Find something else.

The important thing about now is that there is *time*. Try a new language. All that takes is perseverance. What skill do you have? What other skill could ride piggy-back on it? Try a new vacation place. Have you ever been to the Galapagos? You're strapped for funds? Have you ever taken fifteen books with you on a freighter? You were good at tennis but you hurt your knee? What about canoeing in Wisconsin? You've had a hip replacement and don't feel like skiing Aspen anymore? How about Lake Louise on cross country skis or wind surfing in the Caribbean? Better yet, take a scuba course at the Y and go back to the Caribbean, but deeper.

3. WORK SCHEDULES SHOULD BE ADAPTABLE, I.E., TEN TO FOUR, TWO OR THREE DAYS A WEEK.

When I was traveling constantly and getting up at five to catch a plane at seven I was determined to find a job that would let me sleep till ten. When I couldn't travel due to the disintegrating hip, I'd have taken *any* travel hours. Your needs will change just as your tastes do, so don't get hemmed in by one idea. Most of us have dreams of leisure when we are overworked, but I have watched a lot of us: we do fine at nothing for a while . . . and then we start to fidget. Most of us have to do something. We don't necessarily need to be the kingpin, but we do want a say in the matter of ourselves and what we do with our lives. Start now to decide what it is you want to be when you grow up, and—perhaps for the first time ever—plan on making it all come true . . . *for you.*

4. THE PROBLEMS SHOULD BE WELL DEFINED . . . NOT VAGUE.

The problems probably arose in the first place because the principles were vague. Your first task may be to list the essential facts and get your blueprint on the table.

5. THE ASSIGNMENTS SHOULD BE SUCH THAT THEY NEED THE KIND OF EXPERTISE YOU HAVE.

Expertise does not necessarily mean training; a leaning will help. At my school where we train Myotherapists and Exercise Therapists, the ones with a scientific bent do well in one area and the ones with an ear for music do better in the other. They all learn both, and the two sides of themselves complement each other. What you do well allows you to pick up similar skills easily.

Then my friend came to my last question, "Why is joining something like NESC a good idea?" His answer is here, handed out to the after fifty crowd.

UNLESS YOU ARE HALF DEAD . . . OR WANT TO BE, IT . . .
 1. Stirs the old juices . . .
 2. Keeps you in contact with peers . . . lunches, "what's new"
 3. Keeps the phone ringing with peers . . . making dates to interview key personnel on the project, etc.
 4. You are doing on a reduced scale what you always loved doing.
 5. You see worthwhile results . . . YOU ARE MAKING A CONTRIBUTION.

CONSIDER VOLUNTEER WORK

You may want to investigate the GRAY PANTHERS. They are a membership organization working on housing, employment, discrimination, poverty, and other concerns of *the after fifty crowd:* 3635 Chestnut St., Philadelphia, PA 19104.

THE NATIONAL COUNCIL ON AGING, 600 Maryland Ave., Washington DC 20024.

THE NATIONAL COUNCIL OF SENIOR CITIZENS, 1925 15th St. NW, Washington, DC 2005.

If you are looking for recreation services and you really don't know anything about taking vacations, there's an organization called VASCA, VACATIONS FOR THE AGING AND SENIOR CENTER ASSOCIATION, 225 Park Ave. S., New York, NY 10003. They give you information on adult camps in New York, New Jersey, and Connecticut and tell you where to write for other states.

If you are considering volunteer work, try THE FEDERAL ACTION AGENCY, 806 Connecticut Ave. NW, Washington, DC 20525. They sponsor programs like Foster Grandparents, VISTA, and R.S.V.P. (RETIRED SENIOR VOLUNTEER PROGRAM).

A national center for volunteer information is THE NATIONAL CENTER FOR SENIOR INVOLVEMENT, 1111 N. 19th St., Suite 500, Arlington, Virginia 22209.

The NESC, THE NATIONAL EXECUTIVE SERVICE CORPORATION, is at 622 Third Ave., New York, NY 10017. High-level opportunities are offered there both in the United States and abroad.

VOLUNTARY ACTION CENTERS or VOLUNTARY BUREAUS are all over the country. They interview volunteers and refer them to jobs in nonprofit organizations. Some have special services for retirees, such as information on second careers.

Don't forget that volunteer agencies are very happy to get direct applications. In this I should caution you. Don't be discouraged if the interviewer isn't on your wavelength. You have spent upwards of forty years becoming. The interviewer may have been in the job market a couple of years and in that particular job a week. If you don't get "through" the first time you try, and you feel that that's the spot you want to get into, try again in six months and see what's happened in your absence. Nasty, shortsighted, or just plain uninformed people have a way of being replaced.

There's an organization concerned specifically with the problems of the distaff members of the after fifty crowd. THE NATIONAL ACTION FORUM FOR OLDER WOMEN, School of Allied Health Professions, State University of New York, Stonybrook, NY 11794.

And there is NOW, the NATIONAL ORGANIZATION FOR WOMEN, OLDER WOMEN'S COMMITTEE, 425 13th Street NW, Washington, DC 20001.

None of these groups may apply to you. You may know exactly what you want to do. Some things, however, apply to all of us. We are grown up now. We are responsible people and very few of us are still blaming our parents for our shortcomings. Instead, we are probably shaking our heads over being blamed for the problems of our own children. Not only are we finally grown up, we are finally free of a lot of things—not the least being discrimination against the older person.

It's time to be selfish. It's time to plan for us. Let us get to know one another and each other's needs. There is safety in numbers—and now you know how and where to contact those numbers. Go to school; meet, network, share. We are The Last Fit Americans and yes, we will grow older. Dr. Butler says that aging is a part of the body's lifelong growth process. I agree with him, but I want to add something: you can do your aging well or badly. You now have the tools with which to do it well.

Let us help each other.

SOURCES

There will be two books you in the after fifty crowd will need at once:

Pain Erasure: The Bonnie Prudden Way. New York: M. Evans & Co., Inc. 1980 (hardcover). New York: Ballantine Books, Inc., 1982 (paperback).

This is the first book ever written about Myotherapy[sm], a revolutionary method for relieving both acute and chronic pain. Special attention has been given to preparation for and recovery from total hip replacements, often a need for the after fifty crowd. In addition the problems of babies such as colic, teething and growing pains have been addressed. Now grandparents will have an answer that works like a charm. Chair and bed exercises are provided as well as the basics for getting rid of your own pain.

Myotherapy, Bonnie Prudden's Complete Guide to Pain Free Living. New York: Dial 1984 (hardcover). New York: Ballantine Books, Inc., 1986 (paperback).

This is the latest book on Myotherapy[sm] and brings in all the latest discoveries in Myotherapy, including the fact that jaw pain originates in the groin for the most part, that running on cement is leading to pelvic muscle spasm, and that techniques in both sports and the performing arts can be improved with Myotherapy. It describes the dangers deriving from the "Fitness craze" and provides alternatives ways of attaining and maintaining fitness *that do not injure*. This book introduces Quick Fix, a way to temporarily relieve pain such as backache, knee pain, headaches and shoulder and neck pain in minutes. It then provides the instructions for Permanent Fix. This book, written for the lay person, is being used as a text by many professionals in the health care field.

In Doctor Butler's foreword to this book he asks for another book, one designed for the younger Americans who have not had our advantages. The request has been answered with a trilogy for American youth:

How to Keep Your Child Fit From Birth to Six. New York: Harper & Row, Publishers, 1964. Rev. ed. New York: The Dial Press, 1983. Rev. ed. Ballantine Books, Inc., 1986 (paperback).

Fitness from Six to Twelve. New York: Harper & Row, Publishers 1972. Rev. ed. New York: The Dial Press, 1983. Second rev. ed. New York: Ballantine Books, Inc. 1986 (forthcoming).

Teenage Fitness. New York: Harper & Row, Publishers, 1965. Rev. ed. New York: The Dial Press, 1983. New York: Ballantine Books, Inc. 1987 (forthcoming).

The following is something that could help some of your older friends who have difficulty seeing well. While the original talking book was written (or rather spoken) for people who could not see at all, it works wonders for those who need fitness, but who still maintain at least some sight.

Physical Fitness for You (a talking book for the blind) The complete book of exercise for the sight impaired. It can be ordered from The American Foundation for the Blind, 15 West 16th Street, New York, N.Y. 10011.

The next book may not sound like an After Fifty item, but it is. Due to our rugged childhoods, many of us have no fear of water while many of today's parents are afraid of everything where their children are concerned. *Grandparents make wonderful swim coaches.*

Your Baby Can Swim. New York: Reader's Digest Press, 1974. *Teach Your Baby to Swim,* Rev. ed. New York: The Dial Press, 1983. Stockbridge, Massachusetts: Bonnie Prudden Press.

How to Keep Your Family Fit and Healthy. New York: Reader's Digest Press, 1975. Stockbridge, Mass.: Bonnie Prudden Press.

A fitness book that brings in the whole family and can be adapted for every generation.

Exer-Sex. New York: Bantam Books, 1978. Stockbridge, Mass.: Bonnie Prudden Press.

This is a gentle book about feelings and sex, with exercises that improve both. A different, better way of imparting information about sex, sensuality, and loving.

Tapes . . . exercise tapes that provide a high level of fitness without injuring.

Tapes . . . on relieving headaches and back pain.

EQUIPMENT

There are several gadgets that will help you remain pain free whether you live alone and don't have a friend-with-an-elbow in residence or just hate to bother others when you ache.

The Bodo on page 133. That is the little wooden item that helps reach trigger points in hard to get places.

The Shepherd's Crook on page 127. Another gadget that can find trigger points you can't reach with your fingers or are not strong enough to exert the needed pressure.

The Pulley on page 339. You need this whatever your situation is. It will keep the shoulders free and painless and improve your posture by stretching the chest muscles.

WARNING!!!

As with anything else that is successful there will be imitators. There are some people calling themselves "myotherapists" and passing themselves off as the real thing. Some are massage therapists who find that this borrowed technique works when they incorporate it into their practices. That's fine until they start using the title "myotherapist," which they are not. Some imitators are nothing at all, but have read one of Bonnie's two books on pain and decided to hang out a shingle. At best it will cost you, and at worst, you will spend that money *and time* and get worse. Some people who are calling themselves "myotherapists" were certified by Bonnie Prudden, Inc., at one time, but have let that certification lapse. This means that they are not up on the latest developments.

All properly trained Certified Bonnie Prudden Myotherapists^cm study the art intensively (1300 hours) and must pass board exams before they can be certified. In addition, they are required, to update their training every two years with forty-five hours leading to recertification. They have the papers to prove it.

All Certified Bonnie Prudden Myotherapists^cm are listed with the office of Bonnie Prudden, Inc., Stockbridge, Massachusetts 01262, and the name Bonnie Prudden is your guarantee. If you are in doubt, check. If you are offered Myotherapy without a *medical* doctor's referral, that person is not certified. Ask to see papers of certification with certification dates. If you need a Myotherapist^cm, call the office of Bonnie Prudden Inc.

MYOTHERAPY HELP LINE

An annual brochure providing places and dates of pain erasure seminars, workshops and an up to date listing of Certified Bonnie Prudden Myotherapists^cm is sent to people on the Institute's mailing list. For further information, contact the Institute for Physical Fitness, Stockbridge, Massachusetts 01262.

INDEX OF OCCUPATIONS

INDEX OF SPORTS

INDEX

About the Author

BONNIE PRUDDEN has been a world-class authority on physical fitness and exercise since the 1950s. Her research on the fitness of American children helped create the President's Council on Physical Fitness during the Eisenhower administration. She is the director of the Bonnie Prudden Institute for Physical Fitness and Myotherapy in Stockbridge, Massachusetts, and is the author of over twenty books, including *Pain Erasure* and *Myotherapy*.